Introduction to One Health

# Introduction to One Health

An Interdisciplinary Approach to Planetary Health

*Sharon L. Deem*
*Saint Louis Zoo Institute for Conservation Medicine*

*Kelly E. Lane-deGraaf*
*The Center for One Health at Fontbonne University*

*Elizabeth A. Rayhel*
*The Center for One Health at Fontbonne University*

**WILEY** Blackwell

This edition first published 2019
© 2019 John Wiley & Sons, Inc.

The right of Sharon L. Deem, Kelly E. Lane-deGraaf and Elizabeth A. Rayhel to be identified as the authors of this work has been asserted in accordance with law.

*Registered Office*
John Wiley & Sons, Inc., 111 River Street, Hoboken, NJ 07030, USA

*Editorial Office*
111 River Street, Hoboken, NJ 07030, USA

For details of our global editorial offices, customer services, and more information about Wiley products visit us at www.wiley.com.

Wiley also publishes its books in a variety of electronic formats and by print-on-demand. Some content that appears in standard print versions of this book may not be available in other formats.

*Library of Congress Cataloging-in-Publication Data*

Names: Deem, Sharon L., 1963– author. | Lane-deGraaf, Kelly E., 1977– author. | Rayhel, Elizabeth A., 1957– author.
Title: Introduction to one health : an interdisciplinary approach to planetary health / Sharon L. Deem,
    Kelly E. Lane-deGraaf, Elizabeth A. Rayhel.
Description: Hoboken, NJ : Wiley-Blackwell, 2019. | Includes bibliographical references and index. |
Identifiers: LCCN 2018029674 (print) | LCCN 2018031568 (ebook) | ISBN 9781119382836 (Adobe PDF) |
    ISBN 9781119382850 (ePub) | ISBN 9781119382867 (paperback)
Subjects: | MESH: One Health | Ecosystem | Environmental Health
Classification: LCC RA418 (ebook) | LCC RA418 (print) | NLM WA 30.7 | DDC 362.1–dc23
LC record available at https://lccn.loc.gov/2018029674

Cover Design: Wiley
Cover Image: © David Malan/Photographer's Choice RF/Getty Images; © Milosz_G/Shutterstock

Set in 10/12pt Warnock by SPi Global, Pondicherry, India

10  9  8  7  6  5  4  3  2  1

*To our children Aoife, Caleb, Charlie, Laura, and Saoirse, and to the readers of this book, whose actions shape Planetary Health.*

# Contents

# Foreword

## Introduction to One Health: An Interdisciplinary Approach to Planetary Health

*A Foreword by Daniel M. Ashe*

President & CEO, Association of Zoos and Aquariums
Former Director, US Fish and Wildlife Service (2011–2017)

In the introduction to their visionary textbook, authors Sharon Deem, Kelly LanedeGraaf, and Elizabeth Rayhel quote Abraham Lincoln: *"the best way to predict the future is to create it."* With this book, they take a giant leap in creating a future where we recognize and respect, and where our institutions and actions more fully reflect the interrelationships between humans, animals, and the environment – a philosophy called *One Health*.

The twentieth century was marked by tremendous progress in our understanding of the environment, and the effect of human economy and ecology. We built great institutions, framed in academic disciplines like biology, ecology, hydrology, forestry, oceanography, engineering, and the many medical sciences and disciplines. We split the world into wetlands, prairies, forests, farm, ranch, range, rivers, lakes and oceans; and fish, and mammals, and insects, and plants. And we built great corresponding institutions, like the one where I served for 22 years, the last six as its director: The US Fish and Wildlife Service.

Leaders and visionaries, including Aldo Leopold, Rachel Carson, Olaus, and Mardy Murie, and David Suzuki have long inspired us to think beyond our disciplinary training and our institutional boundaries. New interdisciplinary disciplines have emerged, but they suffer a common infirmity. They are disciplines themselves.

*One Health* is more philosophy than discipline. It incorporates human, animal, and environmental health as inherently interrelated, interdependent, and inseparable. The authors, at once, respect and encourage disciplinary scientific expertise, but recognize that evidence-based science is not enough. They recognize that driving societal change requires that science be packaged in ways that fit into a broad milieu of cultural, religious, political, and economic beliefs. Their text is a roadmap to follow in pursuing Leonardo da Vinci's notion of a complete mind: *"Study the art of science; study the science of art. Learn how to see. Realize that everything connects to everything else."*

Their writing is clear, concise, and compelling. It helps us to see that our health, indeed, is connected to everything around us. They use historical examples from Hernando de Soto's 1539 expedition up the Mississippi River, to modern-day Ebola outbreaks. The Lewis and Clark Corps of Discovery is linked to infectious diseases that devastated native peoples, mercury contamination, westward expansion, slavery, economic development, and modern-day environmental inequity and injustice. Their work is a literal melting pot, mixing all the complexity of today's global economy and ecology, pouring it into a conceptual mold that allows us to more effectively aggregate human, animal, and environmental health into *One Health*.

*One Health* is about connection. It is about the recognition that humans, animals, and environment are indivisible. It is about humility, unintended consequences, and the fact that decisions that we make today will shape the immediate and the distant future. It is about finding solutions by looking for something beyond traditional notions of interdisciplinary coordination – what the authors call a *transdisciplinary* approach.

One thing is certain. We cannot address the interrelated challenges of climate change, pollution, extinction, biodiversity loss, invasive species, infectious diseases, poverty, injustice, and inequality with the same approaches of the past. We cannot just continue to seek better coordination between disparate disciplines and institutions. We've known for decades that human, animal, and environmental health are linked. *The canary in the coal mine* is an adage that recognizes it explicitly. Coal miners knew that their environment, and ultimately their health, could be safeguarded by a sensitive, sentinel bird. *One Health* expands this simple concept to reflect twenty-first century complexities and opportunities.

*One Health* is a powerful introductory text. Let's hope it inspires a new generation of *One Health* professionals, in diverse fields throughout the sciences and humanities, to envision and create a future where we link human, animal, and environmental health. Our future prosperity depends on it.

# Acknowledgments

The authors have many people to thank for logistical and personal support of this textbook. We thank the staff, volunteers, and students of the Saint Louis Zoo Institute for Conservation Medicine, with special thanks to Kathy Zeigler, Jamie Palmer, Kathleen Apakupakul, Carol Gronau, and Karen Jordan. Saint Louis Zoo staff members Shawn Lofgren, Kayla Rogers, and Stephen Leard, for providing valuable assistance with recording and editing of the audio interviews, and Fontbonne University staff members Elizabeth Brennan and Anna LeRoy for the cover design, and the Fontbonne University Center for One Health logo. We thank the Fontbonne University students in the Honors Seminar in One Health and the Conservation Medicine courses during the 2016–2017 academic year for providing the case studies presented in the text, and Fontbonne student, Leann Smith for her help in obtaining permissions for use of figures. We appreciate the support and belief in One Health shown by administrators from both of our institutions, especially Adam Weyhaupt and Mike Pressimone of Fontbonne University and Jeffrey Bonner, Eric Miller, and Michael Macek of the Saint Louis Zoo. We also thank Kyle, Harry, and Steve, and our extended families, for supporting us during our One Health journeys and especially during the writing of this book. Lastly, we thank the scientists and civil servants who have dedicated their careers, and in many instances their lives, to advancing a holistic approach to planetary health. In the current uncertain and challenging political climate that many of us face, we encourage them to continue with this invaluable work.

## About the Companion Website

www.wiley.com/go/deem/health

There you will find valuable material designed to enhance your learning, including:

- audio interviews

Scan this QR code to visit the companion website

Part I

An Introduction and Impetus for One Health

1

# Why One Health?

The Mississippi River today is the source of economic strength and cultural movement throughout the USA. The Mississippi reaches more than 2300 miles from Lake Itaska in northwestern Minnesota to the Gulf of Mexico (Figure 1.1). The fourth largest watershed on the planet, it covers 32 states and 40% of the landmass of the USA and reaches from Appalachia to the Rocky Mountains. Pre-dating the European expansion into the Americas, Native American cultures thrived along the Mississippi River Basin. The Ojibwe, the Kickapoo, the Potawatomi, the Chickasaw, the Cahokia, the Choctaw, the Tunica, the Natchez, and many more peoples lived and flourished along the Mississippi River. Culturally diverse and rich in tradition, the peoples of the Mississippi River basin used and respected animals and the environment throughout their traditions. Focused on fishing and hunting, small-scale farming, and foraging, the traditions of the peoples of the Mississippi River are as varied as the people themselves, but importantly, these traditions shared a focus on maintaining a balance between humans, animals, and the environment. The culturally diverse native peoples of the Mississippi River region could truly be considered the first **One Health** practitioners of the region.

In 1539, Hernando de Soto of Spain became the first European to witness the majesty and power of the Mississippi River. In his explorations and quest for gold, de Soto and his men frequently interacted with native peoples. The Spaniards, from their first landfall, exploited native peoples. Language and culture differences, not surprisingly, emerged frequently. de Soto traveled with one translator, who spoke the language of only one tribe. As a result, skirmishes between the Spaniards and the native peoples often broke out while traveling. When the army with which de Soto traveled, numbering approximately 620, encountered a local community, they demanded use of the food stores, preferring this to hunting. As a result, the Spaniards consumed nearly a year's worth of food in only a few days in each community they encountered, with devastating impacts on the survival of these local communities. de Soto and his men also routinely enslaved men, women, and children, demanding individuals carry their equipment and gear, care for their horses, provide cooked food, lodging, and sexual services. Native peoples who resisted were frequently raped, tortured, had their homes and crops burned, and/or were killed. The violence of the initial European arrivals to the Mississippi region resulted in the murder of an uncountable number of native peoples.

The devastation of the communities of Native Americans is not the only devastation de Soto and his men wrought on the Mississippi Basin. The Spaniards were exploring to claim the land for Spain and loot the region of its gold, silver, and other precious metals. In addition to men, de Soto brought with him 220 horses and 100 pigs.

*Introduction to One Health: An Interdisciplinary Approach to Planetary Health*, First Edition.
Sharon L. Deem, Kelly E. Lane-deGraaf and Elizabeth A. Rayhel.
© 2019 John Wiley & Sons, Inc. Published 2019 by John Wiley & Sons, Inc.
Companion website: www.wiley.com/go/deem/health

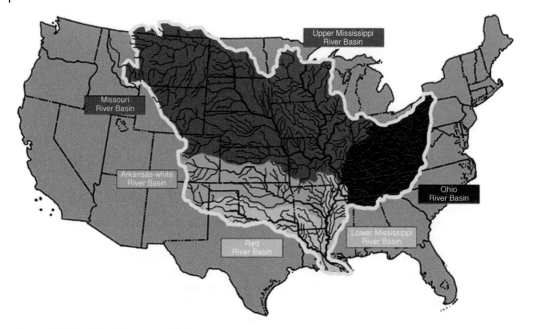

Figure 1.1 Mississippi River watershed.

The movement of this army of people and animals from present day Florida west through Louisiana, north through Arkansas and into Missouri, and then south to Texas left in its trail a swath of deforestation, biodiversity loss, and pollution – all One Health threats. For example, while the Spaniards exploited Native American paths for travel as much as possible, they also carved many new paths through the forests and prairies that they crossed. The livestock brought along also created significant problems for the landscape. Feeding these animals created an additional burden for the land, taxing the ecosystems as the traveling herd of between 300 and 1000 domesticated animals trampled vast swathes of pristine forest and prairie vegetation. Rats and other stowaways from their ships would, in time, become invasive and drive their own ecological catastrophes. de Soto's herd of pigs, which grew from 100 to over 900 by 1542, brought its own unique environmental and ecological threats.

The normal behaviors of pigs – rooting for tubers, wallowing in mud, and trampling vegetation – wreaked havoc on native plant life and, importantly, their feces introduced an entire suite of novel pathogens to an area, contaminating local water supplies as they defecated across the south. An often overlooked consequence of early western explorations was the introduction of lead shot into the Americas; with this, de Soto and his army slaughtered countless native animal species and introduced the potential for lead pollution into the Mississippi River basin.

In what could be considered one of the earliest intercultural One Health threats, the greatest devastation brought by de Soto and his men was not the rape and pillaging of the land and local communities but the introduction of novel infectious diseases into naïve populations. In the wake of de Soto's army, smallpox and measles spread rapidly through the diverse tribes of native peoples of the Mississippi Basin, who were exposed to these pathogens as de Soto and his men traveled through their communities. Smallpox alone killed an estimated 95% of the people with whom the Spaniards came into contact, effectively eliminating entire communities in their wake. This drastically altered the make-up of the Native American landscape well before the French and English returned some 100 years later. de Soto did not survive his expedition, dying on the banks of the Mississippi River of a fever without finding a single piece of gold or silver. More than half of his men perished along the way as well.

Fast forward 150 years to 1682, when, after exploring its reaches and seizing upon the economic and strategic benefit of the Mississippi River system, René-Robert Cavelier, sieur de la Salle claimed the river for France. The southern stretches of the Mississippi Basin briefly fell under the control of the Spanish in 1769; in 1803, the USA, not even 30 years old, purchased the entirety of the Mississippi River watershed as a part of the Louisiana Purchase. When in May of 1804, William Clark, Meriwether Lewis, and 31 others set forth from St. Louis, MO, to find a Northwest Passage, a water route to the Pacific, they were tasked with acting as cartographers, naturalists, and cultural emissaries for the young country. Thomas Jefferson, who commissioned the expedition in 1803, believed that the most critical role for the commissioned explorers was to act as diplomats for the nation among the several Native American tribes the group would encounter. The Corps of Discovery, as the expedition came to be called, ultimately made contact with 55 independent groups of Native Americans and First Peoples, frequently trading for food and medical supplies as well as befriending many tribes people.

Lewis and Clark traversed nearly 8000 miles. Their expedition is touted by many as a model of inclusion – a black man, York, and a Shoshone woman, Sacagawea, were essential members after all. However, their inclusion hints at the exploitative nature of the Corps itself. York was a master hunter, bringing in a large portion of the game that fed the Corps throughout their journey, and acted frequently as the expedition's most stalwart caregiver, providing care to ill expedition members. Still, York was Clark's slave. He was not a paid member of the Corps of Discovery, despite his critical role in its

success. Sacagawea was kidnapped as a teen by the Hidatsa and then sold to her "husband" Charbonneau. As property, neither York nor Sacagawea could refuse participation in the 8000 mile journey. Still, Sacagawea, like York, played a vital role in the expedition, acting as translator and helping with the group's welcome by many Native American peoples.

In all, the Lewis and Clark expedition, while fondly remembered today, was considered at the time as something of a failure. They discovered no Northwest Passage; the northern route chosen by the group was arduous and challenging in a way that the southern route across the Rockies is not and so was not used by later settlers. They mapped lands, documented plants and animals, and improved diplomatic relations with Native peoples, but they also opened the country to western occupation that drastically altered the landscape, replaced the diversity of plants and animals with corn and cows, each with long-term ecological consequences, and ravaged Native American communities through broken treaties, forced migrations, and massacres.

Lewis and Clark's expedition had two additional repercussions in the US West: the spread of sexually transmitted diseases (STDs) and widespread mercury contamination to the environment. STDs were not introduced to Native Americans by the Corps of Discovery; French and Canadian fur-trappers accomplished this. However, STDs spread through the Corps rapidly. As the men traveled west and as they encountered local tribes, it was common for members to trade goods for sex, and frequently, wives of chiefs of several High Plains tribes were shared with expedition members in order to benefit from the men's spiritual power. The result of this was the spread of STDs across the northwest, as the Corps of Discovery shared infections between peoples who would never have otherwise come into contact with each other. At the time, there were few treatments for STDs available, with modern medicine of the day advocating a strong course of mercury pills and bloodletting. As a result of the rampant STDs, members of the Corps of Discovery were also all exposed to toxic levels of mercury. Additionally, heavy use of laxatives, brought on by the lack of plant materials and overconsumption of meats in their diets causing chronic constipation, further increased mercury levels among the expedition's members, as these, too, were mercury-based. As a result, it is possible to retrace the steps of the Corps of Discovery by following the path of environmental contamination of mercury from latrine pits. While not frequently considered through this lens, the Lewis and Clark expedition and its outcomes are a One Health journey, both from the perspective of collaboration and data acquisition, including the detailed accounting of flora, fauna, and people, and from the complex health concerns introduced during their journey.

As the westward expansion of the USA proceeded through the early 1800s, due in part to the doors opened by the Corps of Discovery, one significant question for new territories was whether or not to allow slavery. Resolved by the Compromise of 1850, which settled the issue via a process referred to as **popular sovereignty**, newly established territories were allowed to decide the issue of slavery independently by vote. Voting at this time was, however, limited to white men. Not long after Lewis and Clark departed from Missouri, Dred Scott, a slave born in Virginia, moved with his owners to St. Louis, Missouri. Located south of the **Mason-Dixon Line**, but north of the lines drawn by the Missouri Compromise, Missouri in the 1830s was a slave state. Once there, Scott was sold to John Emerson, a US Army doctor. As a part of his work, John Emerson traveled extensively, taking his slaves with him. As a result of this, Dred Scott and his family found themselves living in Illinois – a free state – and the Wisconsin territory – a territory that, under the Compromise of 1850, had voted to not allow slavery. In 1842, the Emersons returned to Missouri, taking up residence in St. Louis. In 1846, Dr. Emerson died, leaving his slaves to his widow, Eliza (Irene) Sanford Emerson. Upon John Emerson's death, Dred Scott attempted to buy his and his family's freedom from the widow, but she refused. And so, with the help and encouragement of local abolitionists, Dred Scott sued for his freedom in 1846. In total, the Scotts had lived for more than nine years in free territories, and according to the doctrine held by Missouri's courts at the time, "Once free, always free," there was a precedent to support his claim. After 11 years, the case landed before the US Supreme Court, where in a 7-2 decision, the Court ruled against Scott, citing property rights as the justification, and nullifying the 1820 Missouri Compromise in the process. The outrage of this ruling, what has come to be known as the Dred Scott Decision, fanned the flames of civil unrest over "the slavery question" in the USA and came less than four years before the country erupted in war over the issue of slavery in 1861. Dred Scott died a slave less than one year after the Court's ruling, in 1858.

William Clark died in 1838 and was buried in Bellefontaine Cemetery, a beautiful cemetery and arboretum in St. Louis, MO; just 20 years later, Dred Scott was buried in Calvary Cemetery, an equally beautiful Catholic cemetery in St. Louis, MO. A single street separates the two cemeteries. While seemingly disparate, the stories of William Clark, Dred Scott, and the Mississippi River have shaped the region into what it is today. The actions of the past set the path for the realities of today. As such, it is possible to examine how the actions of early Americans shaped the current cultural and environmental health of the region.

St. Louis, MO, now sits as the Gateway to the West. As the second largest city on the Mississippi, it has grown up with the river as a unique part of its cultural identity. The river is the economic and cultural anchor of St. Louis, binding the city to its history in numerous unseen ways. For St. Louis, the cultural reliance on natural resources and the economic and cultural exchange brought by the Mississippi harkens back to Lewis and

Clark's roles as cultural emissaries and naturalists of the Corps of Discovery. Resource extraction, epitomized by long-term iron mining in the area, and the vast loss of habitat through **urban sprawl** are reminiscent of de Soto's approach to exploration. Missourians' love of green spaces, embodied by Forest Park, the largest urban park in the USA, and their ardent support of conservation-minded state agencies, such as the Department of Natural Resources and the Department of Conservation, stem from the values placed on the balance between humans, animals, and the environment. And finally, St. Louis' continued status as one of the most segregated cities in America, brought into sharp focus with the recent events in Ferguson, MO, a suburban area of St. Louis, is a direct result of the country's still-open wound of slavery, as exemplified by the Dred Scott Decision.

The legacy of St. Louis' rich and complicated history is playing out in a myriad of ways today. More than 175 million tons of freight move along the Mississippi River, creating jobs for thousands of people. The river is also the source of rich biological diversity, providing habitat or resources for more than 260 species of fish, 60% of American birds, at least 60 species of mammal, and numerous reptiles, amphibians, and freshwater mussel. The Mississippi is the source of drinking water for more than 18 million people. St. Louis benefits from all of this economic and ecological wealth. The landscape of St. Louis has been shaped physically both by the river and by the social and economic divide between the city residents, established in the years following the Civil War. In the early twentieth century, systemic **redlining** – racist housing policies at federal, state, and local levels – prevented the integration of black and white communities. North St. Louis is now almost exclusively black while south St. Louis is predominantly white. The Delmar Divide – a street that separates north from south, black from white, and frequently, poverty from wealth – spans the city. This Divide has significant consequences for health.

For the people of St. Louis, the zip code into which one was born is the most significant factor for predicting overall health, including rates of heart disease, diabetes, and cancer. City residents living north of the Delmar Divide have an average life expectancy of 12–15 years less than their counterparts living south of the Divide. In some places, this gap stretches to as many as 35 years. The racial and socioeconomic divides, embodied by the Delmar Divide, extend beyond traditional health metrics. Residents in south St. Louis have higher rates of home ownership and a greater access to education, with a rate of college completion at more than twice the rate of residents in north St. Louis. Historic decisions determining where people of color could live, anchored in the state's slave-owning past, have also exposed the residents of north St. Louis to a significant amount of toxic pollutants over time, including heavy metals, from pollution-generating industries, such as lead smelts, refineries, and limestone and iron mines. This long-term exposure to toxic pollutants, which manifests into significant human health costs today, is but one disparity in human and environmental health separating north and south St. Louis.

Surprisingly, this Divide is also significant for the health of urban wildlife. For example, the Camillo laboratory at Saint Louis University has examined bee and other insect pollinator populations across St. Louis and found the diversity of bees is significantly greater in St. Louis than in the rest of Missouri, suggesting that urban ecosystems may promote population diversity. Dr. Gerardo Camillo suggests this is likely due to the loss of habitat in rural areas, where agricultural monocultures dominate the landscape. Wild bees are, more frequently than not, ground-nesting species, and the patchiness of urban green spaces – neighborhood parks and gardens – can promote native wildflower growth, creating small, viable habitats for the insects.

Similarly, the Lane-deGraaf laboratory at Fontbonne University's Center for One

Health has explored the effect of the Delmar Divide itself on urban wildlife populations. Preliminary work out of the Lane-deGraaf laboratory has shown that the Delmar Divide has had profound impacts on populations of urban mammals, resulting in differences in not only physical and population size of raccoons (*Procyon lotor*) but of their **population genetics** as well, suggesting that long-term environmental inequalities throughout the history of St. Louis have the ability to shape the current population dynamics of urban wildlife.

Raccoons are common carriers of the roundworm, *Baylisascaris procyonis*. *B. procyonis* is an important zoonotic parasite that can infect children, who may come into contact with the eggs of the parasite through play in raccoon-feces-contaminated playgrounds or sandboxes. In the work out of Lane-deGraaf's laboratory it is shown that *B. procyonis* is most commonly found in children in areas with high rates of poverty, especially in those areas with high rates of building vacancies. In St. Louis, the **incidence** of *B. procyonis* is increasing only among children living in north St. Louis, where the **prevalence** of raccoon roundworm and vacant buildings is high but available park space is low. In a true One Health synergism, the rise of this parasite is linked to the long-term income inequality of St. Louis, demarcated by the Delmar Divide that drives disparities in environmental health, the effects of which inextricably link human, animal, and environmental health.

This is not just a story of St. Louis. This is a story of connection. Humans, animals, and the environment are indivisible. They are connected not only with each other but with each other through space and time. Decisions made by parents directly affect their children; actions of preservation or pollution done in the past affect the current environment. Acts of health and humanity made locally have global repercussions, with potentially far-reaching, unintended consequences. Decisions made today will shape the future. We are all connected; human health, animal health, and environmental health really is only One Health.

## 1.1 Book Overview

We wrote this book as an introduction to One Health; it is our intention for the reader to acquire a clear understanding of One Health: what it is, why it is important for planetary health and how one may be a part of it. This text has an interdisciplinary point of view that will make it valuable to the growing number of One Health majors, minors, and certification programs in universities throughout the world. The text will also be of value to graduate programs in the sciences, including the health sciences (e.g. veterinary, medical, ecological), serving as an introduction to One Health alongside the more traditional courses in these fields.

What then do we mean by One Health? In this text, we define One Health as the collaborative effort of multiple disciplines – working locally, nationally, and globally – to attain optimal health for people, animals, and the environment. For many of us, as daily news of worrisome health events across the globe from climate change and pollution to infectious diseases in frogs, bats, and people, the One Health approach is a path to start finding solutions, not simply fret over the problems. It may be obvious to some that there is a connection between humans, animals, and the environment, or the **One Health Triad.** What may be less evident to people just starting out in a career is why the need for a **transdisciplinary**, holistic approach. For many decades, there has been division within the sciences, but the incorporation of lessons learned by working across these silos of knowledge is critical for complex problems. After years of creating isolated silos, whether within human medicine or veterinary medicine but also between professions, it is time for experts across disciplines to work together in the increasingly complex and interconnected world of the twenty-first century.

The idea that human, animal, and environmental health are connected has been around, in various renderings, for many years. It is not surprising, then, that many terms have previously arisen evocative of One Health. These include **One Medicine**, first put forth in the 1960s and **Conservation Medicine** introduced in the 1990s. You also may hear of **EcoHealth**, **Ecosystem Health**, and **Planetary Health**. Each has a slightly different definition and/or may have slightly different areas of focus or mandate. However, in this textbook we hope the idea of a need for a interdisciplinary approach for planetary health as an imperative to face real world twenty-first century issues, no matter the term used, is abundantly evident.

Important to a One Health approach are the variety of disciplines associated with health that are necessary for the success of this holistic approach. An often used image to identify One Health, produced by a One Health group in Sweden, shows this diversity (Figure 1.2). However, many of the logos used today display the One Health Triad, with the imagery that shows the interconnections between human and non-human animals and the environment (Figure 1.3). Another way to view One Health is from a thematic point of view. For example, one may identify with the **translational medicine** or ecological viewpoint present within One Health. With translational medicine we see a cross-taxa approach to the health challenges facing humans, which incorporates the shared knowledge of health between animals and humans. Alternatively, the ecological side of One Health focuses more on understanding the relationships of living organisms within their physical environments. This focus

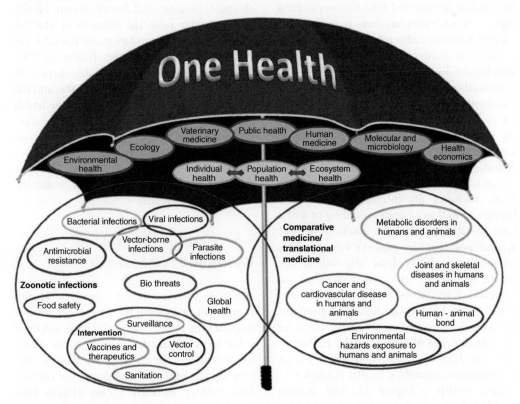

**Figure 1.2** One Health Umbrella, as developed by the group "One Health Sweden." *Source:* Courtesy of One Health Sweden.

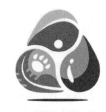

Figure 1.3 Fontbonne University Center for One Health logo, representing the One Health Triad. Be sure to note the person in the white space in the center.

explores how environmental health has direct and indirect impacts on planetary health itself, including human and animal health.

The book is divided into 15 chapters that are further categorized into six overarching themes. In each chapter, there is an abridged excerpt from an audio interview with a One Health Practitioner, whose work is salient to the chapter discussion, and a case study that is co-authored by a 2015–2016 Fontbonne University undergraduate student from either the Honors seminar on One Health or the One Health program's capstone course: Conservation Medicine – One Health in Action.

Part I, *Introduction and Impetus* (Chapters 1–3), includes an introduction to One Health, as well as an understanding of why a One Health approach is essential at this critical point in the planet's history. This introduction shows how dependent the health of all life is to one another. In Chapters 2 and 3, we dive deeper into the connections linking the health of humans, animals, and environments as we consider the "**six degrees of One Health**." In Part II, *The One Health Triad* (Chapters 4–6), we examine environmental health (Chapter 4), animal health (Chapter 5), and human health (Chapter 6) through the lens of One Health. In Part III, *Practitioners and their*

*Tools* (Chapters 7 and 8), we explore the opportunities and necessary skills for One Health practitioners. In Part IV, *How to Start a Movement* (Chapters 9 and 10), we address the challenges involved in educating and communicating with the global public concerning science, risk, and the need to change. In Part V, *The Humanities of One Health* (Chapters 11–13) we explore One Health as it exists within the humanities. All the evidence-based science in the world will not be effective unless it can be packaged through the humanities in a way that people find fits into their cultural, religious, political, and/or economic beliefs.

Finally, in Part VI, we explore *Where We Go From Here*. Thinking about the challenges and opportunities that connect our global environment (Chapter 14), we may also see how this planetary approach opens up new possibilities as we move into a culture of One Health. In Chapter 15, we look at the past, present, and future of One Health and consider how the movement started, where it sits today, and examine the ethics of possible scenarios of the future of One Health. There are many possible directions the One Health movement may take, and the future of One Health is in all of our hands today. As stated by many people, the future is hard to predict. However, Abraham Lincoln reminds us that, "the best way to predict the future is to create it." We hope the readers of this book help to create the future of One Health.

## 1.2 Conclusions and Welcome to One Health

Whether you are new to the One Health movement or looking for a refresher in your current One Health work, this book will be of value to your practice. As the above introductory story exemplifies, we realize that viewing the health challenges of the twenty-first century through a One Health lens, requires an appreciation of the past, awareness of the present, and concern for the future. Only then will we be able to gain a better understanding of, and solve, today's planetary health challenges. Throughout the text it will also be evident that the One Health approach is not only about understanding the twenty-first century health challenges that link humans, animals, and environments, but it is also about finding solutions to these challenges. We live on a finite planet – the only planet in the Universe known to support life – with limited resources and a rapidly growing human population. We must heed the warnings of what the current planetary level health concerns mean for the continued support of life on Earth.

## End of Chapter Questions & Activities

A.  Thought Questions:
   i)  This book starts with a historical perspective of the St. Louis, MO region of the USA. The authors present this as a story of One Health. Do you agree with this assessment, why or why not?
   ii)  There are many terms today that are similar to the term One Health, and with each appreciating the connections of health between humans, animals, and environments. Why do you think there are so many terms? Do you see this as positive or negative for moving the One Health paradigm forward?
   iii)  When you hear news of environmental, conservation, and/or health challenges, do you think you approach these stories with a One Health lens? If not, do you think it would be beneficial to do so moving forward?
B.  In-Class/Guided Activities:
   i)  Consider the history of the area you live in currently or grew up in. Can you retell this story through the lens of One Health? Who are the major players? What are the major events that shape

your region? How has your today been shaped by the past?
   ii)  What events of your area today are shaping the One Health future of your area's tomorrow? How?
C.  At-home Activities:
   i)  Explore the past, present, and future of your region similar to how the authors have done for their region in St. Louis, MO. Write a two to three page essay from the historical to a futuristic perspective through a One Health lens.
   ii)  Consider your career choice. How does a One Health approach fit within this career? Take up to four career choices and for each make a list of what your role in this career would be and how it may help human, animal, and environmental health.
D.  Long-term Action Steps:
   i)  As you become more involved in the One Health movement, you may wish to explore for yourself how these various other terms (e.g. Conservation Medicine, One Medicine, EcoHealth, Ecosystem Health, Planetary Health) movements do or do not fit together.
   ii)  Throughout the coming semester, when you hear any news story (e.g. **social media**, newspaper, T.V.), try to understand how the story ties in with human, animal, and environmental health.
E.  Recommended Reading:

Ambrose, S. (1997). *Undaunted Courage: Meriwether Lewis, Thomas Jefferson, and the Opening of the American West.* Simon and Schuster.

Amsler, K. (2006). *Final Resting Place: The Lives and Deaths of Famous St.Louisans.* Virginia Publishing.

Barry, J.M. (1997). *Rising Tide: The Great Mississippi Flood of 1927 and How it Changed America.* Touchstone.

Gordon, C. (2008). *Mapping Decline: St. Louis and the Fate of the American City.* University of Pennsylvania Press.

Sussman, R.W. (2016). *The Myth of Race: the Troubling Persistence of an Unscientific Idea.* Harvard.

## Interview

*An Interview with Cheryl Stroud, DVM, PhD: Executive Director of the One Health Commission and One Health Practitioner*

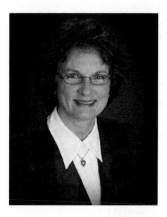

### How did you first hear about One Health?

Like a lot of people, I first heard about One Health in the *Journal of the American Veterinary Medical Association*, which started in 2007 or so, putting articles in about One Health. I followed the formation of the One Health Initiative and how it evolved into a commission. I moved back to North Carolina and was involved in starting up a North Carolina One Health Collaborative, which led to the creation of an inter-institutional course here in North Carolina (NC) between Duke, University of North Carolina (UNC), and NC State; it's a One Health course. And one thing led to another until I was first representing the American Veterinary Medical Association (AVMA) on the One Health Commission Board, and then, in 2013, I was asked to be Executive Director of the One Health Commission.

### Do you see Yourself as a One Health practitioner?

Yes. Totally and completely, and as a veterinarian ... even when I was in practice very early on, I was very intrigued to educate clients about zoonotic diseases. That was in the mid-2000s before we were calling it One Health. So yes, I am absolutely a One Health practitioner; as are many other people who are doing One Health and may not realize it or call it One Health.

### How do your actions reflect One Health, personally or professionally?

I work with the One Health Commission, where we work really hard to create opportunities to form the needed relationships across professions. I tell people in my talks all the time that these collaborations across sectors are not just magically going to happen. Especially in our systems today, where we are so siloed, we cannot even read each other's journals because of our publication system. My mantra these days is, "connect, create, educate." We are trying to connect One Health stakeholders and create opportunities for us to work on One Health issues together, and to educate about One Health and One Health issues.

### What can an individual do to make a difference for planetary health?

Get involved. If there is some issue in the One Health arena, in the space, any issue that falls within the interface of all our professions that you care deeply about, get involved. You can be an active advocate, you can speak to your politicians, and you can educate and nurture the next generation of One Health leaders.

### How can we encourage people to care About planetary health?

I ask people, "Do you care about breakfast, lunch, and dinner?" Then you care about One Health. It includes our food safety and security, and how we care for our soils. Whether food is from plants coming out of the ground or meat coming from our food animal production industries, we have to care about our planet and how we are going to feed the whole world.

### Where is One Health headed?

Toward a tipping point. I really think One Health is being embraced around the world now, in some places a lot more strongly at the government and policy level than in the United States. And it is present more and more loudly. In fact, there's a YouTube recording right now of Matthew Stone, Deputy General Director of the World Organization for Animal Health (OIE), talking about One Health in the OIE. These days the Food and Agriculture Organization of the UN (FAO), the World Health Organization (WHO), and OIE are often referred to as the One Health Tripartite.

### Parting Thoughts?

Oh my gosh, this is urgent! We are losing species at a rate now that is unprecedented. I just read a paper yesterday of how the rate of species loss has escalated from maybe two or three species over a period of 100 years to the present rate 10- or 100-fold greater for species extinctions. The loss is coming from environment devastation, from some of these resource-harvesting processes. It's from encroaching of human populations into some really precious wildlife and species diverse areas in our world. It's just incredibly important for us to actively engage in these conversations that our planet needs, and that our human population needs, and that our animal populations need. From domestics to wildlife to the tiniest microbes and amoeba, we all really need this concept. It is so urgent that we join hands and work on it.

## Works Cited

Charron, D.F. (ed.) (2012). *Ecohealth Research in Practice: Innovative Applications of an Ecosystem Approach to Health.* Springer.

Coughlin, E.K. (2007) The de Soto expedition. *The Chronicle of Higher Education.* http://www.learnnc.org/lp/editions/nchist-twoworlds/1694 (accessed December 15, 2017).

Deem, S.L., Kilbourn, A.M., Wolfe, N.D. et al. (2000). Conservation medicine. *Annals of the New York Academy of Science* 916: 370–377.

Enserik, M. (2007). Initiative aims to benefit animal and human health science to benefit both. *Science* 316: 1553.

Fehrenbacher, D.E. (1981). *Slavery, Law, and Politics: The Dred Scott Case in Historical Perspective.* New York: Oxford University Press.

Fessenden, M. (2015) How to reconstruct Lewis and Clark's journey: follow the mercury-laden latrine pits. *The Smithsonian Magazine.* http://smithsonianmag.com/smart-news/how-reconstruct-lewis-and-clark-journey-follow-mercury-laden-latrine-pits-180956518 (accessed December 15, 2017).

Georgia Historical Society. (2016) Hernando de Soto. http://georgiahistory.com/education-outreach/online-exhibits/featured-historical-figures/hernando-de-soto/contact-with-native-americans (accessed December 15, 2017).

King, L.J., Anderson, L.R., Blackmore, C.G. et al. (2008). Executive summary of the AVMA One Health Initiative Task Force report. *Journal of the American Veterinary Medical Association* 233: 259–261.

Konig, D.T. (2006). The long road to Dred Scott: personhood and the rule of law in the trial court records of St. Louis slave freedom suits. *UMKC Law Review* 75: 1.

One Health Initiative Task Force (2008) One Health: A New Professional Imperative. American Veterinary Medical Association.

Rapport, D. (1998). Defining ecosystem health. In: *Ecosystem Health* (ed. D.J. Rapport), 18–33. Blackwell Scientific.

Sabo, G. (2017) First encounters: Hernando de Soto in the Mississippi Valley, 1541–1542. University of Arkansas. http://archeology. uark.edu/indiansofarkansas/index. html?pageName=First%20Encounters (accessed December 15, 2017).

Schwabe, C. (1984). *Veterinary Medicine and Human Health*, 3e. Baltimore, MD: Williams and Wilkins.

Weaver, D. (2000) Milestones of Missouri's Hidden Hollows. *Missouri Conservationist Magazine*, 2000:3.

Whitmee, S., Haines, A., Beyrer, C. et al. (2015). Safeguarding human health in the Anthropocene epoch: report of The Rockefeller Foundation – Lancet Commission on planetary health. *The Lancet* 386: 1973–2028. doi: 10.1016/S0140-6736(15)60901-1.

2

## Our Interconnected World

*"All things are connected. Whatever befalls the earth befalls the children of the earth."*

Chief Seattle (Figure 2.1)

Have you ever thought of how your health and that of a forest elephant in Africa or a child on the other side of the world are connected? Or maybe you have wondered about the connections that link a potential human influenza pandemic, habitat degradation, and feeding the world's 7.6 billion human inhabitants. These questions ask us to think of how *all* life on Earth is connected. Forest elephants in Africa are **ecosystem engineers,** or forest gardeners, that help maintain the Central African rainforest and the lungs (e.g. trees) of planet Earth. Just like you, all children, no matter where they may live, need fresh water, fresh air, and enough calories to be healthy and survive. The link of habitat loss, food security, and influenza at first may seem harder to grasp. However, humans continue to modify landscapes and destroy wetlands that for millennia have been stopover sites along migrating wild bird flyways. These wetlands are now largely replaced with poultry factories, thus encouraging the mixing of influenza strains so that **spillover** of pathogens, into a growing human population, occurs. In this context, the link becomes evident. *All* life and the health of *all* life are connected.

We may call these connections the "six degrees of One Health." Taken from the six degrees of separation, first set out in 1929 by Frigyes Karinthy but better known from Kevin Bacon, we see that all living things in the world are six or fewer steps away from each other. Today in 2017, we realize that the six degrees of separation applies to the health of *all* life – the six degrees of One Health. We are just beginning to understand the challenges that increasingly threaten human livelihoods and health, the health of domestic and wild animals, and ecosystem health and **resilience**. These extend across the globe and intersect in countless ways. One suitcase of non-human primate **bushmeat** on a plane traveling from Cameroon to Kansas may cause negative health ripples throughout the world, if it harbors **zoonotic** pathogens (e.g. monkeypox virus, simian foamy virus).

Fortunately, the solutions to these health challenges may also reach across the globe. For example, preventive measures that minimize threats to health, such as laws that lower pollutants in the environment, may have significant and positive health impacts over large geographical reaches and across taxa (see Chapter 13). In this chapter, we will explore how the health status of *all* life, from organisms found in the most remote corners of the Earth to the most crowded cities, is connected.

As covered in Chapter 1, One Health is a collaborative effort of multiple disciplines – working locally, nationally, and globally – to attain optimal health for people, animals, and the environment. Fundamental

*Introduction to One Health: An Interdisciplinary Approach to Planetary Health*, First Edition.
Sharon L. Deem, Kelly E. Lane-deGraaf and Elizabeth A. Rayhel.
© 2019 John Wiley & Sons, Inc. Published 2019 by John Wiley & Sons, Inc.
Companion website: www.wiley.com/go/deem/health

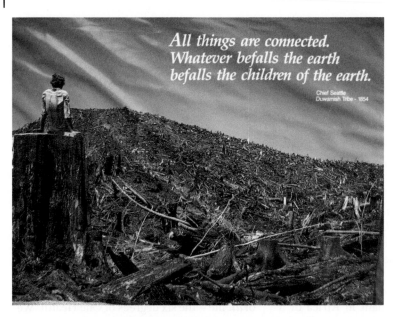

All things are connected.
Whatever befalls the earth
befalls the children of the earth.

Chief Seattle
Duwamish Tribe - 1854

Figure 2.1 Chief Seattle Quote. *Source:* Blanchard, https://creativecommons.org/licenses/by-sa/2.0/. CC BY-SA 2.0.

to this definition is that One Health offers a transdisciplinary approach that strives to ensure the health of human and non-human animals and the environments on which all life is dependent. The emphasis of the One Health initiative is that these three domains of humans, animals, and environments – the One Health Triad – which at first glance may appear disparate entities, are in reality closely interconnected. Therefore, One Health practitioners must fully grasp the why, where, what, when, who, and how of these interconnections. More importantly, we must understand these interconnections if we are to find solutions to the challenges. As the One Health initiative gains momentum across disciplines (see Chapter 7), these collaborative efforts will ensure we are able to better understand, confront, and manage the growing interconnected health challenges.

We are living in the **Anthropocene epoch** in which the 7.6 billion humans alive exert powerful forces that are driving planetary changes and that are increasing connections. These rapid changes provide challenges and opportunities for the One Health practitioner.

To consider these interconnected challenges we may look at how to feed just one species, humans (*Homo sapiens*). As the number of humans rapidly approaches eight billion with approximately 150 000 additional humans added each day, how do we provide food to ensure all people lead healthy lives without destroying the other species that share the planet, or indeed the planet itself?

It is not just the food demanded of the growing human population. Annually, humans as a species use 1.6 "Earths," based on the resources we extract. In fact, "**Earth Overshoot Day**," which has been observed since 1987, shows that humans use more from nature than can be replaced in the entire year. Simply put we overshoot the resources earlier with each passing year. In 1987, the first recorded Earth Overshoot Day was on December 19. Humans used all the resources available without overdrawing the Earth's bounty when there were still 12 days of the year left. In 2017, Overshoot Day was August 2. In other words, by August 2, 2017, humans used all the resources that could sustainably be used in one year without damaging the planet or overdrawing on

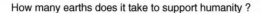

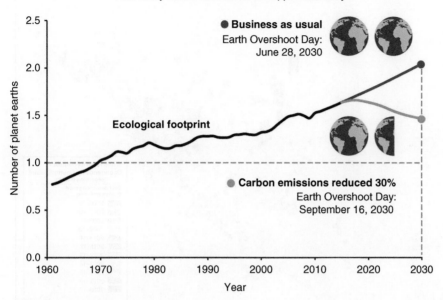

Figure 2.2 Earth Overshoot Day.

resources with 151 days remaining in the year. We borrowed 151 days from the next year. Projections of Earth Overshoot Day, if we continue with "business as usual" is on June 28 by the year 2030 (Figure 2.2). Even with humans consuming planetary resources faster each year, we still have not managed to feed all 7.6 billion of us well, since many people do not get enough calories, and have disease issues of nutritional deficiencies (e.g. starvation, weak immune systems, and vitamin/mineral deficiencies). At the same time many other people get too many calories and have the disease issues of excess (e.g. obesity, diabetes, heart disease). Both present significant public health challenges.

As we dive deeper into our complex connected world and explore what may lie at the core of these concerns across the One Health Triad, we will consider how the 7.6 billion – and counting – human inhabitants are the drivers of these connected health challenges. We will do this by considering the five challenges that connect the health of *all* life and which impact species' survival, including the survival of *H. sapiens*. These challenges,

covered in more detail in Chapter 3, include: (i) **emerging infectious diseases** (EID) and invasive species; (ii) loss of biodiversity and natural resources; (iii) climate change; (iv) environmental degradation and environmental contaminants; and (v) loss of habitat and increased interactions between domestic animals, wildlife, and humans. We are living at a time when the health of all is connected, a time of One Health.

## 2.1 One Health Challenges on a Connected Planet

Let us begin by thinking about bats. When most people think of bats, they may think of rabies, or *Batman*, or vampires. These thoughts, although associated with bats, would miss one of the best One Health examples. With closer consideration of bats, we also may realize the many **ecosystem services** they provide for planetary health. In North America during the past decade, approximately 6 million insectivorous and cave-dwelling bats have died due to an

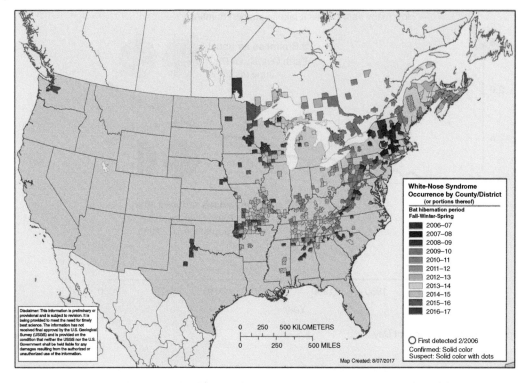

Figure 2.3 White Nose Syndrome Map of USA with spread of disease.

introduced fungus that arrived in the USA in 2006, by – you guessed it – humans. The *Pseudogymnoascus destructan* fungus entered the USA in New York, probably on a spelunker's shoe, and since has moved across the continent (Figure 2.3). The fungus, native to Europe, causes white nose syndrome (WNS) in naïve US bats, which as the name implies causes white noses, and wing webs, from fungal spores that grow on hibernating bats. The fungus irritates and wakes the bats during winter hibernation. Once awake they often starve to death since their diet of choice, mosquitoes and other insects, are not available. In the next warm season, when mosquitoes are back out in force, the bats, which normally eat about 350 mosquitoes per bat per night are no longer present to eat mosquitoes. Other bat ecosystem services, such as pollinating plants, are also lost. Goodbye pest control and pollination!

This loss of bat ecosystem services may result in people using more pesticides to control mosquitoes, or if pesticides are not applied, there may be more mosquitoes present and a higher prevalence of mosquito-transmitted zoonotic pathogens such as West Nile virus (WNV) and Zika virus: two other pathogens recently introduced to the New World; again by humans. Added to this, recent advances in "green" energy with wind farms dotting the land and causing high mortality of tree roosting bats, you have high losses of both cave-dwelling and tree roosting bat species. A six degrees of One Health story of pathogen movement across the globe (e.g. *P. destructan*, WNV, Zika) and the search for solutions to human energy needs (e.g. wind power) leading to a conservation crisis for bats and the associated cost in human health concerns from potential infectious (mosquito-borne diseases) and non-infectious (e.g. cancers and pesticide use) diseases.

## 2.2 Global Challenges for One Health Practitioners

### 2.2.1 Emerging Infectious Diseases and Invasive Species

One of the great challenges today for human, animal, and plant health is the emergence of infectious diseases. Ironically, it was in the 1960s when the US Surgeon General, Dr. William H. Stewart, stated "It is time to close the book on infectious diseases and declare the war against pestilence won." He was echoing the belief that modern medicine had all but conquered infectious diseases. It was soon evident that globalization and the increase in the human population were to bring a very different future. Emerging infectious diseases (EIDs), diseases that have increased in number, have spread to new regions, and/or are found in new species, are a concern for the conservation of all species, including humans. The increase in human EIDs is of global public health significance and largely related to human–animal interactions. In our interconnected world, and possibly of most interest from a One Health perspective, is that 75% of EIDs in humans are zoonotic, shared between animals and humans, and 70% of these are associated with wild animal reservoirs. Many of these approximately 1600 EIDs are now common household names, including avian influenza, WNV, Sudden Acute Respiratory Syndrome (SARS), Ebola, and monkeypox viruses.

We often hear of avian influenza (H5N1) and its impact on human health and livelihoods in Asia, or Ebola outbreaks in animals and humans in Africa. However, EIDs are far from an "over there" disease issue. The USA has experienced multiple zoonotic EIDs with increasing frequency since the last decades of the twentieth century. The arrival in 1999 of WNV, and the subsequent rapid spread across the continent, clearly demonstrates the impact an EID may have on humans and other animals. Ecosystem level impacts associated with the near regional **extirpation**

(local extinctions) of some bird species due to WNV infection, the human health costs from WNV **morbidity** and **mortality**, as well as increased use of pesticides to control mosquito vectors, may be harder to quantify. The introduction of this novel pathogen into the USA, and the presence of suitable mosquito vectors with populations of susceptible amplifying bird species, offered the "perfect storm" for this zoonotic EID to take hold and move across the continent.

EIDs do not just target humans. There are a number of EIDs in non-human animals and plants. White nose syndrome is just one of the many EIDs in wild animal populations that have implications for the health of species beyond the affected hosts. There are countless examples of animal EIDs that are causing population extirpations and in some cases even species' extinctions. These EIDs may be pathogens that infect only animals (e.g. WNS of bats, fungus that cause chytridiomycosis of amphibians) or may be zoonotic with direct infections of non-human and human animals (e.g. Ebola and influenza).

EIDs of food crops, often associated with monoculture agriculture, are another growing health threat. These EIDs may decimate production and lead to the increased development of genetically modified plants to withstand the application of increasingly powerful pesticides and herbicides. Many of these pesticides and herbicides come with health costs for human and non-human animals alike, and the environments where they are applied. There has also been the loss of thousands of acres of forests due to invasive species, from microbes to invertebrates, moved by humans from one location to another. In the USA, these include chestnut disease, Dutch elm disease, Sudden Oak Death, and the emerald boreal beetle.

### 2.2.2 Loss of Biodiversity and Natural Resources

Humans are clearing tracts of land at an unsustainable rate as we make room for the production of food and other products on which humans are reliant. A great example of this is the increased production of palm oil trees in Asia, and more recently in Africa and South America. Palm oil, touted as a heart-healthy oil for people, may be found in products ranging from cookies to detergents. Palm-oil tree plantations cover thousands of acres of monoculture. These monoculture plantations cover land that was once home to many species, including, and most famously, the endangered orangutan (*Pongo* spp.). One can quickly see the One Health connections in that this food source, said to be of a human health benefit, may lead to the loss of other species, both animals and plants, and jeopardize the health of the environment, and ultimately humans themselves.

Today we are living during a time when we are witness to the "**sixth mass extinction**." We are currently losing species at a rate up to a thousand times higher than the background rate, or "baseline norm," and not seen since the age of the dinosaurs. However, unlike the previous mass extinctions, this is the first time in history that one species, *H. sapiens* is the driver of these losses. If one considers the changing composition of the terrestrial **vertebrate biomass**, the total mass of organisms that have backbones, we can understand how biodiversity loss in the context of food, conservation, and public health are connected.

Let's take a trip into the past. Ten thousand years ago, humans were just starting to be successful in domesticating animals, convincing that wolf to sit down next to the village campfire. There were not many humans and fewer domestic animals. Ten thousand years ago, 2% of vertebrate biomass included humans (<10 million) and the few, just domesticated, animals. The other 98% of vertebrate biomass were the non-domestic species – the lions and tigers and bears. Now if we look at the composition of vertebrate biomass today, the percentages flip flop with 2% all the "other animals" that are categorized as neither human nor domestic animal. Humans and our domestic animals now make up 98% of this biomass. This includes the 7.6 billion humans, and the dogs, cats, and other companion animals we invite into our homes. It also includes the approximately 19 billion chickens, 2 billion pigs, 1 billion sheep, 990 million cattle, 450 million goats, and 15 million camels alive on Earth each day, waiting to become human food.

There are many reasons that the loss of biodiversity and resources lead to health costs. One is a recently understood phenomenon called the **dilution effect**, wherein it has been shown that for some systems, infectious diseases may be more likely to emerge in regions that have lost the "normal" suite of species – the biodiversity. For example, Lyme disease, a tick-borne disease of high human health importance and first recognized in the USA in 1976, has during the past 40 years increased in prevalence. Infections are more commonly found in areas that have lost non-human host reservoirs, that may be infested with the tick vector, but which cannot carry the Lyme-causing *Borrelia burgdorferi* bacteria. The loss of other vertebrate hosts has resulted in an increase in Lyme disease in humans as well as domestic animals (e.g. dogs, horses) in these areas.

Second, the health cost from the loss of biodiversity also affects us at the dinner table. The recent loss in bees and other pollinators has created issues for agriculture. For example, bees help to pollinate human food; one of every three bites of food we take is from crops pollinated by bees. The loss of these pollinators, with their ecosystem services, may result in costs to human health, and to environments as the pollination of native plants also rely on bee pollination. This is in addition to the loss of bat pollination, and their pest control abilities, mentioned in the introduction.

With 38% of the arable land on Earth used to produce food for humans, we see there is little space left for the other animals that share our world. This is not that different when looking at the oceans. An estimated 70% of the world's fisheries are fully to overly exploited, or significantly depleted. Further, we also know that the illegal and legal trade in wildlife, taken from lands not dedicated for food production, has become a world-wide enterprise. The numbers are hard to quantify, and harder to comprehend. For example, annually humans take an estimated five million tons of bushmeat just from the forests of the African Congo Basin. This number is a conservation and public health crisis. These five million tons represent both declining wildlife populations and disease threats for *all* life since the animals killed and transported may act as "pathogen packages" as they, and their microbes, move across the globe.

### 2.2.3 Climate Change

It is clear that the climate is changing and that it has impacts on domestic and non-domestic animal, human, and plant health. These impacts may be exacerbated by the inability of animals to emigrate from areas of climatic change or from a mismatch timing of hibernation, flowering, and pollination. Climate change may be the single most significant driver of health concerns that connect all life across the One Health Triad. As the climate changes, there is an increase in vector-borne diseases (VBD), a spread of infectious diseases to new areas, and heat-related non-infectious deaths. Additionally, extreme weather patterns such as more intense El Niños and storm systems create both infectious (e.g. cholera, VBD) and non-infectious (flooding, damage to shelter) health issues.

These climate changes mean that we must develop climate adaptive strategies such as the production of different livestock species, which may add costs to human health while threatening endangered wildlife species. One example of an animal health concern from climate change is occurring in the changing landscape of East Africa in which the semi-arid lands are becoming increasingly arid. The inability of traditional livestock species such as cattle to survive in these regions has led to an increasingly camel reliant human population (see Chapter Case Study).

Similar to the impacts of climate change on human and animal health, these changes create ecosystem damage on unprecedented scales. Floods and droughts associated with extreme weather events lead to significant damage and death of plants. The loss of top soil and vegetation, due to wash away, may also lead to less functional and less resilient ecosystems.

### 2.2.4 Environmental Degradation and Environmental Contaminants

It was in the 1960s with the publication of Rachael Carson's book, *Silent Spring*, that the world was awaken to the dangers of dichlorodiphenyltrichloroethane (DDT) and other environmental contaminants. The near extinction of the American symbol of freedom, the Bald Eagle (*Haliaeetus leucocehalus*), due to egg shell thinning from environmental exposure to DDT, was the first step in the USA for environmental measures to improve the environment. The US Environmental Protection Agency (EPA), created in December 1970, was developed to allow one agency to oversee research and to monitor and set standards for environmental health. Closely following the establishment of the EPA, DDT was banned in the USA. Yet, in the intervening 40+ years, we have seen increasing levels of contaminants that have short- and long-term health impacts for humans and animals. Whether it is the March 2010 BP Deepwater Horizon Oil Spill in which a total of 210 million gallons of oil was released into the Gulf of Mexico (see Chapter 12) or the continuous low-level release of petroleum products added daily to terrestrial and aquatic environments, we are causing severe impacts to human and non-human animal health.

More recently the book *Our Stolen Future: Are We Threatening Our Fertility, Intelligence, and Survival? A Scientific Detective Story* was the next wake-up call on issues of environmental contaminates with emphasis on the endocrine disrupting chemicals (EDCs). Since its publication in 1996, the amount of

EDCs in the environment has continued upward due to the pervasive use of plastics. Studies now confirm that exposure to EDCs, including bisphenol-A (BPA), a common chemical in many plastic products, may cause changes in gonadal tissue in wildlife species, intersex characteristics, and behavioral changes. EDCs may well be the DDT of this generation.

In addition to the toxins discussed earlier, the fragmentation and degradation of large areas across the globe are leading to major health issues. These modifications may create environments that are no longer able to provide ecosystem services for such things as fresh water and oxygen. More specifically, degraded landscapes have been associated with EIDs from disease spillover as humans and their domestic animals move further into previously pristine areas. These landscape changes also include an increase in light and noise pollution, with health impacts that effect species from sea turtles to humans. One need only look at the Great Pacific Garbage Patch (see Chapter 13) to appreciate that these modifications are not just on land. Humans are changing environments, whether on land or sea, and creating many of the threats across the One Health Triad.

### 2.2.5 Loss of Habitat and Increased Interactions of Domestic Animals–Wildlife–Humans

Although human populations are increasingly urbanized, with more than 50% of people now living in cities, the impacts on habitats as mentioned earlier continues unabated. Even if we live in urban environments, we still require shelter, clothes, and food. This takes land and water resources, leading to the environmental degradation touched on earlier. Degraded and fragmented landscapes often trap species on "islands of isolation" surrounded by human change, genetic bottlenecks, and resource limitations. As we know from **island biogeography**, small, isolated populations are more threatened by **stochastic events** and it is more likely these

events will result in population declines and even extinctions.

The growth in livestock production, to feed the 7.6 billion humans, throughout the world also has resulted in an increase at the domestic animal–wildlife–human interface. In today's connected world, this interface allows for disease transmission to occur more often and involving more species. All these changes place stressors, some subtle while others lead to peracute death, to human and non-human animals alike. These multiple stressors (e.g. land degradation, loss of resources, change in predator–prey relationships, invasive species, increased species interface) often lead to declining health and mortality.

## 2.3 Drivers of Our Connected Health Challenges

In the age of the Anthropocene, we humans have a footprint that extends across the globe creating connections near and far. In a few decades, human travel has changed from requiring months to circumnavigate the globe to the present day when we may travel from one continent to another in a matter of hours. Today we travel across the globe rapidly and often. This travel is not just humans physically, but also all the things that travel with us from the organisms traveling within us, and the stuff with us. For example, any one of us could, with little time and money, travel to any country on any continent (maybe not Antarctica but maybe!) by the end of next week. This should scare us, since on the trip, it will not be just us that travels, but also the billions of other life forms (microbes) that call each of our body's home. They too will be traveling across the globe, as will the things we take along in our suitcases.

The global trade in stuff, responsible for many improvements for many humans, also has health implications across the One Health Triad. The simple act of extracting resources at an unsustainable rate (e.g. Earth

Overshoot Day) is part of this cost to health. Possibly of more significance is that this trade provides the potential to transport pathogens and the ability for epidemics to surface anywhere on the planet from a disease event that started somewhere else (see Chapter 14). It may also allow for multiple entrees of an infectious agent. For example, based on genomic epidemiology data, Zika virus most likely arrived into the USA in 2016 from multiple points of entry.

The One Health connection may be most evident when we combine **abiotic** and **biotic** factors in a planetary health approach. In the 1960s, Lovelock, Margulis, and others noted the planet was self-regulating, "alive" in a sense. Their theory, accepted by many and shunned by others, is widely known as the **Gaia theory**, named after **Gaia**, the Greek Goddess of the Earth. They suggested that life on Earth was the creator and regulator of the atmosphere and charged that damage to the Earth, once done, was very difficult to undo. In fact, when we compare Earth with any other planet we have studied, the life force that is Earth is evident (Figure 2.4). Thinking of the Earth's health, we may quickly appreciate the impacts and health threats that humans have placed on it. According to recent scientific reports, humans have transformed between one-third and one-half of the land surface, and now appropriate over 40% of the net primary terrestrial productivity, consume 35% of the productivity of the oceanic shelf, and use 60% of the freshwater run-off each year, primarily to feed our species.

Zoonotic EIDs are also increasing due to human changes to the Earth. EIDs in humans are happening concurrent with **anthropogenic** change that include the over 40% of the land surface exploited by humans, more than half of all accessible fresh water used by humankind, and greenhouse gas and methane emissions escalating annually. Humans may now be the single most dominant driver of planetary health. Today pristine wildernesses may be more of a concept than a reality. We are reaching ever deeper into the most untouched regions of the world with our road networks all but covering the globe. In the USA, it is estimated that roads have impacts on greater than 22% of the land area in the lower 48 states. This network allows the movement of humans, animals, plants, and microbes, making it all too easy to see how infectious and susceptible hosts encounter one another, which may lead to EID events.

The increased demand for protein has resulted not only in major landscape modifications, but also in the use of non-domestic

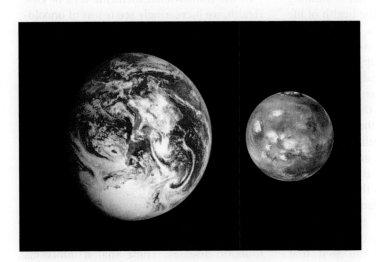

Figure 2.4 Earth next to Mars. *Source:* Courtesy of NASA.

animal products (e.g. bushmeat) which are often moved, along with their associated microbes, between continents. Additionally, as our livestock populations grow across most continents, there is closer and more frequent contact between livestock and wildlife thus allowing for pathogen sharing that may lead to negative results for human health and wildlife conservation. An example of this link, with real world potential global impact, is the Nipah virus epidemic that surfaced among pig farmers in Malaysia in 1999, at a time that pork production was expanding in the country. As pig farms moved farther into forested lands, and the home to fruit bat colonies, the ability to have a bat-associated virus (Nipah) spillover into pigs, and then into humans as a food-borne pathogen demonstrates this One Health link. This bat–pig–virus example is one of many as we see other EIDs in human populations, including Rift Valley Fever, Q Fever, SARS, and Middle Eastern Respiratory Syndrome (MERS) associated with the ever increasing domestic–wild animal links.

## 2.4 Solutions Using a One Health Approach

It is easy to be despondent after examining the challenges that connect the health of life on Earth. However, there is hope. In our complicated and connected world, the One Health initiative may be the approach necessary for solutions to these challenges. Just as in the twentieth century when medical professionals more fully realized the **multifactorial** nature of disease, in the twenty-first century we are more fully realizing the need for a holistic, multifactorial, and transdisciplinary approach to solve these complex issues. The medical doctors that treat their pediatric patients for lead poisoning, without a preventive plan for the environmental factors that created the illness (e.g. lead paint on bedroom walls), know too well that

medicines alone will not "cure" the patients. The same is true of the veterinarians treating herds of cattle for an outbreak of leptospirosis. If they do not look at the whole picture (i.e. reservoir animal sources, water supplies), they will miss the opportunity to solve the problem. No amount of doxycycline will cure the herd without preventive holistic environmental steps incorporated into the treatment plan.

We now have many examples that demonstrate the value of a holistic One Health approach providing benefits and increasingly solutions to the twenty-first century health problems. Disciplines across One Health (see Chapter 7) have teamed together to provide the solutions for many of today's health challenges. For example, once an estimated cost of anywhere between US \$4–53 billion was the price tag from the loss of bats to WNS and wind energy development, people began to care about bats. A One Health team includes those that work to protect caves where bats hibernate from human visitors and potential WNS pathogen **fomites**. Scientists that explore the epidemiology and ecology of the disease and increasingly how to prevent/treat *P. destructan*, while many others that explore methods for more bat- and bird-friendly wind energy.

In the translational medicine arm of One Health, we increasingly see teams of oncologists, from both sides of the human medical/non-human veterinary health professions, working together to find diagnostic and treatment advancements for our efforts against cancer. Both infectious and non-infectious cancers afflict humans and animals, with many of these cancers similar across taxa. Understanding both the environmental causes and mechanisms of cancers in human and non-human patients will lead to advancements for all.

Another important example of the One Health team approach being used to solve the challenges of today is that addressing zoonotic diseases. These shared infectious agents that cross species boundaries, and cause great suffering to human and non-human animals, may be effectively managed if we look at the reservoirs, hosts, and environments together as we work to develop preventive measures. The H1N1 avian influenza epidemics, coronavirus epidemics of SARS, and MERS are prime examples of how a species-spanning approach has helped to avert pandemics.

## 2.5 Connectivity Across the Human–Animal–Environment Interface

It is clear that *all* life modifies other life at some level and that we are *all* connected. There is a reason we call it the "the web of life." Humans are no exception, and indeed, we have been modifying the environment since the first bipedal footsteps of *H. sapiens*. However, our negative global modifications have increased in recent history, with key periods of escalation around 10 000 years ago at the time of domestication and again around the time of the industrial revolution in the 1700–1800s. We are now living in the age of the Anthropocene. With our advanced technologies and communication systems, the rate of change we effect on the planet is ever more evident with environmental harm and resource over-extraction leading to new health hazards for *all* life. We also have never been so knowledgeable of the connections that link health.

As stated earlier, the closest One Health links may be at the dinner Table. A common East African greeting is "Osso saada keriiko?" which means "How are you and your livestock?" Many cultures understand the link that their family's health has with the health of the animals on which they are dependent. The problem of safely feeding the world while preserving the environment and avoiding issues such as **antimicrobial resistance** in animals and humans requires cooperative scientific problem solving – a One Health approach. One area worth exploring may be the ethics of One Health in a connected world. Measures taken to "ensure" human health are often at the cost of animal and environmental health. We must face our desire to provide health care for the 7.6 billion humans while not creating ever greater disease issues and health challenges to *all* other life that share the planet with us.

In today's interconnected world, the human footprint changes climate, fragments and modifies landscapes, moves invasive species, and creates health challenges for *all* life. Understanding these connections and the diseases and health challenges that threaten human, animal, and plant life on Earth is a first step to coming up with solutions. The good news is that One Health teams allow us to do this. After a period in which disciplinary silos were erected, resulting in academic fields becoming insular and disconnected, we now realize that we must bring these disciplines together – again – on One Health teams that work to tackle the challenges of today. We also realize that reacting to health issues, such as an infectious disease pandemic, whether in bats or people, instead of preventing them, is simply bad medicine.

In the chapters ahead, we will more fully explore the challenges and solutions for Planetary Health in the twenty-first century. We will provide tips on how to be a One Health practitioner during the Anthropocene Epoch. These ideas and actions, and the One Health initiative itself, have arrived at the right time since the health and survival of all of us might just depend on this collaborative and transdisciplinary approach. The holistic One Health approach for the health of *all* living beings, on the only planet we know supports life, may be the key to solving the conservation and health crises of today.

# End of Chapter Questions & Activities

A. Thought Questions:

    i) In this chapter, we explore the connections linking all life. Can you think of ways that these connections can be used to the advantage of the One Health practitioner when looking for solutions to the current conservation and public health challenges?

    ii) If you had the ability to make one change on a global scale, what would you choose, why would you choose it, and how would you see it contribute to solutions for conservation and public health?

    iii) In this chapter, we present the world as very connected and assert that humans, animals, and environments influence one another across a continuum. Can you give an example of any situation where this is not true?

B. In-Class/Guided Activities:

    i) Have each student provide one example of how they feel the health of another person, an animal, or their local environment has had direct impacts on their health in the last 24 hours, 7 days, and month.

    ii) Have each student share how they see their health is connected to the health of another student on the other side of the world from where they are sitting. (You can look at a map!)

C. At Home Activities:

    i) Pick a 24-hr period over the past week and consider all the ways that other people, animals and the environment affected your health. Make a list of these connections and indicate for the living organisms (other humans, animals, plants) if they had a negative/neutral/positive impact on your health and conversely if you had a negative/neutral/positive impact on their lives.

    ii) Too often overlooked, a major One Health challenge is created by the products we purchase, and how we consume. Every day in big and small ways, our actions connect us to *all* other life on the planet—the six degrees of One Health. At your next meal, find out where your food originated and what it took to get it on your plate. Think about the clothes, books, furniture, and other items that fill your home. Make a list of all the things you see in front of you right now.

    iii) Visit the website http://www.worldometers.info/world-population/ to visualize how many more humans are on the planet by the second.

D. Long-term Action Steps:

    i) The equation $I = P \times A \times T$ (Impact = population × affluence × technology) is increasingly becoming more understood. Each of us has a global footprint. Going forward, please consider your impact on your health, other humans, animals and the planet. Take measures to minimize your global negative impacts and to increase your positive impacts.

E. Recommended Reading:

Carson, R. (1962). *Silent Spring.* Houghton Mifflin.

Colborn, T., Dumanoski, D., and Myers, J.P. (1997). *Our Stolen Future:Are We Threatening Our Fertility, Intelligence, and Survival? – A Scientific Detective Story.* Plume.

Igo People Pathogens Planet: The Economics of One Health 2010

Lovelock, J. (1991). *Healing Gaia: Practical Medicine for the Planet.* Random House.

Quammen, D. (1996). *The Song of the Dodo: Island Biogeography in an Age of Extinction.* Simon and Schuster.

## Interview

*An interview with Agustin Fuentes, PhD, who is The Edmund P. Joyce C.S.C. Professor of Anthropology at the University of Notre Dame.*

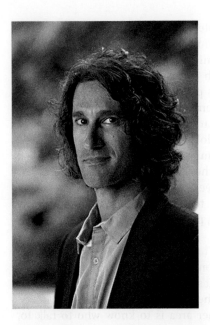

**When did you first hear about One Health?**

Because of my work looking at the interface between human and non-human primates, and humans and some other animals, I have always been working with veterinarians and with medical doctors, plus anthropologists and biologists interested in human biology and exposure to pathogens. The One Health term started emerging in literature quite some time ago, but I became more familiar with the general premise of it as it began to circulate in both anthropological and vet circles.

**How is One Health important to your work?**

I am very interested in integrative approaches to understanding pathogen ecologies and the overall health of humans and other animals. Relevant to my own research, I am impacted by this move for collaborative projects between multiple disciplines as the norm. I think integrative approaches that draw on anthropology, biology, veterinary studies, epidemiological studies, and others are the only way to get at understanding health in the current landscape.

**How do your actions reflect One Health, personally or professionally?**

If you look at my publication record over the last 20 years, a lot of that work has focused on the notion that human-other animal interfaces, in my case particularly human-other primate interfaces, are critical ecologies for understanding what's going on today. In a health context, I think it's even more important because of the commonalities in evolutionary histories and physiologies between human and other primates, and we have got a number of pathogen sharing events that have broad scale implications for humans and other primate health. My actions have been through research and publication, and I'd like to think that I am contributing broadly to the One Health enterprise. We have been pushing an approach called ethnoprimatology, which integrates a kind of primatologist, anthropological, and biological (One Health) approach to trying to understand this interface and pathogen sharing co-ecologies.

**What can an individual do to make a difference for planetary health?**

One of the most important things one can do is to be informed. One of the biggest challenges we have is getting quality information. It behooves individuals to get a good understanding of what their social and pathogen landscapes look like and how an individual is impacted. Education and information acquisition is critical.

**How can we encourage people to care about planetary Health?**

People can think seriously about family planning, community planning, and the infrastructure in which they live. How do we live, how do we consume, how much do we consume, and why do we consume? I am not saying, "Don't consume," people just should be more aware of how their consumption patterns, particularly in the **global north**, affect global patterns.

### Where is One Health headed?

One Health should be going to true integration across the biological and social sciences, and maybe even the humanities and others to develop teams of researchers that have a full complement, or at least a very diverse complement of approaches. This will ensure we look at the complex scenarios across the ecological, biological, historical, political, and economic playing fields.

### What do you see as the top two challenges for global health in this interconnected world?

I will limit this to two. The first would be movement of people and the pace at which we are modifying ecologies. The second big problem is education and information. I think we have to get the data we have in academia and in health research agencies effectively out to the public.

### How do you see a One Health approach may help to minimize the potential danger of movements and trade?

In the most straightforward sense education; we must understand what the primate trade does, not just in the conservation sense, but in the potential to disseminate, and create, pathogens. One Health teams could deploy a fear factor to get people to pay attention to these problems. It can also help with interdisciplinary research in this topic, such as in global trade in animal parts. Humanists can help on how we deal with these moral and ethical dilemmas. We need to take advantage and not be afraid to push into complex, culturally dense, politically touchy topics.

### Parting Thoughts?

Everyone should be bi-lingual or tri-lingual. It's really important that we beef up on the cultural linguistic diversity. Another area is to know who to talk to, since there is just too much data for one person to know. The smart scientist today is a terrific collaborator, not just a terrific investigator.

---

**Case Study: What Does Camel Health Have to Do with Climate Change, Human Health, and Wildlife Conservation?**

Co-authored by Diamond Carroll

The ability to feed the 7.6 billion people that currently inhabit the planet has become increasingly challenging due to climate change and other environmental stressors occurring on a global scale and at an ever-accelerating rate. An example of a One Health program dedicated to looking at these challenges is the Dromedary Camel (*Camelus dromedaries*) Health Assessment Program (Figure 2.5). This program links environmental, human, and animal health. The program is led by the Saint Louis Zoo Institute for Conservation Medicine but located in Laikipia County, Kenya; a region that has experienced significant climatic and demographic shifts in recent decades. During this time, the camel population increased by approximately 75%, while the cattle population greatly decreased. This shift in livestock species is largely due to the semi-arid land becoming increasingly arid (e.g. climate change), and therefore less hospitable for cattle survival. As climate changed in the region, a change in livestock practices also occurred. The shift in livestock has been to a more climate adaptive species – the Dromedary camel.

Camels are an important food source for the 40 million people living in Kenya. Researchers estimate that at least 10% of all Kenyans, an estimated four million people, drink unpasteurized camel milk. The increase in camel milk as a source of protein may have nutritional value. However, it is also a human health hazard since infectious disease causing agents, harbored by camels, may be transmitted when people drink

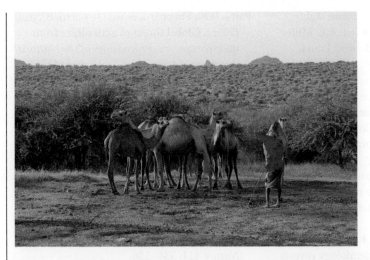

Figure 2.5 Camels in Laikipia County, Kenya, part of the Dromedary camel health program.

unpasteurized milk. Additionally, the increase in camel numbers in Kenya, to approximately three million, is also a concern for wildlife conservation. Laikipia County is one of the regions with the highest camel numbers. It is also a region with some of the best remaining wildlife populations in East Africa. Camels may share pathogens, and compete for resources with these **sympatric** wildlife species.

Many One Health programs focus on stopping the spread of diseases that have negative impacts on humans and animals. This Dromedary camel health program works to understand the pathogens of camels, and to develop methods that prevent the spread of these pathogens from camels to humans, other livestock species, and wildlife. To accomplish this, researchers work to improve biosecurity measures, such as better camel husbandry and veterinary care. This example of camel health in East Africa shows that livestock health has direct impacts for both human and wildlife health in the region. As we search for food security for a growing human population at a time of significant climate changes, we will have new challenges at the animal-human interface on a changing planet.

## Works Cited

Bhandari, R.K., Deem, S.L., Holliday, D.K. et al. (2015). Effects of the environmental estrogenic contaminants Bisphenol A and 17 Ethinyl Estradiol on sexual development and adult behaviors in aquatic wildlife species. *General and Comparative Endocrinology* 214: 195–219.

Boyles, J.G., Cryan, P.M., McCracken, G.F. et al. (2011). Economic importance of bats in agriculture. *Science* 332: 41–42.

Browne, A.S., Fèvre, E.M., Kinnaird, M. et al. (2017). Serosurvey of *Coxiella burnetii* (Q fever) in Dromedary Camels (*Camelus dromedarius*) in Laikipia County, Kenya. *Zoonoses and Public Health* doi: 10.1111/zph.12337.

Crutzen, P.J. (2002). Geology of mankind. *Nature* 415: 23.

Daszak, P., Cunningham, A.A., and Hyatt, A.D. (2000). Emerging infectious disease of wildlife: threats to biodiversity and human health. *Science* 287: 443–449.

Deem, S.L. (2015). Conservation medicine to one health: the role of zoologic veterinarians. In: *Fowler's Zoo and Wild Animal Medicine: Volume 8* (ed. R.E. Miller and M.E. Fowler), 698–703. Saint Louis, Missouri: Saunders Elsevier.

Deem, S.L., Fevre, E.M., Kinnaird, M. et al. (2015). Serological evidence of MERS-CoV antibodies in dromedary camels (*Camelus dromedarius*) in Laikipia County, Kenya. *PLoS One* 10: e0140125. doi: 10.1371/journal.pone.0140125.

Forman, R.T.T. (2000). Estimate of the area affected ecologically by the road system in the United States. *Conservation Biology* 14: 31–35.

Grubaugh, N.D., Ladner, J.T., Kraemer, M.U.G. et al. (2017). Genomic epidemiology reveals multiple introductions of Zika virus into the United States. *Nature* 546 (7658): 401–405. doi: 10.1038/nature22400.

Kahn, L.H., Monath, T.P., Bokma, B.H. et al. *New Directions in Conservation Medicine: Applied Cases of Ecological Health*, 33–44. New York: Oxford University Press.

Kolbert, E. (2014). *The Sixth Extinction: An Unnatural History*. New York: Henry Holt and Company, LLC 319 Pp.

Lovelock, J.E. and Margulis, L. (1974). Atmospheric homeostasis by and for the biosphere: the Gaia hypothesis. *Tellus Series A: Dynamic Meteorology and Oceanography* 26 (1–2): 2–10.

Miller, R.S., Farnsworth, M.L., and Malmberg, J.L. (2013). Diseases at the livestock-wildlife interface: status, challenges and opportunities in the United States. *Preventive Veterinary Medicine* 110: 119–132.

Ostfeld, R.S. and Keesing, F. (2000). Biodiversity and disease risk: the case of Lyme disease. *Conservation Biology* 14: 722–728.

Paini, D.R., Sheppard, A.W., De Barro, P.J. et al. (2016). Global threat to agriculture from invasive species. *Proceedings of the National Academy of Sciences of the United States of America* 113 (27): 7575–7579. doi: 10.1073/pnas.1602205113.

Parashar, U.D., Sunn, L.M., Ong, F. et al. (2000). Case-control study of risk factors for human infection with a new zoonotic paramyxovirus, Nipah virus, during a 1998–1999 outbreak of severe encephalitis in Malaysia. *The Journal of Infectious Diseases* 181 (5): 1755–1759.

Pauly, D. and Watson, R. (2001). Systematic distortions in world fisheries catch trends. *Nature* 414: 534–536.

Postel, S.L., Daily, G.C., and Ehrlich, P.R. (1996). Human appropriation of renewable fresh water. *Science* 271: 785–788.

Robinette, C., Saffran, L., Ruple, A. et al. (2017). Zoos and public health: a partnership on the One Health frontier. *One Health* 3: 1–4.

Rojstaczer, S., Sterling, S.M., and Moore, N.J. (2001). Human appropriation of photosynthesis products. *Science* 294: 2549–2552.

Smil, V. (2002). Chapter 7: the Biosphere's mass and productivity. In: *The Earth's Biosphere Evolution, Dynamics and Change* (ed. V. Smil), 181–198. Cambridge MA: MIT Press.

Taylor, L.H., Latham, S.M., and Woolhouse, M.E.J. (2001). Risk factors for human disease emergence. *Philosophical Transactions of the Royal Society of London. Series B, Biological sciences* 356 (1411): 983–989.

Vitousek, P.M., Ehrlich, P.R., Ehrlich, A.H. et al. (1986). Human appropriation of the products of photosynthesis. *Bioscience* 36: 368–373.

# 3

# Greatest Threats to Planetary Health

As an undergraduate, I read a book entitled *The Sixth Extinction: Biodiversity and its Survival*, by Richard Leakey and Roger Lewin, which spelled out the global extinction crisis in clear and devastating terms, likening the rate of global extinction currently ongoing to prior dinosaur-ending mass extinctions and definitively setting the blame at humanity's collective feet. Gone are the dodo (*Raphus cucullatus*) and passenger pigeon (*Ectopistes migratorius*), of course, but so too, have we lost the Caribbean monk seal (*Monachus tropicalis*), thylacine (*Thylacinus cynocephalus*), Javan tiger (*Panthera tigris sondaica*), West African black rhino (*Diceros bicornis longipes*), the Eastern elk (*Cervus canadensis canadensis*), and thousands of additional species of birds, reptiles, amphibians, insects, and arthropods from all over the globe. For me, it was a call to arms, much like Rachel Carson's *Silent Spring* for scientists, activists, and environmentalists in the 1960s. The idea that we, the people of planet Earth, could so carelessly destroy not just our own environment but the environment of all living things, was horrifying. Even more concerning was the realization that we had already caused the extinction of thousands of species, and we were, effectively, just getting started on our global path of destruction. However, in the nearly 20 years since reading *The Sixth Extinction*, as scientists acknowledge our entry into the Anthropocene, the reality of our **biodiversity** crisis has been clarified. The crisis is not simply the loss of biodiversity (which we will return to shortly). It is a crisis of loss of expertise, of communication, and of humanity's seeming inability to reach out to someone who thinks, speaks, values, and/or looks different from ourselves and work to come to an understanding. While the threats discussed in the remainder of this chapter are real, ruinous, and potentially unrecoverable, the greatest threat to our planetary health continues to be our own inability to communicate clearly and compassionately with others in order to collaborate and solve problems. One Health and its collaborative, interdisciplinary approach to problem-solving is, truly, the best hope we have.

## 3.1 The Climate Crisis

In 2007, Steve Jobs walked on to a stage at Macworld San Francisco in jeans, a black turtleneck, and white sneakers. After approximately 35 minutes, he reached into his pocket, unveiled the iPhone, and changed the world as we know it. Technological advances can be revolutionary and relatively instantaneous; they can also proceed at an almost imperceptible pace. Between the years 1760 and 1850, the world, and specifically the Global North, underwent revolutionary changes in agriculture, textile manufacturing, transportation, metallurgy, social structure, and economics in what we now refer to as the Industrial Revolution.

*Introduction to One Health: An Interdisciplinary Approach to Planetary Health*, First Edition.
Sharon L. Deem, Kelly E. Lane-deGraaf and Elizabeth A. Rayhel.
© 2019 John Wiley & Sons, Inc. Published 2019 by John Wiley & Sons, Inc.
Companion website: www.wiley.com/go/deem/health

Resulting improvements in agriculture, for example switching from wood to metal farming tools, resulted in increased yields in food and in necessary supplies for textile production and livestock feed, which both facilitated human population growth and an expansion in textile production. Mechanization across the fields of textile production, coal mining, and transportation, including the development and expansion of rail roads and steam power, meant an explosion in production in these industries, which in turn resulted in significant changes to the way people spent their time. The developments and discoveries of the Industrial Revolution have improved peoples' lives and livelihoods in a myriad of ways. The unfolding of the Industrial Revolution has led directly to the technological advances we see, use, and take for granted today.

Advances in technology are not without consequence. Today, we face rapidly growing populations, a growing voice of science denialism, and an over-reliance on fossil fuels, mined through increasingly devastating processes (e.g. **fracking** and mountain-top removal) and resulting in an emission of vast quantities of greenhouse gases. As the Global North marched forward from the Industrial Revolution, economic growth was the impetus for large-scale use and destruction of natural resources in developing nations; environmental resources were seen as vast and unlimited, and health was a luxury only the wealthy could truly afford to consider. Alas, while coal and oil barons and shipping and railroad magnates drove the advancement of technology for economic gain, the ongoing legacy of their decisions has led directly to today's climate crisis.

The ongoing climate crisis is real and is caused by human actions. It is considered by many scientists across disciplines to be the greatest threat to human survival today. But what is climate change? In small, backyard greenhouses, light and heat from the sun enter, a portion of which is then retained by the glass of the greenhouse, dispersing throughout the entirety of the greenhouse and warming the soil and air, thus facilitating an ideal climate for year-round plant growth. This **greenhouse effect** is what is driving global climate change today. Our atmosphere acts, in part, to stabilize global temperature and climate by acting as a greenhouse – allowing light and heat to enter and preventing some, but not all, heat escape. Without this, our climate would be similar to the moon's, where daytime temperatures average $106\,°C$ ($224\,°F$) and nighttime temperatures reach as low as $-183\,°C$ ($-298\,°F$). However, as greenhouse gases – carbon dioxide ($CO_2$), methane, and nitrous oxide to name a few – are emitted into the atmosphere, they act as a trap for heat, preventing a significant amount of heat escape. Global fluctuations in temperature and $CO_2$ levels have occurred many times over the millions of years of our planet's history, triggering and ending ice ages and other significant climatic events (See Figure 3.1). However, as early as 1895, scientists had discovered that human action could alter our climate through the release of $CO_2$ into the atmosphere. What sets the current climate crisis apart from past fluctuations in temperature and $CO_2$ levels is that the increase in global emissions of greenhouse gases has occurred rapidly, more than tripling the rate of background emissions since the Industrial Revolution. Non-human-caused emissions of greenhouse gases (e.g. from volcanic eruptions) occur at a much slower rate. Historically, our planet's climate was relatively stable in part because emissions of greenhouse gases were mitigated through the sequestration of these gases by our planet – through carbon fixation by plants and other biological processes and the absorption of carbon into oceans and other reservoirs – before they reached the atmosphere. However, in the current climate crisis, human-caused emissions of greenhouse gases occurs at such a rate that our planet and planet's atmosphere have been unable to respond via the sequestration of these gases through natural biological and geophysical processes.

Evidence of the human causation of the ongoing climate crisis is overwhelming and

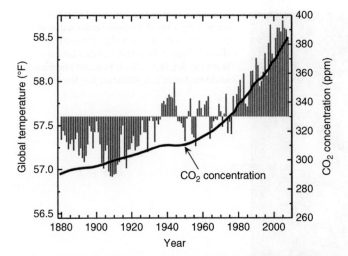

Figure 3.1 Carbon dioxide emissions and temperature over the last 100 years. *Source:* Courtesy of NOAA/NCDC.

based on the coalescing of data from many scientific fields. Of the published, peer-reviewed literature on climate change in any scientific field in 2013–2014, more than 99% of authors agreed that climate change is happening and that humans are the cause. Evidence of human-caused climate change comes from satellite data measurements of global temperatures, greenhouse gases including $CO_2$, methane, water vapor, and ozone, among others, ground-level monitoring of mean global temperatures and mean ocean temperatures, ice core measurements of greenhouse gases, measurement of land ice over the Antarctic, and measurement and monitoring of sea ice levels, among others. Since 1880, there has been a global increase in mean temperature by 0.8 °C, and 15 of the 16 hottest years on record have been in the twenty-first century, despite not receiving any greater amount of solar radiation from the sun, according to NASA scientists. This, coupled with the increase in average ocean temperature, the depletion of the Antarctic and Greenland ice sheets, the accelerated sea level rise since 1960, and the acidification of the oceans (30% more acidic since the nineteenth century), and the stark and dramatic increase in $CO_2$ in the atmosphere since 1950 (Figure 3.1) demonstrate that the Earth is warming and that humans are the cause.

The evidence is clear – the increase in man-made $CO_2$ and other greenhouse gas emissions into the atmosphere is overwhelmingly the cause of the global climate crisis.

As the climate changes, and temperatures warm, the health of the environment is directly impacted. Sea ice and ice covering landmasses at the poles are melting, and glaciers are receding, resulting in an increase in sea levels. This rise in sea levels will devastate coastal communities with far-reaching consequences for human populations. Some communities will be minimally affected, with flooding and loss of shore lines, but even these will have dire consequences to the human populations residing in these areas. Other communities, especially island communities, will be completely eliminated as entire islands are lost to rising sea levels (Figure 3.2). Increases in the strength and frequency of storms, hurricanes, floods, and droughts will also contribute to the devastation of human and animal communities. The frequency of hot days will increase. Extremely hot days are now 100 times more likely to occur than they did between 1951 and 1980, which will, in turn, lead to an increase in heat-related deaths. For example, in India, Pakistan, and Bangladesh, extreme heat waves are already the norm, especially throughout the Indus and Ganges river basins. According to

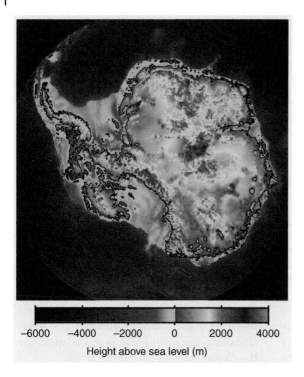

Figure 3.2 Antarctica, represented without current expanse of glaciers. Deglaciation is one predicted outcome of global climate change. *Source:* Robert A. Rohde / Global Warming Art, https://commons.wikimedia.org/wiki/File:Antarctica_Without_Ice_Sheet.png.

recent research, under conditions of unchecked climate change, these heat waves, coupled with the areas' high humidity, are expected to expose approximately 1 billion people to conditions considered dangerous to life and will likely kill approximately 6.4 million people by 2100. Arable land will be lost to desertification, resulting in growing food scarcity issues as human populations grow to exceed the current 7.6 billion.

Compounding the direct effects of climate change to the environment, the impending climate crisis will also result in devastating effects on the health of human populations. First, ongoing civil wars and other strife unrelated to climate change have created a climate of mounting refugees, considered many to be a crisis in its own right. As of June 2015, more than 60 million people have been forced from their homes and homelands due to violence, according to the United Nations High Commission for Refugees, noting that this was the highest since World War II, which was the last time that the number of refugees peaked at just above 50 million. Unfortunately, as global $CO_2$ emissions continue unabated and temperatures climb, the droughts, loss of arable land, flooding, and other climate change-driven destructive events will result in a significant increase in "climate" refugees, or people whose homes and/or homelands have been devastated and now must immigrate elsewhere due directly to climate change. The global nature of the destruction – loss of land to rising sea levels and the increased need for food production in the face of the loss of arable land – in addition to the already existing 60 million refugees, will make the challenge of finding space and resources for these millions of people increasingly dire. Significantly, as more millions of people become refugees, our ability to respond to, and possibly mitigate continuing effects of, climate change will diminish, further antagonizing an already nearly impossible task. Second, an increasing amount of research has shown a direct link between the climate crisis and violence, with the effects documented from fields as diverse as anthropology, economics, psychology, history, and geography, among others. Evidence now links increases in crimes from interpersonal conflicts like domestic violence and murder to larger-scale intergroup conflicts such as minority expulsions, uprising and rebellions, and civil war to the effects of climate change.

Finally, as the climate warms, the range of many plants and animals will expand towards the poles. This range expansion will carry with it an expansion in the range of many infectious diseases as the hosts and vectors move poleward. For example, malaria currently kills more than 650 000 people annually, many of these are children. As the temperatures increase, *Anopheles gambiae*, one of the vectors of the malaria parasite, *Plasmodium* spp., will extend its range, carrying malaria into previously uninfected areas of the world. Compounding this range extension, as *A. gambiae* mosquitoes move poleward, their ranges will begin to overlap with other *Anopheles* species. This overlap will enable an increase in transmission of malaria as additional *Anopheles* mosquitoes become vectors for the *Plasmodium* parasite. In addition to malaria, dengue fever has already expanded its range into the Florida Keys, an area in which it had been eradicated decades ago. Lung worm is flourishing in the Arctic, increasing its incidence and prevalence in musk oxen at alarming rates as the permafrost melts. Thawing permafrost is also exposing ancient viruses as melting reveals prehistoric animals and their infectious agents previously frozen for several thousand years. Warming oceans have resulted in coral die off, leaving remaining coral stands vulnerable to infections. Further, as host ranges expand into more densely populated human areas, the potential for increasing opportunities for **bi-directional pathogen transmission**, or the transmission of pathogens between humans and wildlife as well as between wildlife and humans, also increases.

Unchecked climate change is also reshaping the global economy. Recent research suggests that by 2100, globally, an individual's annual income may be reduced by as much as 23%, with the annual income of the poorest 40% of the world's population reduced by nearly 75% due directly to warming. Increasing population densities, a result of population growth and ecological refugees, will strain resources already in place for the world's poor, limiting their access to food and other resources even more. Importantly, the response to the global climate crisis must be driven by world leaders in both business and politics. A move away from carbon reliance and towards an economy based on renewables will result in a $1.8 billion dollar boon to the global economy. Local government and business leaders, driven by economic considerations alone, have already moved to more carbon comprehensive policies, resulting in commitments to the Paris Accord already in place to be met on time or early for many signatory countries, including the USA, China, and India – three of the world's largest populations and emitters of carbon. Even in the USA, which withdrew from the Paris Climate Accord as this text went to press, is on target to exceed its climate goals through the actions of business leaders and state and local politicians acting on behalf of a concerned populace. Until the climate crisis is addressed in real, sustainable terms, climate change will remain among the greatest threats to human, animal, and environmental health. However, because the climate crisis is caused by us, we have the opportunity and responsibility to alter our actions, mitigating these effects and creating a better future for humanity.

All existing threats to the health of the planet are exacerbated by the climate crisis – the emergence and reemergence of infectious diseases, the loss of biodiversity, the disparity between wealth and poverty and the downstream effects on health, and science denial, to name a few. The actions needed to mitigate the effects of climate change are urgent, and our decisions to engage or not will have far-reaching consequences that have the potential to last long beyond the era of humans.

## 3.2 Emerging and Re-emerging Infectious Diseases

Parasites and pathogens have been a human health concern since before humans emerged onto the African landscape. In fact, evidence from **coprolites** suggests that even dinosaurs had abundant gastrointestinal parasites. The evolutionary importance of parasites cannot be overstated. Parasites and pathogens have been significant evolutionary forces for the development of sexual reproduction, including striking secondary sexual characteristics, the alteration of our own genomes, and the evolution of the immune system. Historically, the impact of most infectious diseases has remained relatively localized, with exposure limited to small groups. However, as population sizes have grown, contact with wildlife and domesticated animals has increased, and global travel has expanded, infectious diseases, and the parasites and pathogens that are their cause, have spread beyond their previous ranges, evolving rapidly in response to the new interconnected world. However, even before the "modern era," infectious diseases had the potential to devastate the health of human populations and reshape the known world. In the biblical story of Moses, five of the ten plagues of Egypt are directly related to infectious diseases. Leprosy, plague, and smallpox have a long, sordid history with humanity: the Black Death (from 1347 to 1351), the Plague of Justinian (in the year 541), and the Antonine Plague (from the 15 years between 165 and 181) each killed millions of people and have permanently left their mark on the human genome. The Black Death, the fourteenth-century outbreak of the bubonic plague, alone is estimated to have killed approximately half of the population of Europe in just four years. More recently, the 1918 Spanish flu pandemic resulted in an estimated 75 million deaths globally, and the emergence of HIV/AIDS has already resulted in more than 30 million deaths worldwide.

Rinderpest, the cattle plague that first emerged in the early eighteenth century and considered to be one of the most deadly animal diseases, killed nearly 100% of naïve populations of cattle and other hooved animals, including goat, sheep, giraffe, wildebeest, and buffalo that were exposed to the virus. Rinderpest was eradicated in 2011, but this came with a five billion dollar price tag.

The emergence of the next devastating infectious disease is inevitable. Human populations, along with the diversity of plants and animals, are at grave risk, with the greatest impact to be faced by those with the fewest resources. Much like in zombie apocalypse movies, if the population of the known world was reduced by 60–80% through the emergence of a global pandemic, as it has in the past, the global economy, political structures, and boundaries, and world aid organizations would be devastated as well, leaving humanity to begin again. The consequences of a novel infection emerging in a major food resource (e.g. cattle, rice, or wheat) would be equally catastrophic as people of the world face the potential decimation of food resources, further challenged by existing wealth inequalities. Emerging infectious diseases (EIDs) are those infectious diseases that are entirely novel in a population. **Re-emerging infectious diseases** are those that have previously been found in a population but that have recently spread to new geographic ranges, new host populations or species, or through novel mechanisms (e.g. development of antimicrobial resistance), or have emerged after previously being eradicated. We will use the abbreviation EID to refer to both emerging and re-emerging infectious diseases generally. The threat of emerging and re-emerging infectious diseases is potentially catastrophic for humans, animals, and the environment alike (Figure 3.3). While changes in news and media access accelerate opportunities for communication and the potential for an immediate global response, globalization also presents challenges for responding to an outbreak of an emerging or re-emerging infectious disease. Global travel can spread

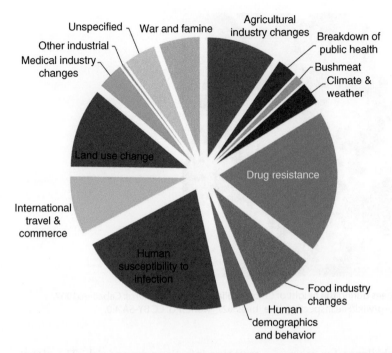

Figure 3.3 The variety of sources of emerging infectious diseases as the world grows smaller with increasing globalization. *Source:* Credit to Colin Butler, BMC Infectious Diseases of Poverty.

pathogens much further and much faster than ever before and political turmoil can complicate the international response.

The potential for infectious diseases to devastate human, animal, and plant populations is evident from the plagues of history. However, the forces underlying opportunities for a novel infectious agent to emerge have drastically shifted from the past. As mentioned, globalization provides new, complex challenges and benefits, including expanded opportunities for international collaborations and the ability to monitor and respond in nearly real time to outbreaks. These collaborations are critical due to ever increasing opportunities for human-animal interactions, resulting in opportunities for novel exposures (e.g. the emergence of zoonotic and **anthropozoonotic infectious diseases**) and a new dynamic of rapid and far-reaching pathogen transmission opportunities as a result of near constant global travel. Importantly, these factors do not act in a vacuum.

The interconnectedness of our world, as covered in Chapter 2, amplifies the occurrence and threat of emerging and reemerging infectious diseases. Habitat destruction and degradation drive people and wildlife into new areas and increase population densities, driving up the risk of exposure to novel pathogens and/or bi-directional pathogen transmission. For example, at least eight outbreaks of Nipah virus, a potentially deadly paramyxovirus characterized by encephalitis and/or respiratory difficulties, have occurred since 2001 in Southeast Asia. These outbreaks are linked directly to exposure to fruit bat saliva, a consequence of growing human populations encroaching into previously undisturbed bat habitat. Habitat destruction also results in shifting exposure to pathogens, including plant-specific pathogens, such as the tobacco and cassava mosaic viruses, the citrus canker, or the Asian soybean rust. The spread of these pathogens through agricultural lands can

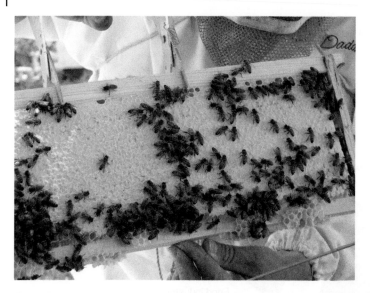

Figure 3.4 A dead colony of bees during the height of Colony Collapse Disorder. *Source:* Caballero1967, https://commons.wikimedia.org/wiki/File:Inspecting_the_bees%27_work.JPG. CC BY-SA 4.0.

result in an increasing challenge for maintaining food biosecurity necessary to feed a growing population. Loss of habitat also affects remaining forest stands through the limitation of population-level resources needed to respond to pathogens. This can result in the decimation of plants important for the stability of remaining ecosystem health (e.g. the etiological agents of sudden oak death, chestnut blight, and Dutch elm disease). Pollutants and other environmental contaminants that degrade habitat can similarly contribute to an increased risk of infectious disease emergence. The most stunning example of this is the resulting emergence of a fungal pathogen in honeybees (*Apis mellifera*) in conjunction with population exposure to neonicotinoids – insecticides intended for insects other than honeybees (Figure 3.4). This association between infectious disease and environmental contaminants needs further research, but the evidence is growing that continued exposure to immune-compromising agents can result in an emergent infectious disease with potentially devastating consequences.

The loss of habitat is but one of many profound variables in the inevitability of future emerging infectious disease risk. The global climate crisis is driving pathogens and disease vectors poleward out of the tropics. As mosquitoes and other vectors encounter novel parasites and pathogens and naïve populations of potential human and animal hosts, the risk of novel disease emergence to occur becomes increasingly inevitable. Importantly, the risk of re-emergence of infectious diseases is even greater as vectors carry pathogens into susceptible, naïve populations. For example, one significant concern of vector biologists is the number of mosquito-borne pathogens that are limited not by their mosquito-specificity, but by the range of their current host mosquito. Mosquito-borne pathogens including Zika, Chikungunya, and dengue virus, which are spread by *Aedes aegypti* and *Aedes albopictus* mosquitoes, may expand their range not only by the expanding range of the *Aedes* spp. poleward but by expanding into the range of other *Aedes* spp. mosquitoes. Further compounding this risk is the likely increase in host density with climate change. As plants and animals migrate poleward in response to climbing global temperatures, population density will also increase, increasing the concentration of people, animals, and disease vectors into limited spaces. Longer storm seasons and increased storm intensity can further complicate the interaction between infectious diseases and climate change as storms move pathogens and hosts, destroy habitat, and damage infrastructure, limiting the effectiveness of potential responses.

Finally, our ability to respond to the threat of infectious disease is being challenged as resistance to antimicrobials continues to develop unabated. Widespread overuse of antibiotics has resulted in the evolution of antimicrobial resistance to nearly every antibiotic developed since the 1940s. The World Health Organization now considers antibiotic resistance one of the most significant public health threats of our time. While over prescription of antibiotics exerts significant selective pressure in the development of antimicrobial resistance, the use of antibiotics in agricultural animals is far more significant, with approximately 80% of antibiotics sold in the USA today used on agricultural animals to promote both health and growth. The US Centers for Disease Control and Prevention (CDC) currently estimates that two million people in the USA are infected annually by bacteria resistant to at least one class of antibiotics, leading to as many as 23 000 human deaths due to infections of previously treatable bacteria. As a result of this growing threat of antimicrobial resistance, the ability of response teams to treat and control emerging or re-emerging infectious diseases becomes more difficult. As resistance to our antibiotic arsenal grows, emerging infections or resistant re-emerging infections may flourish.

Despite the risks, the global response to emerging and re-emerging infectious diseases is frequently awe-inspiring. Scientists and first responders treat people, animals, and plants on the ground and investigate treatments, therapeutics, preventatives, and vaccines. Researchers are actively working to reduce risk, monitor for novel disease emergences, and create fast-acting disease response teams that minimize the health and economic tolls

for humans, animals, and the environment. Disease monitoring networks now exist, spread out across Asia, Africa, and much of Central and South America. Programs foster international collaborations between scientists and community members and focus on outreach, community development, and education as well as training in cutting edge research in some of the world's most recognized disease hotpots.

## 3.3 The Loss of Biodiversity

The global loss of biodiversity has now reached a rate of loss equivalent to major mass extinction events of the planet's past, when between 70% and 90% of species worldwide ultimately went extinct. The most significant difference in the current extinction crisis is that in this event, human beings are the undoubted cause. The loss of biodiversity is a global threat to planetary health for several reasons: the loss of species diversity is irrecoverable. As the saying goes, extinct is forever. Importantly, however, extinction is not simply the loss of an individual species but a loss of the wealth of unique genetic and ecosystem resources that species provides. The interconnected nature of ecosystems means that when pieces are lost, the loss reverberates throughout the entirety of the ecosystem. From direct resources to ecosystem services to indirect, future resource potential, the health of humans specifically and the planet generally is directly tied to the diversity of life. Additionally, natural resources, or those obtained from or inspired by the natural world, are the building blocks of developments in medicine, engineering, bioremediation, and biomaterials. Several medicines, including digitoxin, quinine, and castanospermine, are derived from plants or wildlife. Uses for pharmaceuticals derived from botanicals include major cancer treatment drugs, pain relieving drugs, antivirals, antimalarials, **antihelminthics**, anticoagulants, and many, many more. Finally, the diversity of life is protective of life itself, and the loss of this diversity directly threatens the remaining species. While the climate crisis casts a long shadow on the future of biodiversity, the loss of biodiversity is a result of a myriad of additional human driven forces, including habitat destruction, habitat degradation and pollution, and introduced and invasive species, each with their own systemic concerns for planetary health.

Scientists are just beginning to understand the scope and breadth of the significance of the loss of biodiversity as an environmental health concern. While many scientists have long thought that the loss of biodiversity was an unfortunate side effect of larger, more impactful health concerns, we now understand that the loss of biodiversity will rival the ongoing climate crisis as one of the world's greatest health threats of the modern era. The result of the interconnected nature of our planet's ecosystems is that as individual components of an ecosystem fail, or are destroyed, the larger ecosystem begins to fail as well. For example, the loss of plant biodiversity results in not only loss of genetic variability in an entire phyla of life, but the loss of habitat and food resources for people and animals, contributes additional challenges for addressing climate change, and increases the risk of disease emergence, all of which further contributes to the loss of biodiversity and compound each additional threat. No planetary system is truly independent.

Let's look more closely at how habitat loss, pollution, and invasive species drive the global loss of biodiversity.

### 3.3.1 Habitat Loss

Indonesia is home to approximately 10% of the world's diversity of non-human primates. Ten species of macaque, the slow loris, langurs, gibbons, tarsiers, and orangutans are all native to the archipelago; many of these primate species, including the orangutan, are found nowhere else on the planet. However, Indonesia has quickly become the largest producer of palm oil, the most popular vegetable oil on the planet. Together with Malaysia,

Indonesia exports 85–90% of all palm oil globally. In Indonesia, palm oil is exclusively grown and produced on two islands – Sumatra and Kalimantan – where approximately 13 million hectares of rainforest have been converted into palm oil plantations. This deforestation, often done through slash and burn agricultural practices, devastates local wildlife populations and compounds the climate crisis, by dumping carbon into the atmosphere at the rate of more than 10 million tons of carbon per day during peak burn season. Orangutans, the only great apes native to the islands, have been ravaged by the destruction of habitat associated with palm oil production. As have the Sumatran rhinos (*Dicerorhinus sumatrensis*), now numbering fewer than 100 individuals, the Sumatran tiger (*P. t. sondaica* Sumatra), numerous bird species, including several critically endangered birds such as the rhinoceros hornbill (*Buceros rhinoceros*) and the helmeted hornbill (*Rhinoplax vigil*), and the Borneo pygmy elephant (*Elephas maximus borneensis*), endemic only to Kalimantan. Found nowhere else on the planet, an entire rainforest ecosystem has been brought to the brink of extinction by the destruction of this habitat. In an unfortunate twist, this habitat destruction is now integral to the livelihoods of more than 15 million Indonesians who work and toil on palm plantations. The consequences of unchecked, large-scale destruction of the forests of Kalimantan and Sumatra have placed the lives of Indonesia's most unique biodiversity in peril.

The global loss of biodiversity is intimately linked to the destruction of habitat. While many American school children learn about deforestation of the Amazonian rainforest, coral bleaching of the Great Barrier Reef, or the desertification of the formerly lush landscapes of the Middle East, the destruction of habitat also includes road building and urbanization, encroachment and urban sprawl, and many other localized forms of habitat loss. Large-scale destruction devastates plant and wildlife populations, necessitating either complete relocation or loss of populations. For example, the Amazon rainforest is considered one of the most species rich habitats on the planet. The Amazon is approximately 2.7 million square kilometers in size and is home to more than 20% of the planet's biodiversity and included in this are, at current count, more than 40 000 plant species, more than 450 mammal species, more than 1300 bird species, nearly 1000 reptile and amphibian species, and more than 3000 species of freshwater fish. Quantifying the number of invertebrate species is more challenging, but scientists estimate that the number of invertebrates inhabiting the Amazon of Brazil alone exceeds 100 000 species. While oil and mineral interests expand in the Amazon, cattle ranching and soybean production continue to threaten the rainforest through land consumption. Each hectare of rainforest that is destroyed takes with it countless untold forms of life, threatens the rare and critically endangered species living there, and puts at great risk the lives and livelihoods of numerous local peoples. The rate of deforestation in the Amazon, at its peak in 2014, reached more than 36 football fields per minute, and continues at an astounding rate today (Figure 3.5). Importantly, this deforestation also alters local wildlife population dynamics, resulting in an increase in the number of individuals living in the remaining forest stands. This increase in population density, in turn, makes it more challenging for wildlife populations to find food and other important resources and increases the likelihood of exposure to a novel infectious disease. This irreversible loss of rainforest is drastically altering the climate, local resources, and potentially eliminating future potential benefits for people, both as ecosystem services and future option values, such as medicinal plants. And, while rainforests are at risk of the greatest amounts of biodiversity loss due, in part, to their abundance of available biodiversity, biomes other than rainforests are also at risk. For example, a study published in 2017 found a 76% decline in insect **biomass** over 27 years in protected areas in Germany. The decline

in insects, important for their contributions to food webs and other ecosystem services, happened independent of habitat type, suggesting that loss of biodiversity is not simply a function of habitat loss in ecosystems of high species diversity but is a truly global concern.

Habitat fragmentation can also significantly damage an ecosystem, negatively affecting the health of the people and animals living there and the ecosystem itself. **Edge effects** describe the changes in wind exposure, temperature, light amount, and other climatic variables that differentiate the edge of an intact ecosystem from that of its core. As habitat fragmentation occurs, the increase in edge dramatically reduces the availability of habitat to plants and wildlife species that cannot tolerate the edge. Thus, while fragmentation may leave relatively large patches of habitat available, the actual amount of available habitat may be far less when edge effects are considered. Reduction of habitat into increasingly smaller fragments also limits population connectivity by reducing access to mates and, as a result of reducing gene flow between populations, reduces access to food resources and increases both the likelihood of human–wildlife interactions and wildlife population density in the remaining ecosystem fragments. These increases in potential human–wildlife interactions and wildlife population density in the remaining fragments independently increase the likelihood for disease emergence while acting synergistically to increase population stressors, further amplifying the risk of disease emergence. Landscape degradation, through pollution and other environmental contaminants, can further intensify and complicate human, animal, and environmental health independently and by exacerbating the loss of biodiversity.

### 3.3.2 Pollution

In 1976, the first story describing what is considered by many to be one of the most significant environmental disasters in US history was published in the Niagara Falls Gazette.

(a)

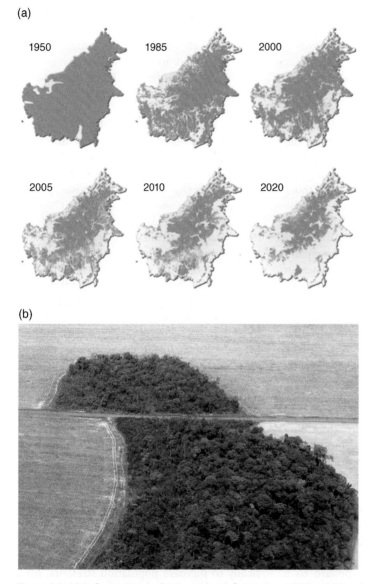

(b)

Figure 3.5 (a) Deforestation in the Amazon rainforest since 1950 and (b) an image of a deforested landscape. *Source:* Pedro Biondi/Abr, https://commons.wikimedia.org/wiki/File:Mato_Grosso_deforestation_(Pedro_Biondi)_12ago2007.jpg. CC BY 3.0.

What unfolded over the next two years was the story of contamination of Love Canal. The community was the country's first **Superfund site** (Figure 3.6), taking more than 21 years and $400 million dollars to clean-up. In the 1970s, the community was a small but thriving working class neighborhood of Niagara Falls, New York. The story of Love Canal begins in the 1940s when the Hooker Chemical Company needed a place to discard toxic waste from the production of polychlorinated biphenyls (PCBs). Between 1942 and 1953, the company dumped more than 22 000 tons of waste and more than 80 industrial chemicals in the unused canal, effectively creating a landfill of waste. In 1953, the company sealed and sold the canal to the Niagara Falls Board of Education, where schools and homes

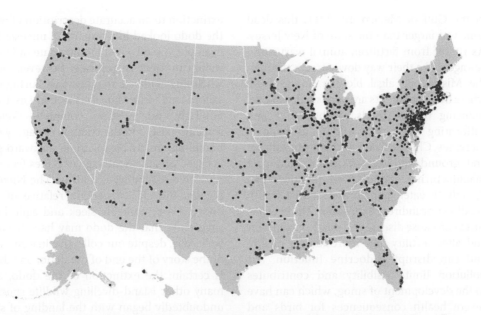

Figure 3.6 Locations of Superfund sites/sites remaining on the NPL as of 2017. Red sites are active, yellow sites are proposed Superfund (future sites), and green sites have been removed from the NPL. *Source:* skew-t, https://commons.wikimedia.org/wiki/File:Superfund_sites.svg. CC BY-SA 3.0.

were later developed. As the industrial wastes began to leak into homes, schools, playgrounds, and the public water supply, community members complained of headaches, respiratory illnesses, hair loss, cancers, kidney and liver failure, epilepsy, and concerns over infertility issues and children born with birth defects. Family pets also suffered, with lost fur, skin lesions, and tumors reported. While the focus of concern in the immediate aftermath of Love Canal was human health and well-being, in the ensuing years, research has focused on the health effects of wildlife in the area. As early as 1983, less than five years after the mandatory evacuation of the Love Canal community, populations of field mice and voles were found to have organ damage and shortened life spans, with those individuals living closest to the canal suffering the most and dying the earliest. Pollution and other environmental contaminants can cause significant human, animal, and environmental health effects, as in the example of Love Canal. Importantly, environmental contamination can be insidious, difficult to mitigate,

and especially difficult to pinpoint any direct resulting health complications.

One significant concern surrounding our ability to mitigate the effects of pollution and other environmental contaminants is the challenge of identifying the source of pollution. In instances of **point sources** of pollution, the cause of environmental contamination is clear. For example, the 2015 ban on microbead production and use in cosmetics in the USA was a significant move to prevent tiny plastic particles from entering surface waters, where they negatively affect the health of the marine environment. In this example, the source of the contamination was clear and a comprehensive solution was available. However, in other instances, identifying the source of pollution is much more complicated. Agricultural runoff, for example, is a major source of water pollution and is considered a non-point source of pollution, deriving from many, often unrelated, locations. While identifying the exact source of the runoff is impossible, the result of this pollution is evident in the growing dead zone in the Gulf of Mexico. By 2011, this dead zone was larger than the state of New Jersey. As runoff from fertilizer, animal waste, and sewage make their way downstream through the Mississippi, algal blooms in the Gulf, where these pollutants are deposited, explode, reducing oxygen levels in the water and suffocating the Gulf's wildlife as hypoxia increases. Chemical contaminants in soil, air, and ground and surface water from past manufacturing and disposal practices can directly threaten human and animal health via direct or indirect exposures. These exposures can cause disease and death, can inhibit and alter fertility and reproductive health, and can disrupt endocrine function. Air pollution limits visibility and contributes to the development of smog, which can have severe health consequences for birds and invertebrates, can contribute to the rise of acid rain, can poison food sources, and can independently result in immunotoxic and reproductive health challenges for humans and animals alike. Noise and light pollution threaten the long-term health of even the most remote landscapes on Earth through the constant exposure to human sounds and artificial lights.

### 3.3.3 Invasive Species

It seems that schoolchildren everywhere know the story of the illustrious dodo bird (*R. cucullatus*) and its extinction. In 1598, Dutch sailors landed on the small island of Mauritius and within a few short decades had eaten the dodo, a small, flightless relative of the Nicobar pigeon (*Caloenas nicobarica*) of Southeast Asia, into extinction. This diet-driven extinction event was aided by the dodo's own lack of fear of humans and the ease with which the dodo was able to be caught. However, this description of the dodo's demise is, at best, an oversimplification. The reality of the demise of the dodo is far more complex, with critical details ranging from the date of discovery (or the first documented sighting from a "white" person from the Global North) to the date of

extinction to an accurate description of what the dodo looked like remaining unclear. For example, the oft-cited landing date of Dutch sailors in 1598 is accurate; however, overwhelming evidence suggests that Portuguese sailors landed in Mauritius as early as 1507. Similarly, no existing complete skeletal remains exist, and the common imagery of a bumbling, portly bird with an awkward gait is based on an assemblage of bones from an unrelated assemblage of birds. The Nicobar pigeon, the closest genetic relative of the dodo, is a remarkably sleek and agile bird, suggesting that the dodo may have been as well. Alas, despite our collective inaccuracies of the story of the end of the dodo, one thing is certain: the extinction of the dodo, and many other island-dwelling wildlife species, undoubtedly began with the landing of sailors from the Global North. If Dutch sailors did not eat the dodo into extinction, what resulted in the dodo becoming extinct so soon after encountering humans? Evidence suggests that the actual reason for the demise of the dodo was the animals that sailors brought with them intentionally or not: pigs, dogs, goats, and rats. These animals both consumed the dodos directly and altered the birds' ecosystems in immutable ways. Exotic species can be introduced into a new ecosystem through a variety of intentional or unintentional means. Many aquatic species are moved around the globe through a ship's ballast water, the water taken in at one port and released at another port in order to maintain stability and balance while loading and unloading cargo. For example, the zebra mussel (*Driessenia polymorpha*), a native of the Caspian Sea, which borders Eastern Europe and western Russia, was introduced into the Great Lakes region through ballast water in 1985. Sometimes, in an effort to solve one environmental problem, people introduce a plant or animal into a new ecosystem as a form of **bioremediation**. For example, several species of Asian carp were introduced into the American south in an effort to reduce local weed and parasite populations within ongoing aquaculture operations, when four species in particular bighead carp (*Hypophthalmichthys nobilis*), silver carp (*Hypophthalmichthys molitrix*), black carp (*Mylopharyngodon piceus*), and grass carp (*Ctenopharyngodon idella*) escaped their introduced confines during a flood and began their spread across the USA. Both the zebra mussel and Asian carp severely affect food chains in their introduced ranges, by outcompeting local wildlife, and both negatively affect human fishing, albeit on different scales. The carp, known for their ability to leap from the water when startled, has become a nuisance for the injuries sustained by local fishers, but more importantly, the speed at which these fish grow and the ability of these fish to outcompete native fish for food resources has resulted in the failures of many native fisheries. Zebra mussels can clog treatment facilities, docks, and boat engines, drastically limiting commercial fishing operations as well as shipping operations. Both the zebra mussel and Asian carp species have spread far beyond their native and introduced ranges, threatening not just the native flora and fauna at their sites of introduction but across the USA. The economic toll of the zebra mussel, as of 2015, has reached an estimated US$ 250–300 million annually while the economic toll of the Asian carp invasion has exceeded US$ 100 million annually and actively threatens the US$ 7 billion dollar Great Lakes fisheries industry. These costs come from loss of direct income from fisheries and other aquatic infrastructure as well as state and federal clean-up and mitigation efforts.

Other examples of **introduced species** gone awry are numerous and as potentially devastating for wildlife and the economy. For example, in 1890, the American Acclimatization Society introduced European starlings (*Sturnus vulgaris*) into the USA in one part of a calculated effort to introduce all of the birds mentioned in the plays of Shakespeare into the USA. The lionfish (*Pterois volitans* and other *Pterois* species) has invaded the coast of the American southeast and the Caribbean Sea from the Indo-Pacific waters through the saltwater aquarium trade, reducing native reef fish diversity by nearly 80%. While many introduced species fail, introductions that do not fail go on to wreak havoc on ecosystems, native species diversity, and local economies. Introduced species that thrive and out-compete native species frequently become invasive. **Invasive species**, like the pigs, dogs, goats, and rats that drove the dodo into extinction, are those introduced species that become established and go on to spread rapidly throughout their introduced range, often at the expense of native plants and wildlife.

Beyond simply outcompeting for resources or growth outpacing native species, invasive species also present an unexpected health challenge for the local ecosystem. Parasites and pathogens are frequently species-, or genus-, specific infections, meaning that it is difficult, albeit not impossible, for parasites to reproduce outside their evolved host. Host-switching events are, therefore, relatively rare. In successful host-switching events, typically the original and novel hosts are closely related (e.g. humans and non-human primates). For invasive species, this can result in two opposite effect forces that each benefit the invasive species – **parasite escape** and **pathogen introduction**. In a parasite escape, the introduced species is not a known host to local parasites and pathogens; thus, the introduced species can grow, reproduce, and consume resources in the local ecosystem without the cost incurred by native species through parasitism. Compounding the benefits of parasite escape mechanisms, introduced species often bring their own compliment of parasites and pathogens with them. Pathogen introduction, then, occurs when naïve populations are exposed to non-native parasites and pathogens. If these naïve populations are exposed and susceptible to the novel parasites, then a pathogen introduction occurs alongside the host invasion, compounding the potential ecosystem health consequences. In much the same way, introduced and invasive species may act as a novel predator, altering the ecosystem further. Finally, an interesting argument for the beneficial value of introduced species is that the introduction results in an increase in local species diversity. However, this is misguided at best. While short-term local species diversity does increase, the long-term consequences of invasive species can be dire, and ultimately, the result is likely to be the loss of biodiversity and a global homogenization of species.

## 3.4 The Anthropocene and Inequality

Scientists mark the beginning of a new era, the Anthropocene, by the radioactive elements spread across the globe by nuclear tests, by plastic pollutants in the environment, and the marked increase in chicken bones in human waste bins. In a seminal paper, published in *Nature* in 2000, Crutzen and Stoermer suggested that humankind has altered our world so significantly and so irreversibly that it signaled the end of the previous geologic era and the beginning of the Anthropocene. While the date of the onset of the Anthropocene is still under debate – did it begin during the Scientific Revolution in 1610 or at the onset of the nuclear world in 1950? The evidence of the Anthropocene is now undeniable. It could be argued that a change in language is insignificant; however, this renaming signals the importance of the largest threat to planetary health – humans. As suggested by Crutzen and Stoermer, the evidence of the Anthropocene include a marked rise in the extinction of biodiversity far above **background extinction rates** driven by human destruction of habitat, a dramatic rise in levels of atmospheric carbon dioxide driven by the burning of fossil fuels, the near ubiquitous nature of plastics in our environment such that they will likely leave an indelible mark in the fossil record, and the distribution of a layer of black carbon in the records of sediment and glacial ice. While the markers of the Anthropocene should serve as a warning of the impact of human activities on the health of the planet, three additional human

actions exacerbate the already troubled system – wealth and resource inequality, food insecurity, and environmental racism.

### 3.4.1 Wealth and Income Inequality

In 2017, Gary Cohn, the then US President's chief economic advisor, suggested that Americans would benefit dramatically from a proposed tax reform. In his statement, Cohn, whose net worth at the time was more than $266 million, proposed that a family of four with an income of approximately $100 000 would save $1000 under the newly revised tax plan, allowing these families to "renovate their kitchen, buy a new car, take a family vacation." Industry estimates placed the average cost of an American kitchen remodel at nearly $22 000 and the cost of a new car around $35 000. This is a striking example of how out of touch the world's wealthiest 1% is with the economic reality of most Americans. The reality of this inequality is put into even more stark contrast when considered against the backdrop of the relative wealth of the average American versus some of the world's most impoverished communities.

Across the globe wealth is now more unequally distributed than ever before, with more than half of the world's wealth in the hands of less than 1% of the world's population. The middle class, which in the USA represents individuals with wealth between $50 000 and $500 000 in assets, represents 14% of the global population. As such, this concentration of the wealth results in more than 80% of the global wealth being accessible to less than 15% of the individuals on the planet. Wealth inequality has enormous consequences for global health but so, too, does **income inequality**. Income inequality is the difference in annual income earned from salary and investments between, for example, a CEO and the employees of that CEO's company. On average, in 2016, CEOs of companies publicly traded on the Standard & Poor's Index earned more than

354 times the income than the average employee in the same companies. To put this into perspective, if the average employee earns a wage of $60 000 annually, the CEO of the company he or she works for is likely to earn more than $21 million annually. **Wealth inequality**, however, is the difference in accumulated income, assets, and investments over time. Wealth is driven, in part, by income, but wealth also includes investments in property, stock, education, and other assets. It may seem obvious, but the simplest way to amass wealth is to be born into it: wealth begets wealth. Therefore, if one considers the impact of the existing inequality in wealth distribution, with more than half of the planet's wealth concentrated with 1% of the population, this challenges the concept of individual economic mobility (Figure 3.7). And, wealth and income disparities have a further divide – a racist divide. For example, the average white family in the USA has more than 16 times the wealth of the average black or Latino family. This racial wealth gap will continue to exacerbate human, animal, and environmental health through the mechanism of wealth accumulation over generations and the historic effects of racism through unfair housing and zoning policies,

access to education, and disparity in access to jobs, quality food, and health resources.

Wealth affords individuals many things, including access to power. Therefore, it is important to acknowledge that, for most of the world, this inequality in wealth and income results in economic and political power being concentrated into the hands of a very small number of individuals. This has enormous consequences for planetary health. Decisions of resource acquisition, of consumption, of access to clean air and water, of access to quality education and decisions of curriculum content, individual healthcare access, of access to homes far from sources of pollution and other environmental contaminants, and more are made by those with wealth, often to the detriment of those without. The global disparity in wealth and resources results in the consumption of resources in even more inequitable ways. For example, according to research published in 2011, the average citizen of the USA emits more carbon than 500 citizens of Ethiopia, Chad, Afghanistan, Mali, or Burundi. And, the citizens of the state of New York consume more energy than the 900 million people living in sub-Saharan Africa combined. Powerful companies, buoyed by political interests swayed by corporate lobbies, exploit resources in the most impoverished nations, often at the cost of human, animal, and environmental health. For example between 1964 and 1992, the Chevron Oil Company, going by the name Texaco then, drilled for oil in a remote northern region of the Ecuadorian Amazon. In doing so, the company made millions of dollars by exploiting the natural resource of a developing nation and exposing the indigenous people living in the area to toxic waste and polluted water. At the height of its operation, Texaco dumped more than four million gallons of toxic waste directly into rivers as a cost-saving measure. The result of this environmental recklessness was hundreds of deaths from cancers, respiratory illnesses, spontaneous abortions, and worse. In response to the $18 billion dollar judgment levied against Chevron in Ecuadorian court

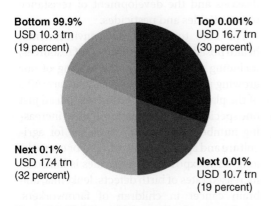

**Bottom 99.9%**
USD 10.3 trn
(19 percent)

**Top 0.001%**
USD 16.7 trn
(30 percent)

**Next 0.1%**
USD 17.4 trn
(32 percent)

**Next 0.01%**
USD 10.7 trn
(19 percent)

**Figure 3.7** Global wealth inequality demonstrating that 0.1% of individuals hold more than 80% of global wealth. In the USA alone, 80% of the population has access to just 7% of the financial wealth. *Source:* Guest2625, https://commons.wikimedia.org/wiki/File:Global_Distribution_of_Wealth_v3.jpg. CC BY-SA 3.0.

for their environmental and human health offenses, the lawyer for Chevron said in his explanation that Chevron would appeal the decision, "The plaintiffs are really irrelevant. They always were irrelevant." This is the power of wealth inequality.

### 3.4.2 Global Food Insecurity

In the spring of 2006, professional and hobby beekeepers across the globe noticed an abundance of empty hives and a new health scare, **Colony Collapse Disorder**, began. Threatened by the environmental contamination of a new class of insecticides, the neonicotinoids, bees that did not simply die frequently lost cognitive function, impeding their ability to return to the hive. Neonicotinoids are now ubiquitous in the environment. As of 2015, it was estimated that neonicotinoids are used on more than 150 million acres of US farmland, including nearly all corn and soy fields and more than a third of cauliflower, cherry tomato, and bell pepper fields. Initially, the research on Colony Collapse Disorder was complicated, with evidence that suggested that neonicotinoids alone were not the sole cause of the decline of healthy bee populations. The insecticide also acts to increase susceptibility to the varroa mite, which can interfere with the queen's reproductive capacity. However, in 2016, the US Environmental Protection Agency has recognized that neonicotinoids, even in small doses, are enough to harm bees and destroy previously thriving hives. We rely on bees to pollinate more than 10% of the global food harvest, and the loss of this resource cost an estimated $200 billion in 2005, but more importantly, Colony Collapse Disorder demonstrated the fragility of the global food market.

The rate of human population growth increases annually, and it is estimated that by 2050, the human population will have exceeded 10 billion. Globally, 842 million people live in a state of food insecurity. In the USA alone, which is the most food secure nation on Earth, 42 million people, including 6.5 million children, live in food insecurity, and annually, malnutrition causes almost half of the deaths of children under five globally. As significant a global health problem as this is, food insecurity will only be worsened by the threat of global climate change. Climate change is altering the growing season, and the risk of desertification of current arable land grows with increasing temperatures. Climate change will also create additional challenges related to water scarcity. Nearly 30% of global agricultural lands exist in already water-stressed regions, and climate change will further stress these regions. Growing food consumption as a result of growing populations will require addressing the issue of water scarcity. This issue will be exacerbated by changing food tastes that frequently come with increased wealth. Consumption of beef, pork, and chicken increase with wealth, and the water and land needed to produce these is significantly greater than that needed to produce wheat, corn, rice, or other plant staples. For example, a kilogram of wheat requires 1500 liters of water for growth while a kilogram of beef requires 16 000 liters. Finally, large-scale agricultural monocultures, especially under the changing conditions of global climate change, can be susceptible to novel infectious diseases and the development of resistance to insecticides and pesticides.

The cost to animal and environmental health posed by the consumption of resources, including arable land, by the feeding of our growing population is significant. Nearly 40% of the planet's land currently goes to feed just one species – us. This can result in an increasing number of chemical exposures for agriculture and agricultural workers. For example, long-term exposure to pesticides is linked to increased rates of birth defects, leukemia, and brain cancer in children of farmworkers. Migrant workers are especially at risk, as these populations frequently lack access to quality, affordable healthcare and education and, in the USA, often face the threat of deportation when reporting violations in proper handling or exposure to pesticides.

Additionally, the increase in pesticides and herbicides associated with feeding growing human populations can negatively affect animal health, including the pollinators we rely on for food production. An increase in non-point source pollution entering our waterways can contribute to exposure of environmental contaminants to aquatic animals and lead to **biomagnification**, or the concentrating of a toxic chemical as it progresses through the food web. Pesticide exposure in birds has been linked to declining ability for song, resulting in loss of reproductive capabilities, and to a decreased interest in fledglings, often resulting in nest failure. Pesticides have also been shown to have endocrine disrupting effects in reptiles and amphibians. Finally, the increased requirement for land for agricultural needs frequently results in habitat destruction, as is evidenced by the destruction of rainforests in Indonesia and Malaysia for palm oil plantations and in the Amazon for soybean and cattle.

### 3.4.3 Environmental Racism

In 2014, the residents of Flint, MI, began to complain about the taste, smell, and color of the water coming from their taps. Less than one year prior, Governor Rick Snyder and the State of Michigan had taken over control of the city's finances after declaring it to be in a state of financial emergency. As a result of this decision, the governor and his staff implemented a money-saving strategy in which the city of Flint would no longer receive water from Lake Huron filtered and pre-treated with corrosion inhibitors through the city of Detroit, 70 miles to the south. The city would, instead, receive water via pipeline directly from Lake Huron. Since this pipeline was still under construction, however, the back-up water source to be used was the Flint River, a body of water renowned for its filth by local residents and considered by researchers to be so contaminated and corrosive that it could damage community water lines and household plumbing. This decision would ultimately result in the poisoning of the people of Flint, MI, a predominantly black community with more than 40% of its population living below the poverty line.

In October 2015, the city reverted to using Detroit's Lake Huron water, but the corrosive nature of the Flint River's water had already permanently damaged the community's water pipes, almost all of which were old and made of lead and galvanized steel. Unfortunately, the leaching of lead from the metal pipes into water cannot be reversed, and even with Lake Huron water flowing through the pipes, the lead continued to leach into the water. In 2017, only about one-third of the lead pipes in Flint had been replaced. Until that effort is completed, which will likely take four additional years and cost upwards of $1.5 billion, Flint's water will continue to be toxic to the community members that require it to live. Already hard hit by the economic downturn following the decline of manufacturing jobs associated with the US auto industry, the lead contamination of the water of Flint, MI resulted in every single child under six being exposed to dangerous levels of lead, a potent neurotoxin, with potentially devastating consequences that will continue to unfold over decades, an increased rate of infertility and fetal deaths in the immediate aftermath, and the death of at least 12 people due to an outbreak of Legionnaire's disease, also due to the contaminated water. According to Dr. Mona Hanna-Attisha, the pediatrician who uncovered elevated lead levels in the blood of Flint's children, "If you were to put something in a population to keep them down for generations and generations to come, it would be lead. It is one of the most damning things that you can do to a population. It drops IQ, it affects behavior, it's been linked to criminality, it has multigenerational impacts. There is no safe level of lead in a child."

Racism is an insidious, corrupting power, which in the USA continues as a result of the still unaddressed, horrific, historic wound of slavery. In the USA in 2017, advocates fight for the value of black lives while simultaneously white supremacists march in protests around the country. Cities and states have begun removing Civil War monuments to leaders of the southern insurgency, but black men and women are shot and killed by police at alarming rates. Since the end of the Civil Rights era of the 1960s, many Americans, although not many black Americans, believed that the issue of race was largely laid to rest. However, racism in America has been systematically instilled and enforced through a series of institutionalized, racist policies limiting equal access to jobs, pay, homes, education, and healthcare for people of color. These institutionalized, systemic policies have allowed covert racism to endure, marginalizing generations of communities of color and forcing populations of color into the jobs no one else wanted, housing on land that was already polluted or near to sources of pollution, and worse.

In the field of Conservation Biology, the concept of NIMBY, or Not In My BackYard, is not new. For example, when construction of a new power plant is proposed, the plant's location is thoughtfully considered. Land use, through zoning and other regulations, is evaluated and a cost–benefit analysis is conducted. The ideal power plant location is one that displaces the fewest number of individuals during construction, is located on inexpensive land, with the greatest access to necessary resources for producing power once online. The NIMBY concept explains why large power plants are not, typically, found in wealthy, white enclaves. These individuals have the resources to petition zoning commissions, hire lawyers to sue if necessary, and/or to simply move. Wealth inequality and environmental racism, however, work synergistically to limit the ability of certain individuals in our community to be able to equitably access resources, wealth, and health.

While the USA can be painted with the brush of environmental racism, it is naïve to think that the USA is unique in this. The story of Chevron/Texaco dumping in Ecuador, described earlier, is an example of environmental racism. However, the Union Carbide disaster in Bhopal, India, in December 1984 stands out as a particularly devastating example of international environmental racism. Union Carbide manufactured methyl isocyanate (MIC), an extremely toxic chemical used in pesticides. Due to a lack of regulatory oversite, a shanty town developed around the chemical plant, encroaching to the point of leaning on the walls of the plant for structural support. When a leak of MIC occurred, allowing MIC to enter the water of Bhopal, the poorest of the poor – living in the shanty town in the shadow of the plant itself – were the most affected. More than 500 000 people were exposed to MIC and more than 3787 people died in a span of three days after the leak. Delays in notifying and receiving medical care in the wake of the disaster compounded the devastation, with the worst affected, again, being the residents of the Bhopal shanty town.

The impact of human activities, the depth and scale of which is now recognized as the Anthropocene, had and continues to have the potential for dire consequences for humanity and, indeed, for the planet itself. However, as we have been the force of destruction, we too can be the force of change for good. For example, The Bill and Melinda Gates Foundation actively works to promote and fund research into health issues, including emerging infectious diseases, women's health issues, water and sanitation resources, sustainable agriculture, and wealth and income inequality. Importantly, Bill and Melinda Gates have already donated more than $28 billion to the Foundation and have encouraged others of great wealth to do the same. And the Gates Foundation is not alone; scientists, community members, and charitable organizations across the globe are working cooperatively to address the issues of planetary health in the Anthropocene. While much work remains to address the challenges discussed here, we can choose to work collaboratively, embracing One Health as a path for improved progress towards human, animal, and environmental health.

## 3.5 Science Denial

In 2004, the Dover, PA, school board altered their biology curriculum to include the teaching of "intelligent design" alongside the teaching of evolution, requiring teachers to read a statement challenging the validity of evolution in advance of any lesson on the subject. As a result of this decision, school board members resigned, science teachers refused to participate at the risk of their own jobs, and ultimately, 11 parents, with American Civil Liberties Union representation, sued the district. In December 2005, US District Judge John E. Jones ruled on the case, after months of testimony, finding that including the intelligent design curriculum in a public school classroom was unconstitutional as it violated the Establishment Clause of the First Amendment, which prevents the government from establishing a religion. His decision was broad, stating "To be sure, Darwin's theory of evolution is imperfect. However, the fact that a scientific theory cannot yet render an explanation on every point should not be used as a pretext to thrust an untestable alternative hypothesis grounded in religion into the science classroom or to misrepresent well-established scientific propositions." Evolutionary biology has, historically, been a special case of science denialism in the USA. Despite the field being supported through evidence from fields across the sciences – paleontology, chemistry, genetics, and molecular biology, to name a few – the study of evolution via natural selection has challenged the religious origin story for many people. As such, it has faced repeated criticism and challenges in state and local school boards, beginning as early as 1925 with the Scopes Monkey Trial. However, in recent years, there has been a profound shift in how we, as a culture and as a world, value the contributions of science and scientists that reach far beyond the perceived religious conflict that challenges the fundamental understanding of evolution in the USA.

The rise of science denial is linked with the rise of anti-intellectualism. In the USA skepticism in intellectual elites began before the founding of the country. However, in recent years, due in large part to the shift in the way in which many people receive their news, there now exists a filtering bubble, in which it is possible to only receive information that already supports an individual's world view. Science deniers use several strategies to discredit evidence and scientists alike. These include creating conspiracy theories, such as suggesting that the moon landing was a hoax, manufacturing experts, and cherry-picking data. The result of the denial of decades of evidence of human-caused climate change has been global economic and health consequences that are just beginning to be understood. The safety of genetically modified foods and the safety and value of vaccines are also frequently challenged by science denialism. Genetically modified foods (GMOs) have the ability to save millions of lives annually (e.g. through the creation of beta-carotene enhanced Golden rice). In 2016, the National Academy of Sciences issued a report evaluating hundreds of peer-reviewed papers and hours of testimony by experts, activists, and the general public that found no substantive evidence of safety concerns from GMO foods. Further, several recent advances in agriculture, including the development of grown "meat" products, would allow a significant increase in food growth in a much smaller land footprint. Yet, almost 90% of scientists consider GMOs safe while less than 40% of the general public shares that view. In much the same way, the denial of vaccine safety is rapidly approaching epidemic status. In 1998, Andrew Wakefield and colleagues published a manuscript in *The Lancet* linking the MMR vaccine to the development of autism in children. Despite the subsequent retraction of the paper due to evidence of fraudulent data, personal financial conflicts of interest, and ethical violations on Wakefield's part resulting in the loss of Wakefield's medical license in the years following this publication, and the dozens of papers, examining thousands of children, which found no evidence of a link between any vaccine component and autism or autism symptoms, science deniers continue to advocate against routine childhood vaccinations. As a result of this, measles – an infectious disease previously considered extirpated from the USA – and measles-related deaths are on the rise, as are pertussis, mumps, and chickenpox. The rise of vaccine-preventable infectious diseases puts children and the immune-compromised at unnecessary risk. Each of these examples illustrates a scientific discovery that has had enormous benefit to global health and has saved millions of lives, and yet, science deniers, with cherry-picked evidence and anecdotes in hand, challenge scientists and other experts who have spent their lives working for the greater good.

One unexpected consequence of the development of the internet and personal computer, technological advances that have directly benefited society in real and expanding ways, is the loss of expertise. While these two technological advances have opened up avenues of communication between scientists and non-scientists in ways that were previously unimaginable, the equalizing ability of an individual voice to reach a large audience has created a scenario in which everyone has an opinion and every opinion is perceived as equally valued. Moreover, the loss of expertise is exacerbated by the false positioning of expert versus "expert" across many traditional news media platforms. This dichotomy in voice perpetrates the myth of false equivalency, lending credibility to those with no credible expertise, only personal agenda. For example giving voice to a climate change scientist and a climate change denier suggests that the evidence on both sides is roughly equivalent. A more accurate presentation of voice in this example would be to interview 99 climate scientists for every single climate denier interviewed. Accessibility to data, transparency in reporting, and public accountability are all important in science and beyond, but the perceived loss of

expertise, in conjunction with the rise of science denial, challenges the nature of global health and scientific advancement. In the USA and across the globe, policy decisions are made by politicians who cannot distinguish the voice of scientists from the voice of science deniers, with devastating consequences for human, animal, and environmental health.

While the consequences of the denial of science are only now beginning to be fully understood, a new global reckoning has begun. Scientists are more and more entering the political arena, running for elected offices at all levels in the USA – from school board to US Senator. Women and people of color are demanding that their voices be heard in unprecedented ways. The denial of science is beginning to be countered by curricular changes at the earliest levels of education and the increasingly ardent voice of scientists in the media. Social media has opened the doors of accessibility and encouraged a dialogue between scientists and the general public, and these conversations will grow in time to drown out the voice of denial.

## 3.6 Conclusion

Despite the current state of planetary health (as discussed throughout this chapter), scientific advances, and the scientists that strive to achieve them, have positioned the planet to be in the best position for the most number of people alive today: there is greater access to healthcare for more people than ever before, there is greater access to education for more people than ever before; there is greater wealth available to more people than ever before, and science has given the world amazing advances that have enabled us to solve complex, global problems like never before. However, simultaneously, there are significant threats to planetary health that challenge us like never before. Human, animal, and environmental health are intrinsically connected. The creativity of scientists and the work of science – collaborative, holistic, peer-reviewed solutions to complex problems – is what is needed to solve the greatest threats to planetary health. This is One Health.

## End of Chapter Questions & Activities

A. Chapter Thought Questions

   i) Why One Health?

   ii) In your opinion, what is the Greatest Threat for life on our planet? Why? What evidence supports your argument?

   iii) Consider the Greatest Threats discussed in this chapter. What can you most immediately affect through changing your own actions?

   iv) The threat of science denial, in particular, poses significant challenges in addressing all other threats discussed. Evidence suggests that a simple presentation of fact does little to change an individual's mind on any issue. What specific strategies can you identify to encourage the acceptance of science?

B. In-Class/Guided Activities:

   i) Using Twitter, investigate #OneHealth daily over the course of a week (or two) to identify trends and patterns in #OneHealth conversations. Use NodeXL to map out #OneHealth networks, identify #OneHealth practitioners, and #OneHealth issues. Contribute to the conversation!

   ii) Calculate your Ecological Footprint. This will give you an idea of the number of Earths needed to support resource consumption if everyone on the planet lived as you do. There are a number of calculators available online.

C. At-home Activities

   i) Consider becoming an invasivore. Identify invasive species that are problems in your local community, and then expand your palette. Many invasive species are edible and, with some creativity, can be an interesting new adventure in eating.

   ii) Meet with your local school board and advocate for sustainable practices to be implemented in your own school. This can include school-level recycling, composting, and gardening as well as larger-scale improvements such as a green energy audit.

D. Long-term Action Steps

   i) Work to identify ways to reduce your carbon footprint in significant ways. Start small – recycle if you don't already. Begin composting your food waste. Plant a small garden to grow your own vegetables. Give up meat (even for 1 day per week). Walk and/or cycle more and drive less. Work to larger, more impactful changes – give up driving in favor of cycling or public transportation. Move closer to your work. Invest in solar panels. Strive for a Zero Waste household. Decide to have one less child.

   ii) Act to improve your world. Do not wait for someone else to take the lead.

E. Recommended Reading:

Egginton, J. (2009). *The Poisoning of Michigan*. Michigan State University Press.

Farmer, P. (2001). *Infections and Inequalities: The Modern Plagues*. University of California Press.

Garrett, L. (1994). *The Coming Plague: Newly Emerging Diseases in a World Out of Balance*. Penguin.

Al Gore (2007). *An Inconvenient Truth: The Crisis of Global Warming*. Bloomsbury Press.

Leakey, R. and Lewin, R. (1995). *The Sixth Extinction: Biodiversity and its Survival*. Weidenfeld & Nicolson.

Rothstein, R. (2017). *The Color of Law: A Forgotten History of How our Government Segregated America*. Liveright Publishing Corporation.

Zimring, C.A. (2015). *Clean and White: A History of Environmental Racism in the United States*. New York University Press.

## Interview

*What is the greatest threat to planetary health? A panel of experts weighs in.*

**Cheryl Stroud, PhD, DVM, Director of the One Health Commission:**

I think our greatest threat to planetary health is our human attitude as a species towards our planet. It's our home, our only home, and our attitude is that the planet's here for our use, and we are just sucking up big resources, and sometimes doing it to the great detriment of human populations in the locations that we are sucking these resources out of the Earth. Our greatest threat is that attitude, our failing to include people at the table to really address some of our most wicked challenges (a term coined by Lonnie King). I used to think very early on of One Health as a three-legged stool with the human domain, the animal domain, the environmental domain, and it makes total sense if you leave one of those domains (legs) out, that stool is going to fall over. I have kind of expanded that a little bit now because we specifically are trying to include plants. I think they were being lumped into the environmental domain very early on, but plants and soil health are going to be incredibly important for how we are going to feed the nine billion people that we are looking at feeding eventually, and how we are going to do it without further destroying our planet. So that's our greatest threat to planetary health.

**Agustin Fuentes, PhD, University of Notre Dame:**

You know, there are the general threats, which are rapid and relatively unplanned habitat conversion, increasing contact between organisms that had not had extensive or prolonged contact before, rapidly expanded travel opportunities and movement, all of which can actually have beneficial outcomes. But on average, because they are generally unplanned, increase the risk for novel pathogen transmission or novel complexities in health for both humans and other organisms.

**Barbara Natterson-Horowitz, MD, University of California, Los Angeles:**

It's hard to offer a single answer. Certainly, the many potentially catastrophic consequences of climate change and related phenomenon has to be first. But hand in hand with climate change or connected to it is the problem of human exceptionalism and a kind of blindness to a collective human responsibility.

**Christine Fiorello DVM, PhD, Rio Grande Zoo and Aquarium at the Albuquerque BioPark:**

People are a pretty big threat, but that's a pretty vague answer because people are the cause of a lot of different types of threats to the planet. If you are going to be a little more narrow, I would say global climate change because it is global and we are definitely approaching the point of no return. Soon, we are not going to be able to stop and the planet is not going to be able to recover from the amount of change that we have already caused.

**Dawn Holliday, PhD, Westminster College:**

The greatest threat I think is climate change. It's the single biggest, most pervasive issue affecting all species, including humans. And there's a myriad of direct and indirect consequences that I really think are grossly underestimated. And, then just a lack of understanding by the general public as to the immediacy of the impact and the necessity of the changes and sacrifices that we should be making. Climate change is going to affect my little branch in environmental toxicology, especially with reptiles, who are poikilotherms and so any change in temperature affects whether they produce males or females, which affects what the population of the next generation looks like. And we see it affecting humans and where humans are living and losing land and the ability to farm like they used to. Climate change, because of its pervasive impacts, is the biggest issue.

**Lise Saffran, MPH, MFA, University of Missouri, Columbia:**
  Climate change.

**Philo Mbong, PhD, 500 Women Scientists:**
  I live in California. It is unseasonably warm, and today it is 80° outside. It should not be this hot in December. Climate change is real, and it is something that is affecting us right now. Unfortunately, as much as scientists step up and say that climate change is real and that it is affecting our planetary health, people in power are not taking it seriously enough. I would say that is the major threat that we have right now.

**Louise Bradshaw, MS, Saint Louis Zoo:**
  Climate change.

**Natalia Reagan, MA, Anthropologist and Comedienne:**
  Climate change and Congressional Republicans of 2017, who exemplify and exacerbate wealth and health inequality.

**Julienne Anoko, PhD, World Health Organization:**
  For me, the best thing we want to do for the planetary health is to apply the concept for One Health in the respect of people's culture, equity, and a real communication. This gives opportunity to each one wherever he's from, whatever his religion, color, and socioeconomic status to be heard in our intercultural global world. For me, this is the greatest threat. This is my threat as a social anthropologist and implementer in the field.

**Martin Meltzer, PhD, US CDC:**
  Our first and primary focus, and what we are tasked for and what we are given

resources for, is human health. And I think the biggest risk to human health, in terms of infectious diseases on a global scale, is outbreaks of diseases such as influenza pandemics that still are novel strains of influenza virus that spill out of animals. The whole planet is vulnerable to outbreaks of infectious diseases, no matter where the origin is from. And to rapidly diagnose, understand the degree of risk, and get in and respond is the biggest challenge.
  It's a global problem. It is not a country by country or local community problem. The Ebola epidemic and the Zika epidemic clearly demonstrate what happens in one country across the ocean can rapidly impact countries that have never heard of this disease before but suddenly it is possible that it could be on their doorstep tomorrow.

**Keith Martin, MD, PC, Consortium of Universities for Global Health:**
  I am going to respond to your question in two parts. The destruction of ecosystems from several anthropogenic causes including climate change poses the greatest threat to the health of the planet, ourselves, and indeed all species.

**Gary Vroegindewey, DVM, MSS, Lincoln Memorial University:**
  Identifying the greatest threat to planetary health is so challenging because, like One Health, all the parts are interrelated. One of the biggest concerns that I have is loss of biodiversity. Loss of biodiversity does not stand alone because it may be the proximate concern, but loss of biodiversity is attached to loss of habitat. And so, if we look at loss of habitats, then we are looking at our use of land and how that encroaches upon habitats that affects biodiversity. Ultimately, we are looking at our consumption and our population. My proximate concern is biodiversity, but my long-term concern involves loss of habitats, including destruction of habitat and climate change.

**Martyn Jeggo, PhD, DVM, Deakin University:**

It would be totally naïve not to consider climate change and the effects of humans, the anthropomorphic effects on climate change, which are having a profound effect on all sorts of things, and that includes infectious diseases. We are seeing a change in distribution of a number of vector-borne diseases associated with changing climate. From my perspective, climate change is one crucial element.

Another crucial element is our continuous invasion of our environment. As we do that, more of these viruses change hosts. The fact that we are seeing more bat-borne diseases is associated with our movement into areas where bats have previously lived without much human interaction. And I think we have still got a lot of viruses we do not understand in the rodent population as well, like the Hantavirus group, which might become important in time.

From an infectious diseases point of view, climate change and environmental invasion are probably the two key threats. From a broader perspective, there's no doubt that food security and food safety these days are crucial elements that have a strong One Health component. And so as we think about how we create a global food-secure environment, particularly for the many people in developing countries, we start to see that as a serious threat.

And then finally, you cannot have this conversation without talking about antimicrobial resistance and understanding all the issues that are involved in that. When we talk about the misuse of antibiotics in livestock, as a livestock growth promoter, then you have another significant threat.

**Sharon Deem, PhD, DVM, Institute for Conservation Medicine, Saint Louis Zoo:**

The four word answer is "the loss of biodiversity." We are losing species at an unprecedented rate and one not seen since the end of the dinosaurs. We are living at a period of the sixth mass extinction. Unfortunately, humans are driving these extinctions. It is estimated that we loss species at a rate of 100–1000 × above baseline levels. E.O. Wilson estimates that we loss 27 000 species per year which is 3 species per hour. This is tragic. Of course along with this loss in biodiversity I would list human population explosion and overconsumption (especially of animal protein sources) that have created the other big evils such as climate change, ocean acidification, and habitat destruction.

**Kelly Lane-deGraaf, PhD, Center for One Health, Fontbonne University:**

The greatest threat to planetary health is the inability of people to communicate clearly and with compassion for others. This, combined with things like racism, greed, and the inability to care about people different from yourself, fundamentally prevent collaboration and the exchange of ideas. If we could work together, hear, and engage with a diverse spectrum of people, and communicate without agenda, the greatest threats to our health could be resolved.

**Elizabeth Rayhel, PhD, Center for One Health, Fontbonne University:**

Climate change.

## Works Cited

Acevedo-Whitehouse, K. and Duffus, A.L.J. (2009). Effects of environmental change on wildlife health. *Philosophical Transactions of the Royal Society, B: Biological Sciences* 364: 3429–3438.

Bloom, D.E., Black, S., and Rappuoli, R. (2017). Emerging infectious diseases: a proactive approach. *Proceedings of the National Academy of Sciences* 114 (16): 4055–4059.

Burke, M.B., Miguel, E., Stayanath, S. et al. (2009). Warming increases the risk of civil war in Africa. *Proceedings of the National Academy of Sciences* 106 (49): 2670–2974.

Carter, C., Finley, W., Fry, J. et al. (2007). Palm oil markets and future supply. *European Journal of Lipid Science and Technology* 109 (4): 307–314.

Ceballos, G., Ehrlich, P.R., and Dirzo, R. (2017). Biological annihilation via the ongoing sixth mass extinction signaled by vertebrate population losses and declines. *Proceedings of the National Academy of Sciences* doi: 10.1073/pnas.1704949114.

Chick, J.H. and Pegg, M.A. (2001). Invasive carp in the Mississippi River basin. *Science* 292 (5525): 2250–2251.

Ellis, J.D., Evans, J.D., and Pettis, J. (2010). Colony losses, managed colony population decline, and Colony Collapse Disorder in the United States. *Journal of Apicultural Research* 49 (1): 134–136.

Fowlkes, M.R. and Miller, P.Y. (1987). Chemicals and community at Love Canal. In: *The Social and Cultural Construct of Risk* (ed. B.B. Johnson and V.T. Covello), 55–78. Dordrecht: D Reidel.

Gilligan, C.A. and van den Bosch, F. (2008). Epidemiological models for invasion and persistence of pathogens. *Annual Review of Phytopathology* 46: 385–418.

Goldman, L.R., Paigen, B., Magnant, M.M. et al. (2009). Low birth weight, prematurity, and birth defects in children living near the hazardous waste site, Love Canal. *Hazardous Waste and Hazardous Materials* 2 (2): 209–223.

Hanna-Attisha, M., LaChance, J., Sadler, R.C. et al. (2016). Elevated blood lead levels in children associated with the flint drinking water crisis: a spatila analysis of risk and public health response. *American Journal of Public Health* 106 (2): 283–290.

Hansen, J., Sato, M., and Ruedy, R. (2012). Perception of climate change. *Proceedings of the National Academy of Sciences* 109 (37): e14720.

Henry, M., Beguin, M., Requier, F. et al. (2012). A common pesticide decreases foraging success and survival in honey bees. *Science* 336 (6079): 348–350.

Hodges, E. and Tomcej, V. (2016). Is there a link between pollutant exposure and emerging infectious disease? *Canadian Veterinary Journal* 57 (5): 535–537.

Hsiang, S.M., Burke, M., and Miguel, E. (2013). Quantifying the influence of climate on human conflict. *Science* 341 (6252): 1235367.

Im, E.S., Pal, J.S., and Eltahir, E.A.B. (2017). Deadly heat waves projected in the densely populated agricultural regions of South Asia. *Science Advances* 3: 1–7.

Jerde, C.L., Chadderton, L., Mahon, A.R. et al. (2013). Detection of Asian carp DNA as part of a Great Lakes basin-wide surveillance program. *Canadian Journal of Fisheries and Aquatic Sciences* 70 (4): 522–526.

Jones, K.E., Patel, N.G., Levy, M.A. et al. (2008). Global trends in emerging infectious diseases. *Nature* 451: 990–994.

*Kitzmiller v. Dover Area School District* (2005) US District Court, case 4:04-cv-02688-JEJ, 139 pp.

Long, J.L. (2003). *Introduced Mammals of the World: Their History, Distribution, and Influence*. CSIRO Publishing.

Luby, J.L., Barch, D.M., Belden, A. et al. (2012). Maternal support in early childhood predicts larger hippocampal volumes at school age. *Proceedings of the National Academy of Sciences* 109 (8): 2854–2859.

Lymbery, A.J., Morine, M., Kanani, H.G. et al. (2014). Co-invaders: the effects of alien parasites on native hosts. *International Journal of Parasitology. Parasites and Wildlife* 3 (2014): 171–177.

Mellor, J.M. and Milyo, J.D. (2001). Income inequality and health. *Journal of Policy Analysis and Management* 20 (1): 151–155.

Messenger, A.M., Barnes, A.N., and Gray, G.C. (2014). Reverse zoonotic disease transmission (zooanthroponosis): a systematic review of seldom-documented human biological threats to animals. *PLoS One* 9 (2): e89055.

Morens, D.M. and Fauci, A.S. (2013). Emerging infectious diseases: threats to human health and global stability. *PLoS Pathogens* 9 (7): e1003467.

Murtaugh, M.P., Steer, C.J., Sreevatsan, S. et al. (2017). The science behind One Health: at the interface of humans, animals, and the environment. *Annals of the New York Academy of Sciences* 1395: 12–32.

Myers, S.S., Gaffikin, L., Golden, C.D. et al. (2013). Human health impacts of ecosystem alteration. *Proceedings of the National Academy of Sciences* 110 (47): 18753–18760.

Narain, S. and Bhushan, C. (2015). *Capitan America-US Climate Goals: A Reckoning*. New Dehli: Centre for Science and Environment.

Olsen, J. (2001). Environmental problems and ethical jurisdiction: the case concerning Texaco in Ecuador. *Business Ethics: A European Review* 10 (1): 71–77.

O'Neill, C.R., and Dextrase, A. (1994) The introduction and spread of the Zebra mussel in North America. *Proceedings of the 4th International Zebra Mussel Conference*, Madison, WI.

Panko, B. (2017) Scientists now know exactly how lead got into Flint's water. Smithsonian Magazine. http://www.smithsonianmag.com/science-nature/chemical-study-ground-zero-house-flint-water-crisis-180962030 (accessed October 30, 2017).

Pickett, K.E. and Wilkinson, R.G. (2015). Income inequality and health: a causal review. *Social Science and Medicine* 128: 316–326.

Poinar, G. and Boucot, A.J. (2006). Evidence of intestinal parasites of dinosaurs. *Parasitology* 133 (2): 245–249. doi: 10.1017/S0031182006000138.

Rothstein, R. (2017). *The Color of Law: A Forgotten History of How Our Government Segregated America*. New York, NY: Liveright Publishing.

Rowley, M.H., Christian, J.J., Basu, D.K. et al. (1982). Use of small mammals (voles) to assess a hazardous waste site at Love Canal, Niagara Falls, New York. *Archives of Environmental Contamination and Toxicology* 12 (4): 383–397.

Sherwood, H. (2014) Global refugee figure passes 50m for first time since Second World War. The Guardian. https://www.theguardian.com/world/2014/jun/20/global-refugee-figure-passes-50-million-unhcr-report (accessed August 13, 2017).

Torchin, M.E. and Lafferty, K.D. (2009). Escape from parasites. In: *Biological Invasions in Marine Ecosystems* (ed. G. Rilov and J.A. Crooks), 203–214. Berlin: Springer-Verlag.

United Nations (2015). *Paris Agreement*. New York, NY: United Nations.

WHO (2017) Annual Review of diseases prioritized under the Research and Development Blueprint. *World Health Organization*, Geneva, Switzerland.

Wicke, B., Sikkema, R., Dornburg, V. et al. (2011). Exploring land use changes and the role of palm oil production in Indonesia and Malaysia. *Land Use Policy* 28 (1): 193–206.

Wilts, A. (2017) Trump economic adviser worth $266m thinks a car costs $1000. *The Independent*. www.independent.co.uk/news/world/americas/us-politics/gary-cohn-trump-tax-reform-cost-new-car-home-improvement-a7974731.html (accessed September 14, 2017).

Wuebbles, D., Fahey, D., and Hibbard, K. (2017) U.S. Global Change Research Program Climate Science Special Report (CSSR). National Science Foundation, National Oceanic and Atmospheric Administration, and National Aeronotics and Space Administration.

Zenni, R.D. and Nunez, M.A. (2013). The elephant in the room: the role of failed invasions in understanding invasion biology. *Oikos* 122: 801–815.

Part II

The One Health Triad

# 4

## Environmental Health as One Health

Ghost towns are part of the cultural heritage of Americans. Throughout the Westward Expansion, small towns frequently blinked in and out of existence. As the first transcontinental railroad joined the eastern and western coasts of the USA, the ability to move goods to market shifted drastically and limited economic growth for many communities. This shift signaled the beginning of the end for many small towns in the American west, as the railroad passed by without stopping. The gold rush of 1849 also resulted in the creation of boomtowns, many of which now stand abandoned. Environmental disasters can also create ghost towns. The catastrophic meltdown of the reactor core at a nuclear power plant in Chernobyl in 1986 resulted in the forced, immediate evacuation from a radioactive exclusion zone 18 miles in diameter, leaving the once bustling community of Pripyat, Ukraine, home to nearly 50 000 people, now standing abandoned. For the people of St. Louis, MO, the most infamous ghost town known was Times Beach, a small community not far from St. Louis entirely surrounded by tall fences and deep lore.

Times Beach, MO, was an idyllic, American small town, located about 20 miles southwest of St. Louis. Now a state park, the community began as a summer resort for St. Louisans looking to escape the summer heat and humidity. The town's first plot was sold in 1925 for $67.50, which included a newspaper subscription. The Meramec River quietly flowed through the community, providing cooling breezes and easy access to opportunities for summer fun in the river: river floats, fishing, and swimming in the shallow waters. However, the town remained a resort town for only a short while. The Great Depression, followed quickly by World War II, left the community facing economic challenges, as interest in summer homes dwindled. Times Beach was also extremely flood-prone because of the close proximity of the river. In time, the community transitioned from a resort town of summer homes for St. Louis' wealthy to year-round homes for working class families. By the early 1970s, Times Beach remained unable to pave a large number of roads throughout the community and as a result, was facing a significant dust problem. The city hired waste hauler, Russell Bliss, to spray motor oil onto the roads to help control the dust. From 1972 to 1976, Russell Bliss sprayed the roads of Times Beach with motor oil. Unbeknownst to the people of Times Beach, this motor oil was contaminated with toxic waste.

Russell Bliss began his career as a waste hauler. He worked hard and succeeded in an unpopular job, becoming a millionaire by age 48. He frequently sprayed the roads on his own farm with a fine mist of motor oil in an effort to minimize dust kicked up by equipment, and soon, he was hired by local horse farms for this service. In a stroke of genius, Bliss recognized an opportunity to combine the two arms of his business – waste hauling and dust management – into one, by

*Introduction to One Health: An Interdisciplinary Approach to Planetary Health*, First Edition.
Sharon L. Deem, Kelly E. Lane-deGraaf and Elizabeth A. Rayhel.
© 2019 John Wiley & Sons, Inc. Published 2019 by John Wiley & Sons, Inc.
Companion website: www.wiley.com/go/deem/health

mixing the toxic waste collected with the oil sprayed on the land. This combining of motor oil and toxic waste allowed him to double his income by being paid to collect toxic waste and then being paid to spray it on the land. One of the companies that Russell Bliss was contracted with for waste removal was Northeastern Pharmaceutical and Chemical Company (NEPACCO). NEPACCO had been a large scale producer of Agent Orange, a chemical defoliant used widely in the Vietnam War. The waste from this facility was a sludge contaminated with concentrations of dioxins at more than 2000 times greater than the dioxin concentration of Agent Orange. Dioxin is a lethal material that is environmentally-persistent and capable of biomagnification in wildlife; the World Health Organization considers dioxins to be one of the most toxic chemicals known. Dioxins can cause reproductive and developmental problems, damage the immune system, interfere with hormones, and are known carcinogens.

In the early 1970s, local horse farms began reporting sick and dying animals at unusual rates. One farm – Shenandoah Stables – reported the deaths of 62 quarter horses. As a result, in 1971, the Centers for Disease Control and Prevention (CDC) began testing soil and blood samples for chemical contaminants. The reports were inconclusive, detecting low levels of polychlorinated biphenyls (PCBs) and insecticides, but not in amounts enough to conclusively identify the offending chemical or source. While the CDC investigation continued, the owners of the Shenandoah Stables blamed Bliss despite his protests. Rabbits and sparrows also began dying at these horse farms, and as a result, the CDC expanded the testing and ultimately found evidence of significant concentrations of trichlorophenol, PCBs, and dioxin in the samples taken from horses and local wildlife.

While the CDC was investigating the deaths of horses and wildlife in the farms outside St. Louis, MO, Russell Bliss began spraying a mixture of motor oil and toxic waste on the unpaved roads of Times Beach.

Over the four years of dust-suppressant activities, Bliss sprayed an estimated 160 000 gal of contaminated oil throughout Times Beach. CDC testing was incomplete until 1974, but by that time, the damage to Times Beach was done. In 1982, after an increasing amount of complaints, the US Environmental Protection Agency (EPA) intervened, testing soil and water samples throughout Times Beach. The results showed that sediments in Times Beach were contaminated with dioxin at concentrations more than 100 times higher than what the agency considered safe for human or animal exposure. The day after the results were revealed in 1983, the Meramec River overflowed its banks, resulting in the largest flood to date that the community had experienced. Community members who had not already fled in advance of the flood were told to leave immediately and to leave behind all belongings. The town was fully evacuated and declared a Superfund site, a federal designation for a site that has been previously contaminated by toxic waste and has become a priority for clean-up by the EPA often at the expense of taxpayers. By 1985, Times Beach was a ghost town. The widespread contamination with lethal toxic contaminants took almost 20 years to clean up and included removal and disposal of more than 900 truckloads of contaminated soil and approximately 2000 barrels of toxic waste from Bliss's own property.

Times Beach was removed from the National Priorities List (NPL) as a Superfund site in 2001. As of 2016, other large areas that Bliss sprayed remain on the NPL as active Superfund sites managed by the EPA. As of December 1, 2017, there are 1319 sites remaining on the NPL as active Superfund sites in the contiguous USA.

There exists an indisputable connection between human, animal, and environmental health. However, in the early 1970s, while the disaster in Times Beach was unfolding, the separation between how we consider human health, animal health, and environmental health was still a deep gulf, entrenched by a lack of communication and collaboration between practitioners across disciplines. As a consequence of this gulf, the residents of Times Beach were exposed to potentially lethal concentrations of toxic waste after more than 62 horses and numerous wild animals died and the CDC began its investigations. The connection between human, animal, and environmental health, however, is increasingly recognized. For example, in 1999, one of the first practitioners to note that West Nile virus had reached the USA was the head pathologist at the Bronx Zoo, a wildlife veterinarian by training, who grew concerned with the number of crows and other corvids who were unexpectedly dying that summer while simultaneously noting an unusual rash of Zoo collection animals also dying including a cormorant, flamingos, and a bald eagle.

Intuitively, most people prioritize the health and well-being of people over the health of animals and the environment. And, historically, our research efforts have reflected this concern, with a focus on human health often to the exclusion of research on the environment and environmental health. However, this emphasis on human health has left us poorer in terms of our understanding of the context through which the environment directly affects our own health. While the effects of human activities are more evident on the health of the environment, environmental health also impacts human and animal health. All of our actions have consequences. Frequently, the actions of humans have a myriad of direct and indirect consequences for the environment, which result in countless unintended consequences for the health of humans and animals.

Humans now sully every ecosystem on earth. There is no longer a patch of earth that can be described as pristine; even if humans have not yet touched a spot of land (or sea), our noises, pollution, and global presence have altered that spot in an unassailable way. The greatest concern for environmental health is undoubtedly the overwhelming and long-term contamination of our environment through the dumping of chemical pollutants and waste. This includes pollution of air, water, and land, which degrades habitat for wildlife and potentially devastates resources available for any future use. The resulting alteration of our environment has systemic effects on planetary health. Here, we will explore the threat to environmental health from pollution and other environmental contaminants as well as examine the effects of the **anthropogenization** of landscapes on environmental health. In doing so, we will also analyze how these environmental health threats create and exacerbate human and animal health threats, such as when a toxic chemical is sprayed directly into the environment, as in the case of the Times Beach contamination with dioxin. We have the ability to create novel, life-changing responses to human, animal, and environmental health; however, our impetus to act for the health of the environment depends, in part, on our own ability to comprehend fully the intrinsic value of the environment as well as the long-term costs and benefits of environmental health for humans and animals.

## 4.1 Threats to Environmental Health

Threats to environmental health are numerous, but most share a specific set of common characteristics. Frequently, threats to environmental health are diffuse and widespread; present challenges for clean-up and containment; and are difficult to pinpoint the exact, original source or sources of the threat. For example, when a chemical pollutant leaks into a river, the damage to the environment is likely to occur downstream, and potentially far downstream, of the original site of contamination. While it may appear less challenging to determine the cause of habitat loss, that is not always the case. For example, the transition from oak-hickory forest to farmland throughout the American Midwest has resulted in numerous landscape-level alterations to the environment. However, the honeybee (*Apis mellifera*) has continued to thrive. In 2006, when Colony Collapse Disorder was first detected, the threat to the survival of honeybees was clear, but the cause of the honeybees' population collapse was unknown; complicating the investigation was the long-term alteration of the native habitat. Finally, while it is difficult for many to consider large-scale consequences of their actions, the diffuse and widespread nature of many environmental health threats suggest that local actions have global consequences. For example, in China, the levels of air pollution in urban areas results in an estimated 1.2 million premature deaths annually. Winds that blow across the Pacific Ocean, called the westerlies, carry with them air pollution as far as the western USA. As much as 24% of the sulfate-based air contaminants and approximately 9% of the carbon monoxide contamination in Los Angeles can be traced back to industrialized areas in China. However, the USA drives much of the global market for inexpensive, Chinese-produced goods, suggesting that the purchasing power of consumers in the USA fuels the manufacture of industrial pollutants in China, which in turn find their way back to the USA as air pollution. Threats to environmental health can have far-reaching, unexpected consequences.

## 4.2 Pollution and Environmental Contamination

According to a report published in *The Lancet*, more than nine million people died in 2015 due to diseases caused by the effects of pollution. This sobering number is more than three times the number of people who died from malaria, HIV, and tuberculosis combined, according to the same report. To suggest, then, that pollution is not a global health threat is indefensible. While we have already touched on the emission of greenhouse gases as it relates to the climate crisis, pollution is a much broader problem for

health than simply air pollution driving up global temperatures. Pollution contaminates the air, the water, and the soil of the planet, can be large-scale or small-scale, accidental or intentional, and can originate from **point sources** or **non-point sources**. While numerous examples of threats of pollution and other environmental contaminants exist that are limited in scope and scale, short-term, and attributable to a single, non-repeating event (e.g. an individual dumping motor oil on the ground after changing their car's oil), these examples tend to be the exception. As such, entities and processes that threaten environmental health by polluting often indirectly threaten human and animal health as well. For example, while most people would not knowingly add lead contamination to their family's drinking water, many corporations, and the people that work for them, knowingly make decisions that result in lead contamination eventually entering drinking water systems. The reasons for this are numerous and complex and include economic incentives, lack of awareness of the environmental health costs, lack of understanding of the connections between environmental health and human and wildlife health, among others.

In the USA, the mining of precious metals involves the extraction of resources through underground mines. However, many precious metals are not easy to extract. Gold, for example, is often found co-occurring with pyrites (including arsenopyrite, chalcopyrite, and sphalerite), galena, bournonite, jamesonite, and tetrahedrite. Silver is frequently found in close co-association with sulfur, arsenic, antimony, or galena. If a precious metal, such as gold or silver, is found as an alloy with another metal or as a compound with another element, then an additional step is needed – amalgamation or electrolysis – in order to isolate the metal from the mineral context. This process ravages the surrounding environment. From the increased opportunity for erosion and contamination of soil to the creation of sinkholes and dumping of mine tailings, mining for precious metals

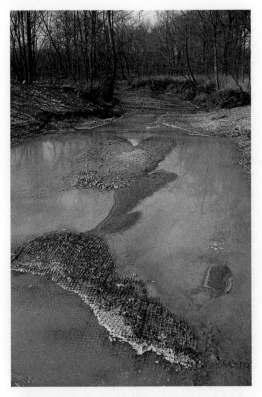

**Figure 4.1** Water pollution as a result of leaching from mine tailings.

creates lasting damage to the environment (Figure 4.1). In the US West, it is estimated that there are now more than 500 000 metal mines abandoned and no longer in use. This estimate includes both pit mines and subsurface mines, and the estimated cost of remediation of these is more than $35 billion. For example, the Berkeley Pit Mine had a long history of producing gold and copper. Open from 1955 until 1982, the pit mine reached a vertical depth of almost 1800 ft and produced more than one billion tons of material. Groundwater began seeping back into the mine after its closure, rising at the rate of about one foot per month. This presents a significant threat to human, animal, and environmental health.

As water enters the mine pit, pyrite and other sulfide minerals react with the dissolved oxygen in the water, creating an increasingly dangerous lake of acid over time that also carries significant concentrations of heavy metals leached from the mine. In November 2016, thousands of snow geese died after the flock landed in the lake in Berkeley Pit. **Necropsies** revealed internal burns due to exposure to high concentrations of heavy metals, including copper, cadmium, and arsenic, as well as numerous skin lesions from contact with acidic waters. The critical water level for the Berkeley Pit, or the point at which the water level in the mine, resulting from rain and snowmelt, reaches the natural water table, is expected to occur sometime between 2020 and 2023. Once this occurs, the waters from the mine will flow into the area's groundwater and contaminate the Silver Bow Creek, headwaters for the Clark Fork River. The Clark Fork is the major source of drinking water for nearby Butte, MT, which is home to almost 40 000 people, and feeds into the Columbia River system, which covers 14 million acres across Montana and Idaho and provides drinking water to more than 350 000 people. Water in the Berkeley Pit mine is currently so contaminated with heavy metals that it is possible to mine the water directly for copper. In 2017, Butte, MT, began the development of a massive water treatment facility to mitigate future environmental damage and prevent groundwater contamination from the Berkeley Pit. In 2017, the EPA estimates that in the USA, more than 40% of watersheds in the West have been polluted as a result of mining practices.

Importantly, mining is only one example of a specific land use that despoils the land, and as a result, contaminates local waters that carry pollution far beyond the original source. Agriculture, oil and gas production, and fashion are also industries that result in significant pollution entering the environment, and like pollution from mining, pollution from these industries can also poison widespread areas of ground, air, and water far beyond the site of the initial contamination.

Ground pollution is frequently cryptic, or hidden from view, for most people. Many people do not fully appreciate agricultural lands, roads, and urban areas as sources of ground pollution at the scale of mining, for example, but the actions needed to alter the environment into agricultural lands, roads, and urban areas created large-scale ground and soil pollution. Air pollution, however, may be visible, as in the example of smog in Los Angeles, New Delhi, or Beijing, but, as in the example of greenhouse gas emissions, may also be invisible to the unaided eye. Importantly, air pollution has significant health effects for humans and animals that are exposed to it. Air pollution can come from volcanic eruptions and other naturally occurring biogeochemical processes, but human actions now account for the greatest amount of chemical and particle contamination of the earth's air and atmosphere.

In 1952, London was shrouded in a thick blanket of smog for four days. When the blanket had lifted, more than 4000 people had died. Over the following two months, more than 150 000 people were hospitalized. In all, more than 12 000 people and many thousands of domesticated animals died as a direct result of the Great Smog of London, as the incident has come to be known (Figure 4.2). Smog was a relatively common part of London life in the 1950s, and as such, the devastation of the 1952 smog confounded scientists, doctors and veterinarians,

politicians, and community members for years. It was 2016 before scientists fully understood the mechanism of the lethal effects of the pollution from the London Smog of 1952. Nitrogen dioxide and sulfur dioxide, both products of coal burning, combined with water droplets in fog to form aerosolized droplets of sulfuric acid, which were then inhaled by the city's residents and wildlife, ultimately poisoning them. As a result of the Great Smog, in 1956, the British Parliament passed the Clean Air Act. Unfortunately, the acid fog side-effect of coal-burning has not been limited to 1950s London and occurs frequently throughout China, where as recently as 2015, 16 of the 20 most polluted cities can be found. Additional health risks from air pollution include loss of lung capacity and function, damage to the heart and cells of the respiratory system, development of diseases including bronchitis, emphysema, and cancer, and ultimately, early death. Air pollution also creates serious health effects for wildlife: pollution has been linked to physiological changes in amphibians; birds' respiratory systems are damaged; evidence links an increased rate of cancers in birds to the proximity of nests to coal plants; and acid rain has been shown to result in significant fish kills. Air pollution in all its forms

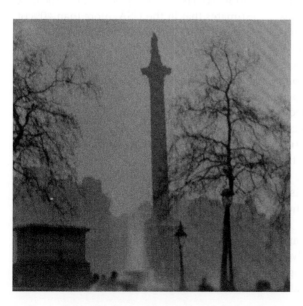

**Figure 4.2** Great London Smog of 1952 in which thousands of people died due to the significant air pollution that blanketed the city for days. This image is of Nelson's Column, a prominent landmark in London. *Source:* N.T. Stobbs, https://commons.wikimedia.org/wiki/File:Nelson%27s_Column_during_the_Great_Smog_of_1952.jpg. CC BY-SA 2.0.

is persistent in the environment and poses a demonstrably significant threat to human, animal, and environmental health.

Water pollution is pervasive in our environment and is often compounded by run-off from soil and ground pollution as well as by the settling of particles from airborne pollution. For example, groundwater leaching of heavy metals and arsenic and cyanide pollution from mine tailings are a significant environmental health threat resulting from the mining of precious metals. However, in addition to run-off from agricultural lands and contamination from mining operations, water pollution is worsened by two notable human actions: the use of plastics and of pharmaceuticals. Plastics degrade and enter the water stream after being discarded, resulting in the breakdown of these plastics into microscopic particles. As a result, small, micro-particles enter the food chain, endangering fish and other aquatic life. In addition to the longevity of these micro-plastics in the environment, many plastics contain bisphenol A (BPA), which is an estrogen mimic. As a result of its estrogen mimicking properties, BPA can act as an endocrine disruptor. As plastics break down in the environment, BPA can leach out directly into the surrounding air and water. BPA has a relatively short half-life of between 1 and 10 days, but the prevalence of BPA in manufactured products results in an estimated 15 billion pounds of BPA produced annually, much of which finds its way into the environment. BPA can contribute to a number of health problems among individuals who are chronically exposed to it – from mild skin blisters to cancer. However, its role as an endocrine disruptor presents more prolonged concerns for human and animal health. For example, recent work in turtles suggests that exposure to BPA is capable of disrupting the development of tissues involved in sexual differentiation. Possibly more concerning, research on the effects of BPA on the reproductive physiology of the California mouse (*Peromyscus californicus*), small mammals with remarkably similar

mating strategies as people, found a decrease in long-term reproductive fitness over several generations among individuals with prenatal exposure to BPA and found an increase in the feminization of males, resulting in challenges in finding mates and reproducing. It is clear, then, that our reliance on plastics is directly impacting our own health and the health of wildlife through both the physical contamination of the environment with plastic micro-particles and through the chemical contamination of the environment with hormonal mimics, which can have long-term consequences and possibly multigenerational effects.

The introduction of pharmaceuticals into our waters poses a multiplicative challenge for human and animal health. Pharmaceuticals enter our water through a variety of sources, but two stand out: improper disposal of unused medicines directly into water (typically via flushing) and non-metabolized medicines excreted into water systems through human waste products (also typically via flushing). In recent years, researchers sampling water systems have found evidence of blood-pressure medications; pain-relieving medications, such as oxycodone, acetaminophen, and ibuprofen; hormonal birth control; and antimicrobials, to name a few. The development of antimicrobial resistance continues to be one of the greatest health threats, as identified by the World Health Organization in 2002, and environmental pollution of medicines, including antibiotics, in our waters compounds an already alarming and complex threat to human and animal health. The threat of antibiotic resistance is likely to continue to rise as additional antibiotics are used or over-used. In addition to pollution via human flushing, antibiotics are provided to large numbers of agricultural animals in order to promote growth, and contamination from their waste products can be easily carried into drainage ditches and waterways. Recent evidence has shown an increase in the amount of antimicrobial resistance in environmental soils can put human and animal health at risk. In addition to the threat from antibiotics in the environment, the large number and variety of pharmaceuticals entering the water is a significant health threat. Water treatment facilities are unable to filter out the small, trace compounds, resulting in a growing number of pharmaceuticals present in drinking water of more than 40 million Americans. According to a recently published work in the *New Republic*, Nick Schroek, executive director of the Great Lakes Environmental Law Center, was quoted as saying, "The scary thing for me is not one particular drug, although do I want to be drinking Viagra in my water? No. It's potentially hundreds or thousands of compounds interacting with each other and how that affects aquatic life and human health."

## 4.3 Habitat Loss and Land Use Alterations

The global loss of biodiversity, as discussed in Chapter 3, is one of the greatest threats to planetary health. This loss is profound, resulting in the extinction of thousands of species, and sometimes entire **phyla**, of plants and animals. One of the most significant, demonstrable causes of the global loss of biodiversity is the destruction of habitat. Habitat degradation, through pollution, fragmentation, and introduction of invasive species, can result in the decline of biodiversity; habitat destruction devastates entire populations and eliminates the possibility of recovery in any reasonable timeframe. Habitat loss occurs through a number of processes, including **deforestation**, **desertification**, and urban sprawl.

*Deforestation* is the permanent destruction of forested lands. It can occur for several reasons, including creating space for housing and urban development, cattle ranching, and agriculture; to create goods, such as paper and furniture; and to generate resources to be extracted and used in other products, such as palm oil. Deforestation is a complete destruction of the landscape and comes about through **clear cutting** and **slash and burn clearance**, although **selective logging** can be damaging to forest ecosystems as well. Clear cutting is the removal of large swaths of forest by cutting down entire plots of trees, allowing the wood from the trees to be used for wood and paper products while simultaneously clearing the land for urban development or agricultural uses. Slash and burn clearance, typically for agriculture, is the removal of large swaths of forest by the cutting down of the largest trees and using fire to burn out all remaining vegetation. Both clear cutting and slash and burn agriculture leave the land completely devoid of trees and are devastating to ecosystems. According to the National Resources Defense Council, clear cutting is akin to "an ecological trauma that has no precedent in nature." Slash and burn agriculture further degrades the environment by adding vast quantities of greenhouse gases to the atmosphere. In contrast to these large-scale, destructive clearance practices, selective logging is a much less destructive form of forest clearing wherein individual trees are chosen and removed from large patches of forest, leaving the majority of the forest intact. However, the process of removing individual trees from intact forests can damage forest habitat. Road building is still an important part of selective logging, which opens up forests to the risks associated with edge effects. Importantly, gaps in forest cover, created from the removal of these trees, can degrade habitat for existing wildlife and can alter the growth dynamics of the overall forest.

An estimated 80% of the world's terrestrial biodiversity resides in a forest. In addition to the devastation to biodiversity from deforestation, the result of global destruction of forests results in a reduction in the amount of **carbon sequestration**, or the absorption of greenhouse gases from the atmosphere, that can occur, further contributing to climate change on a global scale. Deforestation also results in an increase in air and water pollution, a disruption of the water cycle, and rapid soil degradation. Currently, approximately 30% of the planet's surface is forested, but the rate of deforestation today, about 36 football fields destroyed every minute, puts their existence in jeopardy.

*Desertification* is the transition of fertile land into desert, as a result of drought, deforestation, and/or the overuse and inappropriate agricultural methods, such as overgrazing. Ecosystems that have undergone desertification are characterized by the total depletion of previously available water sources and the loss of native flora and fauna; as a result, desertification drastically reduces the biologic and economic value of the land (Figure 4.3). Dryland ecosystems are spread over nearly half of the planet's lands, and as much as 20% of existing dryland ecosystems has already undergone some form of desertification. While the loss of habitat for plants and wildlife alone is a significant environmental threat, more than two billion people live in dryland ecosystems. Approximately 90% of these populations also face extreme poverty and a challenging sociopolitical climate, intensifying the threat to survival in the face of increasingly extreme environmental conditions. And, importantly, while the people, animals, and environment of dryland

ecosystems are the most vulnerable to desertification, this process can result in the loss of arable land in any biome – from lush tropical rainforests to diverse temperate prairies.

In 1931, as the Great Depression was spreading beyond the USA to ravage the world's economy, a massive drought devastated the American Midwest. Drought coupled with decades of overgrazing and over-plowing resulted in "black blizzards" blowing for days at a time. And so began the American Dust Bowl. By 1934, more than 40 large-scale dust storms had blown through the Midwest, and the drought had become the most devastating drought in American history – severely affecting 27 states and more than 75% of the population. As a result of the "black blizzards" that swirled through the plains, human and animal health was severely affected. Horses, cattle, and other domesticated animals were frequently found dead in the fields after dust storms. Respiratory illnesses were common, including a new diagnosis of "dust pneumonia." Reports of asthma, strep throat, and measles also increased dramatically, and deaths reported from respiratory and other infections skyrocketed. Infant mortality was the highest

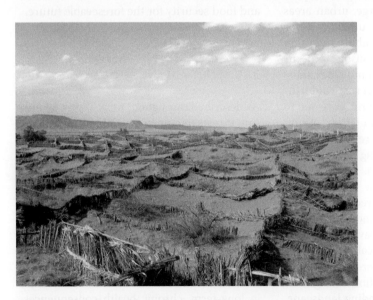

Figure 4.3 The effects of desertification and the attempts to keep back the desert through anti-sand fencing in Morocco. *Source:* Anderson sady, https://commons.wikimedia.org/wiki/File:Anti_desertification_sand_fences_south_of_the_town_of_Erfoud,_Morocco.jpg. CC BY-SA 3.0.

on record in the affected states during the summers of 1934–1937. And, evidence now demonstrates that in communities directly impacted by dust storms, there exists a significant risk of long-term chronic health challenges associated with exposures to heavy metals, which were likely breathed in as dust particles. The increase in airborne dust throughout the decade of the Dust Bowl resulted in an increase in sunlight being reflected back into space, which in turn, drove down local surface temperatures and reduced evaporation, further exacerbating the drought conditions. As the current climate crisis worsens, the opportunity for desertification to expand grows. In response to humanity's mounting food needs, agriculture and grazing has vastly expanded into ecosystems previously considered unsustainable for these tasks. As a result, the likelihood of future dust storms and the growing threat of desertification globally have grown significantly. Currently, equivalent dust bowl events are occurring in rural China and in the Sahel region of northern Africa, both due to the effects of long-term overgrazing.

The world's population is growing at an alarming rate. As a result of this growth, people living in and around large, urban areas frequently look beyond the urban core for housing. While urban and suburban design has allowed for growth in housing to occur that is largely sustainable and mitigates many environmental health concerns, unfortunately many areas of the world have yet to embrace urban and suburban design principles. *Urban sprawl* is the result of rapid, unplanned growth in housing and development outside urban areas. Due to the unplanned nature of urban sprawl, these expansive communities are frequently low in population density with limited public transportation infrastructure, leaving residents dependent on cars for local travel. This results in an increase in water and air pollution from traffic congestion, limits to agricultural capacity of the surrounding landscape, and local deforestation or habitat loss. Urban sprawl can also interrupt flight patterns for migratory birds and other long distance migrators as well as limit access to mates and resources for wildlife with large home ranges, especially if their range abuts new developments. Human health is put at risk, as well, as a result of urban sprawl. In addition to the increased incidence of high blood pressure and chronic hypertension, linked to the creation of **food deserts**, urban sprawl increases the likelihood that people will have frequent interactions with wildlife, which can have devastating consequences for wildlife and can create opportunities for bi-directional pathogen transmission. Examples of urban sprawl in action abound, with cities like Los Angeles, CA, Atlanta, GA, and Nashville, TN, frequently being cited as some of the most sprawling cities. American and Australian cities tend to be the worst for sprawl, according to research published in 2017, while cities in East Asia and South America exhibit minimal sprawl. Annually, the equivalent of a one kilometer wide strip of land, stretching from San Francisco to New York is lost due to housing development growth and urban sprawl. The result of this growth in land consumption will threaten human and animal health, wildlife habitats, and food security for the foreseeable future.

## 4.4 Environmental Health and Health of the Future

As described throughout this chapter, significant threats to human and animal health exist as a result of the contamination or destruction of the environment. However, there are two additional, significant concerns to human health, in particular, stemming from the devastation of our environment. Long-term consequences of threats to environmental health can extend into future generations via two mechanisms. First, children are an especially vulnerable population and exposure to environmental contamination as a child can result in long-term, chronic health consequences. Second, threats to environmental health can result in significant changes to future generations, with potentially devastating consequences, as patterns of gene expression are altered through exposure to environmental contaminants and stresses. These **epigenetic** consequences can be profound and multigenerational.

For many health threats, children are considered a vulnerable population. This is unequivocally true for environmental health threats. Environmental health threats result in the deaths of more than three million children under five annually, and children comprise approximately 40% of the population suffering from environmental health threats, despite making up only about 10% of the world's population. Both outdoor and indoor air pollutants have driven up the incidence of asthma in children across the planet. Lack of access to clean drinking water has left more than two million children under the age of five suffering from malnutrition and diarrheal diseases, many of which are fatal. And, across the planet, more than 350 million children between the ages of 5 and 17 work to provide income for their families, often including unpaid or illegal work. It is estimated that nearly 50% of these children work in conditions where they are regularly exposed to environmental health contaminants, including toxic chemicals, such as lead, mercury, arsenic, and a variety of pesticides, or that leave them vulnerable to an increased risk of exposure to infectious diseases. The long-term global health effects of the disparity in access to wealth and resources are heightened when the stark contrast between the health of children living in poverty is compared to the health of children living in relative wealth.

Threats to the environment can also threaten the health and well-being of human populations in ways that result in unintended consequences and span generations by changing the timing of when our genes turn on and off. Research into these epigenetic effects has shown that exposure to certain chemical pollutants can **methylate** genes, which results in heritable changes to the expression patterns of our genes, specifically the timing of when genes turn on or off. Exposure to pollutants and other environmental contaminants can result in methylation-driven epigenetic effects, but so too can chronic stress. Chronic stress can result from a number of sources in today's world including threats to the environment, such as exposure to toxic pollutants, the loss of diversity in our foods, and, for some, the loss of livelihoods through erosion, desertification, and degradation of the land. For example, a link has been found between exposure to high levels of polycyclic aromatic hydrocarbons, a common air pollutant found in car emissions, with the development of asthma in children. However, researchers found that the development of asthma in these children was not associated with direct exposure to contaminants, but instead developed as a result of *in utero* exposure. In examining the saved cord blood of these children, the mechanism of this was uncovered – asthma had developed in children where methylation had occurred at a specific gene ($ACSL_3$) and not in children where this gene remained unmethylated. Our understanding of the mechanisms of epigenetics is still unfolding. However, evidence of the heritability of the alteration of genetic expression patterns is mounting. And these epigenetic effects can occur via exposure to environmental contaminants and stressors in humans and wildlife alike. The potential multigenerational consequences for planetary health cannot be underestimated.

## 4.5 Two Things Exacerbate Everything

### 4.5.1 Population Growth and Consumption

Each year, the global population grows by more than 76 million people, adding more people to the world's population every year than the current populations of London, New York, Mumbai, and Beijing combined. This incredible global growth rate is a result of, among other things, a lack of family planning resources, declining infant mortality rates, and medical advances resulting in a doubling of the global life expectancy in the last 100 years. Human overpopulation, coupled with effects of global wealth inequality, has far-reaching consequences not only for environmental health but threatens the very concept of applying One Health solutions. For example, in addition to intensifying the existing challenges specific to human health as a result of the world's more than 7.6 billion people – malnutrition, starvation, infectious disease, and increasing global conflicts over access to resources, the rapid growth rate of human populations has contributed to global consequences for environmental health concerns – increased contamination of water, the loss of nonrenewable resources, such as oil and natural gas, an increase in desertification, and an increase in greenhouse gas emissions and related climate change disasters. The consumption of resources by an ever-growing human population alone is considered by many a global health crisis irrespective of all other environmental health concerns. However, unsustainable consumption, coupled with growing human populations, presents a challenge to global health that, left unaddressed, has the potential to exacerbate all other existing threats to planetary health far beyond the scope of any environmental threat acting independently.

### 4.5.2 Climate Change

All existing threats to the planetary health are intensified by the ongoing climate crisis: the emergence and re-emergence of infectious diseases, the loss of biodiversity, the disparity between wealth and poverty and its downstream effects on health, among others. In focusing on environmental health specifically, climate change magnifies the threat of habitat loss, speeding the conversion of quality habitat into unusable habitat, and amplifies the effects of pollution and other environmental contaminants. As discussed in Chapter 3, greenhouse gas emissions are not only a significant cause of concern for global climate change but are also,

independently, a significant source of air pollution, resulting in air quality declines across the globe. For example, evidence now suggests that in addition to the nine million people who die early from the effects of pollution, 800 000 deaths annually can now be directly linked to the burning of coal. And importantly, the actions we take that result in the destruction of habitat and the pollution of our air, water, and land are the same actions that exacerbate the effects of climate change. For example, when vast areas of forest are destroyed in slash and burn agriculture in the tropics, the air is polluted with carbon and other fine particulate contaminants, local water sources are polluted with ash and potentially heavy metals that are leached from the soils, erosion results in additional pollution entering the water, and the ability of the forest to sequester carbon from the atmosphere is destroyed. Climate change must be addressed. The threat of the climate crisis and the threats of and to environmental health are inextricably linked.

## 4.6 Things Can Get Better

Environmental health concerns are complex and both climate change and our growing human and animal populations work synergistically to increase the potential risk of these threats beyond the scope of the environment, directly affecting both human and animal health. The scale at which threats to environmental health occur can present significant challenges to finding solutions; the immensity of the problems can be daunting. However, this does not mean that the problems cannot be solved or that even small actions cannot result in significant improvements to environmental health.

Climate change is considered by many to be the most significant threat to planetary health today. Cattle production has skyrocketed in recent decades due to the rapid increase in human population sizes and the growing demand for beef in our diets, as we shift away from a predominantly

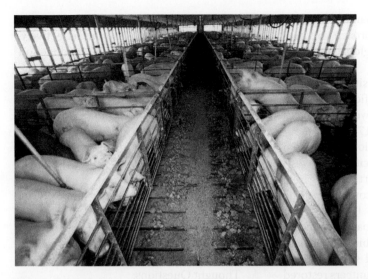

Figure 4.4 Confined-animal feeding operation (CAFO). Hogs waiting for slaughter in a large CAFO building.

plant-based diet. Large **confined-animal feeding operations (CAFOs)** represent a significant contributor of emissions of greenhouse gases into the atmosphere (Figure 4.4). However, several companies in recent years have worked to develop plant-based "meats" that match the taste, texture, and "mouth feel" of real meats, with the goal of reducing or eliminating livestock use. The result of a switch from meat to vegetable-based "meat" by a significant portion of the population would result in a drastic reduction in greenhouse gas emissions, improving planetary health outcomes. Other advances in farming and agriculture that can improve health outcomes for the environment include moving towards carbon-neutral chicken farming by, for example, using food waste that would have previously been discarded as animal feed and powering the farms with solar panels, as is currently being done by Kipster Farms in the Netherlands. Solar panels are not only for chicken coops or rooftops, however. Transparent solar cell technology is becoming increasingly available, and according to research published in *Nature Energy* in 2017, these small, transparent solar devices could replace windows on buildings and cars, tapping a currently unavailable source of solar energy and in the process meet nearly

the entire US demand for energy, drastically reducing the US's reliance on fossil fuels.

Desertification has previously been considered irreversible. However, recent successes in Jordan and other locations have begun to challenge this idea. In the Bani Hashem community in Jordan, a government-supported effort to replant the desert has had success in reclaiming desert land by embracing holistic, traditional agricultural techniques that integrate nature, community, and animal welfare. The results have been astounding. In one year, indigenous flowers, shrubs, and grasses are returning, with more than 36 restored native plant species recorded. And, successes in reclaiming land from desert extend beyond Jordan. In Burkina Faso, where individuals have returned to traditional agricultural practices, called Zai, large swathes of forest have also returned. In Senegal, the planting of a wall of trees has been successful in reclaiming land from the desert. And in Mongolia, for more than 15 years, Korean Air has been working with local communities to plant more than 110 000 poplar, buckthorn and Siberian elm trees in order to reclaim land and prevent further desertification. Efforts like these, which include actions by individual concerned citizens to corporate-sponsored programs to government mandates, which embrace the One Health approach, are having success in responding to global threats to environmental health.

The loss of global biodiversity is also considered one of the most significant threats to planetary health today. However, research published in *Nature* in 2017 has demonstrated the benefit to global biodiversity from conservation spending. Specifically, investment in conservation efforts from 1996 through 2008 by signatory countries to the Convention on Biological Diversity and Sustainable Development Goals resulted in an average 30% reduction in biodiversity loss per country. At a more local scale, in Peru, one team of scientists and volunteers restored the El Cascajo marshland by employing nanotechnology and biological filters to remove high concentrations of bacteria and toxic pollutants, completely reviving the waters in about two weeks. This same team is now expanding their work to other marshlands throughout Peru in an effort to significantly improve the environmental, human, and animal health throughout the region.

These, and other creative ideas like them, are driving improvements for environmental health, and as a result, for planetary health. It will take continued creativity and hard work, advances in science and technology, funding, and most importantly, a desire to act for our global environment.

## 4.7   Conclusion

Our ability to respond to the global threats to human and animal health is astounding; so too is our ability to respond to threats to environmental health. However, responses to human and animal health threats are frequently considered a greater priority than the need to respond to threats to environmental health. Threats to environmental health are often complex issues, spanning many years potentially and widespread in scope and scale. Frequently, it is challenging to identify the exact source of and responsibility for the threat, complicating our ability to respond effectively. However, evidence of the connection between environmental health and the health of humans and animals is now overwhelming and unambiguous. Ignoring the threat to the environment will result in devastating consequences for not only human and animal health but for planetary health as well.

## End of Chapter Questions & Activities

A.  Thought Questions:
   i)  How is environmental health important for answering One Health questions?
   ii) What policies do you think must be put in place for environmental health? What should the role of regulations be in maintaining and protecting environmental health?
   iii) What are the ethical considerations of urban sprawl, meat eating, or our continued reliance on fossil fuels? How can we ameliorate these problems to minimize the negative effects to environmental health?

B.  In-Class/Guided Activities:
   i)  Identify a relevant environmental law and evaluate the effectiveness of this on environmental health. Consider the Clean Water Act, the Clean Air Act, the Comprehensive Environmental Response, Compensation, and Liability Act (Superfund), or the Resource Conservation and Recovery Act.
   ii) Consider the effects of air, water, or ground pollution. Choose one and investigate the myriad of health outcomes for humans and animals exposed to these pollutants.

C.  At-home Activities:
   i)  Compost and recycle everything that can be composted and recycled. Avoid consuming things that are disposable

after single uses. Invest in quality belongings that can be repaired instead of discarded.

ii) Avoid harming wildlife and biodiversity in your vacations and local outings. Do not buy souvenirs made from endangered wildlife, such as ivory, and do not take selfies with animals.

iii) Reduce your reliance on plastics. Use reusable products made from recyclable products, such as paper, glass, or metals, as much as you can.

D. Long-term Action Steps:

i) Prevent erosion. Apply mulch in your gardens, carefully position gutters and downspouts to let water seep into your lawn.

ii) Avoid letting your car idle. Invest in a hybrid. Or, even better, go carless.

iii) Give up meat. Even reducing meat consumption for one day a week can significantly reduce greenhouse gas emissions and reduce other air pollutants.

E. Recommended Reading:

Egan, T. (2006). *The Worst Hard Time.* Mariner Books.

Pachirat, T. (2011). *Every 12 Seconds: Industrialized Slaughter and Politics of Sight.* Yale University Press.

Steinbeck, J. (1939). *The Grapes of Wrath.* Viking Press.

Taylor, D.E. (2014). *Toxic Communities: Environmental racism, industrial pollution, and residential mobility.* New York University Press.

## Interview

*An Interview with One Health Practitioner Dawn Holliday, PhD: Associate Professor in the Department of Biology and Environmental Science at Westminster College in Fulton, MO*

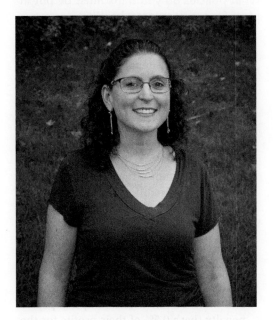

**When did you first hear about One Health?**

I was first introduced to One Health by Sharon Deem. She was giving a presentation at the University of Missouri's College of Veterinary Medicine. My background is as a broadly trained ecologist, and so I was aware of all the individual components but had never really heard of them within that One Health framework. And so that was my first introduction to it.

**How is One Health important to your work?**

It has actually set the framework for much of the research that I have been doing. My research colleagues and I examine how environmental chemicals affect the anatomy, physiology, and behavior of turtles. My focus has always been with turtles, but environmental chemicals are clearly not only affecting turtles. Within that One Health framework, it enables all of the researchers to view the impacts in a broader context, and therefore generate some additional hypotheses within that concept. We can look across taxa to figure out how the different components, the ecosystem, animals, and people, which are really just animals, are interacting and how it's changing the effects that we are seeing.

### Do you see yourself as a One Health practitioner?

I have always lived within that framework but never really saw myself in that role until recently. I would not call myself a One Health practitioner yet, but maybe a practitioner in training.

### How do your actions reflect One Health, personally or professionally?

My undergraduate institution (SUNY ESF) was an absolutely phenomenal place, fostering and promoting the idea of One Health without specifically naming it. Most of our forest biology courses looked at human stewardship and how that affected the different individual topics that we were studying. I was immersed in this community that respected the planet and saw the interconnectedness among humans, animals, and ecosystems. I have tried to expose my kids to that same sense, by helping them understand how their actions will affect the environment, how they affect other animals that share our same space.

Professionally speaking, at Westminster College, one of my colleagues, Dr. Irene Unger, and I recently designed an interdisciplinary major in One Health. We are starting to expose our students to that idea. The major combines some natural science, so biology, chemistry, environmental science. It also involves human health classes that are in the human and exercise science program as well as some ethical perspectives.

### What can an individual do to make a difference for planetary health?

Many people go about their daily business without stopping to question something that's happening or providing assistance to something that they see. There are little things that we can do to really make a difference, but if you are not noticing them, you do not know that you can act on them. It really takes the idea of caring about something bigger than yourself and being aware of the world around you. If someone sees you doing something, especially if a child sees it, that can really make them stop and then maybe they it too, and this can become organically a self-propagating effect. It's important to consume information and think critically about it.

### Where is One Health headed?

It's hard to see where things are going, but momentum is gaining. My colleagues and I received a grant that was specifically a One Health, One Medicine study. Having funding specifically in this framework is important. Recently, I was at a conference with a special symposium focused on One Health, which was new. And Elsevier even has a One Health journal. In the academic sense, we see momentum. However, despite the fact that the CDC and the AVMA have campaigned for One Health, I have not seen much change in public awareness. I think that's the next greatest hurdle: showing the interconnectedness to the public.

### What policies do you think must be put in place for environmental health?

I worry that recent changes at the EPA will result in a reversal or weakening of key regulations that impact clean water, clean air, and environmental integrity. That does not mean the political climate will not change, and the regulations can't be reinstated later, but I think that we need to focus on the long-term. It's really not business versus the environment. Both can find a compromise that's appropriate for everyone involved.

### What is the role of regulations?

Regulations should be enforceable guidelines, but that does not seem to be the way it works in practice. Perhaps they are not as sufficient a deterrent as they should be. If a multi-billion dollar company pays a penalty that's 0.5% of their profits for the year, I am not sure that's deterring them. If they do not have a sense of interconnectedness already, then regulations are definitely not going to be deterrents. They are hard to enforce because there's so much uncertainty.

## How is environmental health important for answering One Health questions?

Environmental health is important because it provides the context. We look at animal and human health, but we are not looking at them in a vacuum. We are looking at them in the context of the environment in which individuals are living. In all cases, even though we build walls and houses and try to close ourselves off from the environment, we still share that environment. It provides the context. The lab bench research that I have been doing lately certainly needs to be ecologically relevant, and we have strived to make sure everything we are doing can be translated to what we see in the field. Field research needs to examine the parameters within that ecological context so that we can provide usable data. If we have usable data, then we can actually enact meaningful change.

## Parting Thoughts?

Communication is needed in every aspect of life and tends to be the downfall of any system. If environmental scientists can effectively communicate with health practitioners, who can then effectively communicate with the public and politicians, we are likely to see change. If we just communicate among ourselves, we are going to miss those broader intersections, and regardless of whether we get it right or wrong, no one will be listening.

---

## Case Study: Baia Mare Cyanide Spill

Co-authored by Diamond Carroll

On January 30, 2000, a dam broke in a small mining community along the Săsar River in Romania. The resulting spill contaminated the dominant source of fresh water for five European countries with cyanide, resulted in the death of nearly all aquatic life in the contaminated waters (Figure 4.5), and has come to be known as the worst environmental disaster in Europe since the Chernobyl disaster in 1986.

The people of Baia Mare, Romania, a small community in northwestern Romania, have been mining since the mid-1700s. Baia Mare

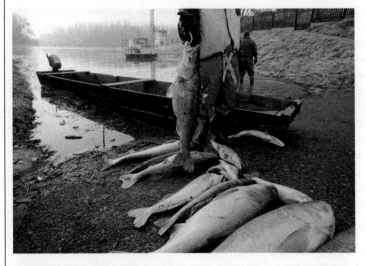

Figure 4.5 Baia Mare cyanide spill kills thousands of fish. Romanian fishermen pull dead fish out of boat after cyanide release.

has been the site of multiple gold, silver, lead, zinc, copper, manganese, and salt mines, resulting in long-term pollution to the community's air, soil, and water. By the 1990s, gold mining was the dominant industry in Baia Mare.

Waste from gold mines is typically stored in ponds and isolated from the rest of the water supply by a series of **tailings dams**. A tailings dam is an earthen structure that is specifically built to contain waste from mining operations and is designed to grow over time as waste is generated throughout the life of a mine. At the time of the spill, approximately 215 tailings dams were in use in Romania. When the Aurul SA Company offered a newer and more effective means of storing waste in exchange for opening a new mining plant, the Romanian government was very supportive. Aurul SA would pipe waste into tailings 6.5 km away to the town of Bozanta Mare. Before opening the Baia Mare operation in 1999, the pipeline suffered two leaks. However, the Baia Mare mine was expected to produce more than 1.6 tons of gold and 9 tons of silver annually, and as a result, the company was allowed to proceed with operations.

Cyanide is frequently used in gold mining to separate metals from rock. It is extremely toxic and can be deadly. Its most dangerous form was used by the Nazis as a tool for genocide during World War II. Cyanide poisoning can be a result of drinking, eating, breathing, or touching anything containing the chemical. Exposure to even a small amount of cyanide can result in dizziness, headaches, nausea, vomiting, rapid breathing or heart rate, restlessness, and weakness. Exposure to large amounts can lead to convulsions, loss of consciousness, low blood pressure, lung injury, respiratory failure, and slowed heart rate. Cyanide is toxic to both humans and animals and can bioaccumulate, making cyanide contamination of fish – a significant food source for people and other animals – particularly devastating. In addition to cyanide, heavy metals are frequently leached into water as a result of the mining process, sometimes with devastating health effects. Copper and zinc can both be linked to anemia, decrease in high density lipoprotein (HDL) cholesterol, and damage to the pancreas, liver, and kidneys. Cadmium is a

known carcinogen and, with a half-life of 30 years, can be dangerous for years following a spill. Lead is also a carcinogen and can negatively affect the liver, kidneys, spleen, and lungs.

In the months preceding the spill, there had been an abnormally large amount of rain and a significant snowmelt from an unusually warm winter. The increase in water pressure, due to the added water from rain and snowmelt, caused the new dam to begin leaking, although later government agencies from neighboring countries found evidence the dam was not built to meet the correct standards. The resulting spill discharged more than 100 000 $m^3$ of liquid waste waters into the Săsar River and surrounding agricultural lands. These waste waters contained more than 70 tons of cyanide and were also contaminated with heavy metals, including lead, mercury, copper, and zinc. Over the course of four weeks, the cyanide pollution spread from the Săsar River to the Somes River, which crosses into Hungary. Cyanide-contaminated waters next reached the Tisza River, before ultimately reaching the Danube River and entering the Black Sea, resulting in cyanide-contaminated waters reaching beyond Romania, where the spill occurred, and into Hungary, Ukraine, Serbia, and Bulgaria.

The concentrations of cyanide and other heavy metals in the affected waters came under surveillance starting January 31, just one day after the spill began. By February 1, contamination had reached Hungarian waters. On February 2, the first reports of dead fish were made in Baia Mare. On February 3, the contamination reached the Tisza River. On February 12, contamination reached the first municipal water supply (Szolnok). On February 15, contamination reached the Danube. On February 16, fishing and drinking water from the Danube was banned. By February 25, contamination had reached the Black Sea. During the incident, sanitation and industrial plants were shut down, and wells near the spill tested positive for cyanide at levels more than 100 times higher than considered acceptable for human exposure and high concentrations of cadmium, copper, manganese, iron, and lead. Dead fish were reported in Hungary, Romania, and Serbia, with Hungary alone claiming an estimated 1240 tons of dead fish. There were also reports of dead waterfowl, eagles, and otters being found near affected bodies of water. Although there were no human deaths, there were more than 100 hospitalizations, mainly from children who had eaten fish laced with cyanide.

This Baia Mare cyanide spill resulted in a One Health catastrophe that cost an estimated US\$ 10 million in damages. The fish industry was at a standstill when 38 species were killed off across three countries; the aquatic population has since recovered, with microorganism populations having recovered within days and fish populations taking years to fully recover. Because of the bio-accumulative nature of heavy metals, heavy metal concentrations still have to be monitored in water, produce, and fish in the Baia Mare area. With homes being within 50 m of waste sites, the lead concentration for adults in Baia Mare is about 2.5 times higher than acceptable and 6 times higher in children. Respiratory problems have always been common in the area, and the life expectancy of citizens is about 12 years below the national average. A study done in 2013, years after the Aurul SA dam break, found unsafe levels of these chemicals can still be found in several fruits and vegetables grown in the Baia Mare region, with root and leafy vegetables being most affected due to high heavy metal concentrations in soil. As a result of the spill, stricter environmental standards have been implemented, resulting in a short-term halt to the industry locally and the implementation of required Environmental Impact Assessments to meet EU standards long-term. However, mining is still commonplace in the Baia Mare region and in 2007, permits were issued for Romaltyn, a new mine that will resume ore processing using the same cyanide-based extraction techniques and the same tailings dam as at Baia Mare, suggesting that the consequences of this disaster are poised to be repeated.

## Works Cited

Antal, L., Halasi-Kovacs, B., and Nagy, S.A. (2013). Changes in fish assemblage in the Hungarian section of River Szamos/Someş after a massive cyanide and heavy metal pollution. *Northwestern Journal of Zoology* 9 (1): 131–138.

Baccarelli, A. and Bollati, V. (2009). Epigenetics and environmental chemicals. *Current Opinion in Pediatrics* 21 (2): 243–251.

Baia Mare Task Force. (2015) The Cyanide Spill at Baia Mare Romania. Baia Mare Task Force, June 2000. http://archive.rec.org/REC/Publications/CyanideSpill/ENGCyanide (accessed January 9, 2015).

Bell, M.L., Davis, D.L., and Fletcher, T. (2004). A retrospective assessment of mortality from the London smog episode of 1952: the role of influenza and pollution. *Environmental Health Perspectives* 112 (1): 6–8.

Boxall, A.B.A. (2004). The environmental side effects of medication. *EMBO Reports* 5 (12): 1110–1116.

Bushnell, M.C., Case, L.K., Ceko, M. et al. (2015). Effect of environment on the long-term consequences of chronic pain. *Pain* 156 (1): S42–S49.

Canesi, L. and Fabbri, E. (2015). Environmental effects of BPA: focus on aquatic species. *Dose-Response* 13 (3): e1559325815598304.

Chance, G.W. (2001). Environmental contaminants and children's health: cause for concern, time for action. *Paediatrics & Child Health* 6 (10): 731–743.

Clay, K., and Wright, G. (2011) Gold Rush Legacy: American Minerals and the Knowledge Economy. *Lincoln Institute Conference on Property Rights and Natural Resources*, Cambridge, MA.

Das, P. and Horton, R. (2017). Pollution, health, and the planet: time for decisive action. *The Lancet* doi: 10.1016/S0140-6736(17)32588-6.

Eisler, R. and Wiemeyer, S.N. (2004). Cyanide hazards to plants and animals from gold mining and related water issues. *Reviews in Environmental Contamination and Toxicology* 183: 21–54.

Flint, S., Markle, T., Thompson, S. et al. (2012). Bisphenol A exposure, effects, and policy: a wildlife perspective. *Journal of Environmental Management* 104: 19–34.

Frumkin, H. (2002). Urban sprawl and public health. *Public Health Reports* 117: 201–217.

Geist, H.J. and Lambin, E.F. (2002). Proximate causes and underlying driving forces of tropical deforestation. *Bioscience* 52 (2): 143–150.

Hileman, B. (2009) Are contaminants silencing our genes? Scientific American. http://scientificamerican.com/article/silencing-genes-chemical-contaminants-cancer-diabetes (accessed August 13, 2017).

Ho-jung, W. (2016) Korean Air works to stop desertification. *The Korea Herald*, December 28, 2016.

Jandegian, C.M., Deem, S.L., Bhandari, R.K. et al. (2015). Developmental exposure to bisphenol A (BPA) alters sexual differentiation in painted turtles (*Chrysemys picta*). *General and Comparative Endocrinology* 216: 77–85.

Johnson, M.P. (2001). Environmental impacts of urban sprawl: a survey of the literature and proposed research agenda. *Environment and Planning A* 33 (4): 717–735.

Lin, M., Ning, X., Liang, X. et al. (2014). Study of the heavy metals residual in the incineration slag of textile dyeing sludge. *Journal of the Taiwan Institute of Chemical Engineers* 45 (4): 1814–1820.

Liu, Y., Wu, J., and Yu, D. (2017). Characterizing spatiotemporal patterns of air pollution in China: a multiscale landscape approach. *Ecological Indicators* 76: 344–356.

Malhi, Y., Timmons Roberts, J., Betts, R.A. et al. (2008). Climate change, deforestation, and the fate of the Amazon. *Science* 319 (5860): 169–172.

Namrouqa, H. (2017) Jordan wins anti-desertification policy award. *The Jordan Times*, Aug 27, 2017.

Neira, M., Pfeiffer, M., Capbell-Lendrum, D. et al. (2017). Towards a healthier and safer environment. *The Lancet* doi: 10.1016/S0140-6736(17)32545-X.

Roba, C., Rosu, C., Pistea, I., et al. (2015). Heavy metal content in vegetables and fruits cultivated in Baia Mare mining area (Romania) and health risk assessment. *Environmental Science and Pollution Research* 27: 6062–6073.

Rochester, J.R. (2013). Bisphenol A and human health: a review of the literature. *Reproductive Toxicology* 42: 132–155.

Straskraba, V. and Moran, R.E. (1990). Environmental occurrence and impacts of arsenic at gold mining sites in the western United States. *International Journal of Mine Water* 9 (1–4): 181–191.

Traverse, C.J., Pandey, R., Barr, M.C. et al. (2017). Emergence of highly transparent photovoltaics for distributed applications. *Nature Energy* 2: 849–860.

*United States v. Bliss* (1987) US District Court, no. SC85652.

Waldron, A., Miller, D.C., Redding, D. et al. (2017). Reductions in global biodiversity loss predicted from conservation spending. *Nature* doi: 10.1038/nature24295.

Walsh, J.F., Molyneux, D.H., and Birley, M.H. (1993). Deforestation: effects on vector-borne disease. *Parasitology* 106 (S1): S55–S75.

Whitford, W.G. (1995). Desertification: implications and limitations of the ecosystem health metaphor. In: *Evaluating and Monitoring the Health of Large-Scale Ecosystems*. NATO ASI Series, vol. 28 (ed. D.J. Rapport, C.L. Gaudet and P. Calow), 273–294. Berlin: Springer.

WHO (2009). *Improving Children's Health and the Environment: Examples from the WHO European Region*. Geneva, Switzerland: World Health Organization.

Zhang, S. (2016) The goose-killing lake and the scientists who study it. The Atlantic. http://theatlantic.com/science/archive/2016/12/berkeley-pit-geese/510089 (accessed September 9, 2017).

5

## Animal Health as One Health

"Lots of people talk to animals," said Pooh.
"Maybe, but...."
"Not very many *listen*, though," he said.
"That's the problem," he added.

The Tao of Pooh

How many ways will your life and the life of a non-human animal intersect today? How will these interactions occur? Maybe the first animal you see will be your dog or cat staring at you as you open your eyes to start the day. She may simply want you to get up and let her out for a pee; or maybe he is staring at you just because he is a cat and that is what cats do. Or will your first interaction with an animal be at the breakfast table as you consume some type of animal product – eggs, milk, cheese, bacon. Perhaps when you are heading to school or work, you will notice a bird of prey hunting in a field, or a bee pollinating a plant. It is nearly impossible for anyone to go 24 hours without some interaction with an animal. This fact has been true since the first *Homo sapien* walked across the African savannah. There may be more variety today in the types of human–animal connections, with people living in a Manhattan high rise possibly feeling less animal contact than a hunter gatherer hunting in the rainforest of the Congo. However, humans have a need for animals in ways often overlooked. The links our species have with non-human animals may be the most important One Health connection for us to understand in

the context of why healthy animals are important for healthy people and a healthy planet.

The ties that bind human and non-human animals come in many forms, and often may be in ways that you have not yet considered (Figure 5.1). As omnivores, most people eat animals while others may keep them as companions. Animals have worked alongside humans since the early days of domestication when we first convinced animals to hunt alongside us or when we domesticated animals as beast of burdens or food sources. We have increasingly utilized animal parts for human medicines, in both unscientific ways such as the false use of rhino horn and tiger bone as supposed aphrodisiacs, to the scientifically proven use of animal-derived insulin and organs that help extend human life.

We also use many species as service animals that help people with disabilities, from a quadriplegic person with limited mobility, to someone with debilitating anxiety. Maybe less appreciated by most people are the roles that animals play in providing ecosystem services for planetary health. Animals, across the globe – from oceans to deserts – provide services that may at times be hard to quantify, but that nonetheless are imperative for healthy ecosystems. From pollination to pest control, landscape modifications (think elephants moving trees) to predation, seed dispersal to fertilization, animals are busy 24/7 providing health care for the planet.

*Introduction to One Health: An Interdisciplinary Approach to Planetary Health*, First Edition.
Sharon L. Deem, Kelly E. Lane-deGraaf and Elizabeth A. Rayhel.
© 2019 John Wiley & Sons, Inc. Published 2019 by John Wiley & Sons, Inc.
Companion website: www.wiley.com/go/deem/health

(a)          (b)          (c)

(d)          (e)          (f)

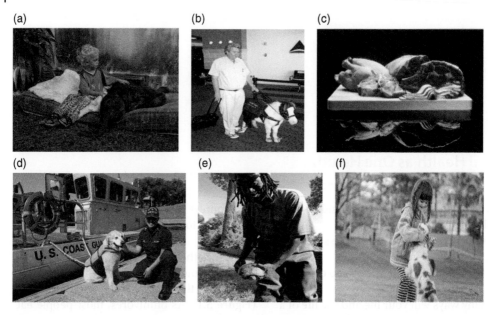

Figure 5.1 How many ways will you interact with a non-human animal today? (a) child with orphaned African forest elephant (*Loxodonta cyclotis*); (b) blind person with guide pony. *Source:* Courtesy of Dan Morgan; (c) meat from various animal species; (d) coast guard with working dog. *Source:* Courtesy of US Navy; (e) biologist with painted turtle; (f) child with pet dog. *Source:* Courtesy of Kai-Chieh Chan, Pexels.

These ecosystem engineers have impacts on human, animal, and environmental health.

As the utilization of animals has expanded along with a growing human population, we also see that the numbers of domesticated animals have increased at an alarming rate. This change in animal biomass on the planet should be of concern for all of us, especially as we think as One Health practitioners. Taken from a historical perspective, if one considers the changing composition of the vertebrate biomass, the total mass of organisms that have backbones, we can start to understand why the One Health approach is so important for conservation and public health. As covered in Chapter 2, there has been a dramatic switch in numbers of non-domestic to domestic species. The world is now largely dominated by the 7.6 billion humans and the billions of domestic animals alive that serve humankind as food, working and companion animals. However, just as important, and probably more commonly overlooked, is that 97% of the Animal kingdom is made up of **invertebrates** (Figure 5.2).

It is true that when most people think of animal health they immediately consider the health of vertebrate species. However, during this time of the Anthropocene, we see that invertebrate losses and challenges to their health may pose as great a threat to life on Earth. Losses in invertebrate species from **coral bleaching** to Colony Collapse Disorder create conservation and public health challenges that span from the health of oceans to food crops on which humans are dependent. We have recently seen documentation of catastrophic declines in insect biomass. This loss, calculated in one study at 76% over 26 years, was shown irrespective of habitat type. And, a loss of insects is much larger than just a loss of insects and speaks to a greater concern from a One Health perspective. Insects are often central within a food web. Additionally, insects serve a diversity of ecosystem functions. With the loss of insects, we are just now realizing the cascading ecological effects for human, animal, and environmental health. Therefore, we must consider animal health whether that animal is a yet to be

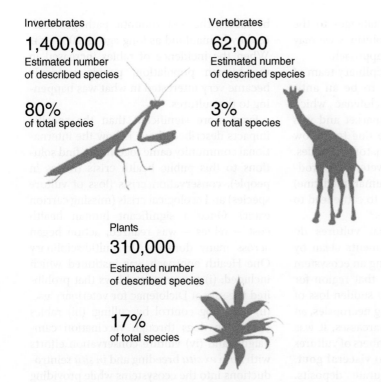

Invertebrates
**1,400,000**
Estimated number
of described species

**80%**
of total species

Vertebrates
**62,000**
Estimated number
of described species

**3%**
of total species

Plants
**310,000**
Estimated number
of described species

**17%**
of total species

Figure 5.2 Invertebrate animal numbers compared to vertebrates. *Source:* Baillie (2012). Reproduced with permission of Zoological Society of London.

identified coral species, an insect that is the main food source for birds and bats, an elephant providing ecosystem services within the forest of Asia, or a chicken in Paraguay that will soon be on a family's dinner table.

In this chapter, we will explore how we provide health care for animals: from pigs on a farm to polar bears in Alaska. We also will consider the connections that link animal health to the health of people and environments. We will consider those events that threaten animal health, how these may have disease implications across taxa, and how using a One Health approach to guide us, we may provide health care for animals by both preventive and therapeutic means. Before we delve deeper into the chapter, a real life event that has played out over the past three decades provides an excellent example of the One Health link, connecting food animals, wildlife and human health within a changing ecosystem.

## 5.1 Vulture Declines and One Health

The Indian subcontinent was once home to several million vultures. These **raptors**, from the Latin word rapere meaning to grip or grasp, play a vital role in the ecosystem, cleaning up carcasses of dead animals, which helps reduce disease-causing agents and toxins in the environment. However, since the 1990s there has been evidence of vulture population losses on a scale never before seen in recorded history. The three most abundant species – the oriental white-backed vulture (*Gyps bengalensis*), the Indian vulture (*Gyps indicus*) and the slender-billed vulture (*Gyps tenuirostris*) declined by more than 95% in Pakistan, India, and Nepal between 1990 and 2001. The reason for these losses, and the **multidisciplinary** epidemiological studies that helped to unravel the cause of these near species' extinctions is an excellent example of the challenges to the One Health Triad and the solutions we may develop using a One Health approach.

Findings from an interdisciplinary team of experts showed the culprit to be an anti-inflammatory drug called Diclofenac*, which had recently come on the market and was being administered to cattle due to its low cost and great anti-inflammatory qualities. You may wonder, how did a veterinary product (which is also used in human medicine) that was being administered to cattle lead to a catastrophic loss of vultures?

Vultures were doing what vultures do best – keeping our environments clean by eating carrion – and providing an ecosystem service as they had done in that region for millennia. But, why then the sudden loss of so many vultures? Performing necropsies, an animal autopsy, of vulture carcasses, it was determined that massive numbers of vultures had kidney failure that led to **visceral gout**, or the accumulation of urate deposits. However, microbiological and toxicological studies failed to pinpoint the cause of the kidney failure and gout. It was not until an investigation of the primary food source of the vultures, livestock carcasses, that the source of the die-off was determined to be Diclofenac. The use of a veterinary product in a livestock species was having a significant impact, near extinctions, on free-living wildlife species. But, how could we have known that the add-on effect of Diclofenac in the meat (e.g. the dead cattle) the vultures consumed would lead to kidney failure in the birds at such a catastrophic level?

Had the loss of vulture species been the end of the story, three raptor species may have gone extinct without attracting much attention. However, with the vultures' niche empty a new predator took the role of carrion eater. In the regions of vulture losses, feral dog populations increased significantly. This increase in feral dog numbers may not seem too bad on first inspection, unless you think as a One Health practitioner. What is the first disease that comes to mind when thinking of feral dogs? That of course would

be rabies, the first zoonotic pathogen realized by humankind as long ago as 2000 BCE. When the incidence of rabies increased in the human population, people suddenly became very interested in what was happening to the vultures.

Even more significant than the specific impacts described above is how the international community came together to find solutions to this public health crisis (rabies in people), conservation crisis (loss of vulture species) and ecological crisis (missing carrion eater). Once a significant human health cost – rabies – was realized, action began across many domains. A multidisciplinary One Health approach was instituted which included: (i) governmental laws that prohibited the sale of Diclofenac for veterinary use; (ii) feral dog control by culling; (iii) rabies control in dogs through vaccination campaigns, and (iv) vulture conservation efforts with both *ex situ* breeding and *in situ* reintroductions into the ecosystems while providing untainted meat via "vulture restaurants."

This real world multi-decade event exemplifies not only the challenges identifying the connections between environmental, animal and human health, but of more importance, it provides an example of a One Health approach to provide solutions to the growing health and conservation challenges. Although it would be nice to end this story on a positive note, unfortunately a different type of vulture loss is playing out in Africa due to intentional poisoning. Poachers now intentionally poison vultures in hopes there will be none present to circle poached wildlife, which is one way law enforcement agents are clued into the site of wildlife kills. This creates two conservation challenges; one for the loss of vultures themselves and the other since the poached animals are often endangered species.

With the decline of vultures, including a number of species now on the brink of extinction, there is one positive from these losses. The world is starting to realize how interconnected life is on Earth, and how important animals are for our own species' health. The loss of these ecosystem carrion eaters, "garbage collectors," and the realization that this loss may translate into significant human health issues (e.g. rabies from feral dogs) has given conservationists and veterinarians a platform for discussing these links and the need to conserve **umbrella**, **flagship**, **and keystone** species.

## 5.2 Animals that Share Our Planet

Before we look at how we provide health care to animals, it would be valuable to define an **animal**. The simplest definition is that animals are living organisms that feed on organic matter, typically having specialized sense organs, and they are able to respond to stimuli. Animals are also classified as eukaryotic, multicellular organisms that constitute the kingdom Animalia, just a single branch of the larger tree of life (Figure 5.3). The word animal comes from the Latin *animalis*, meaning having breath, having soul or living being. We may think of animals in the biological sense, encompassing creatures as diverse as sponges, jellyfish, corals, insects, and humans. Yes, we humans are part of the kingdom Animalia. This one fact might be

the "gorilla in the room" when animal and human health are artificially divided, as we do in Chapters 5 and 6.

*Homo sapiens* are indeed members of Animalia in the class Mammalia, along with the other approximately 5500 mammal species that science has identified to date. In the medical professions, one branch of medicine focuses on human health whereas another branch, veterinary medicine, focuses on non-human animal health. We humans often feel a bit special and different and thus place ourselves in our own "human" category. However, as should be evident the deeper you move into One Health, there are great benefits to be gained for humans and other animals if we consider health care, and the threats to health, from a more holistic view that includes *all* life.

Let us consider all those animals that are not humans. This includes the vertebrate **taxa** of birds, amphibians, reptiles, and mammals. There are also the invertebrates, such as sea stars, sea urchins, earthworms, sponges, jellyfish, lobsters, crabs, insects, spiders, snails, clams and squid. One dichotomy in health care might be that we most commonly think of the vertebrate species as those we "treat" and the invertebrates as those we fear, eat, or admire during scuba

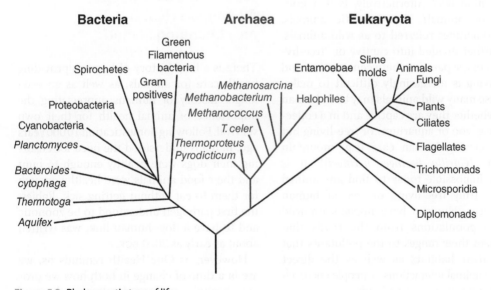

**Figure 5.3** Phylogenetic tree of life.

dives. However, this narrow approach is changing as veterinary medicine is applied to corals, spiders, and other animals, with an entire textbook dedicated to invertebrate medicine. Additionally, it has become clear that the full biome is important for life and that if we lose one species, it may have major ramifications across taxa. For example, the rise in human allergies in much of the developed world may be related to a lack of parasite loads (tapeworms and hookworms) in humans due to improved hygiene and preventive medicines. This "**hygiene hypothesis**" contends that the proper development of the immune system depends upon at least some exposure to parasites. Therefore, the rise in allergies, particularly in young people in developed nations may be due to the lack of parasitic exposure and thus a suppression of the natural development of the immune system. Improved health care in one way (e.g. hygiene and antihelmintics) may lead to a different human health concern (e.g. allergies).

Another way to view animals is the more traditional one, in which we consider the animals that exist in our everyday space, and how they integrate into our lives. This perspective includes the role an animal plays; is it domesticated for food, work, or as a companion pet? Alternatively, is it a non-domestic animal? Non-domestic animals, also sometimes referred to as wild animals, are further divided into captive or "free-living." This separation between captive and free-living is increasingly difficult to make, because many wild animals may be in human care whether they are captive and in a collection (e.g. zoo or aquarium) or free-living but still receiving human care (e.g. mountain gorillas [*Gorilla beringei beringei*]). It is nearly impossible today to find any animal that is truly free-living or free of human influences. Humans have impacts on wild animal populations from the roads that fragment their ranges to the pollutants that enter their habitats as well as the direct human-animal interactions as people encroach farther into once pristine lands.

Unfortunately, as is evident by the changing percentage of domestic and non-domestic species, the dominant animal species today are domestic animals with a shift to a potentially unsustainable level. We are seeing the implications of this shift as regards health and welfare for animals as well as humans and environments. When we add the 7.6 billion people along with the billions of domestic animals produced solely to feed our own species we can see how this makes for the increasingly complex health challenges facing humanity. We also create conditions that change invertebrate species numbers and distributions as humans help to move these species into new regions and to change habitat suitability following anthropogenic impacts such as climate change. In addition to the shear loss in insect numbers, one example of this is the spread of mosquitoes as the climate warms, which has led to the spread of malaria (i.e. *Plasmodium* spp. carried in mosquitoes) into new regions with increased temperatures. This leads to the emerging diseases of animals and humans discussed in Chapter 3 and elsewhere in the text.

## 5.3 How Do We Keep All Animals Healthy on a Changing Planet?

There is a long history of humans providing health care for animals, as well as an even longer history of humans appreciating the importance of animal health for their own survival. Following domestication 10 000 years ago, humans understood the need for ensuring their dogs were healthy enough to hunt and their food animals were healthy enough for them to eat without getting sick. Rabies, the first pathogen understood to be zoonotic and to have a dog–human link, was written about as early as 2000 BCE.

However, as One Health reminds us, we are in a time of change in both how we provide health care for animals as well as of the interconnected impacts that animal diseases have for human and environmental health. When it comes to health care, it is not a "one size fits all" approach. For example, there may be a difference in health care provided to species produced as a human food source versus health care provided for the last remaining individuals of an endangered species. This may be especially true if we know that the species in peril is a keystone species and key to the stability of the ecosystem in which it lives. Approaching animal health within a One Health context therefore requires broad thinking for application across the animal kingdom.

**Veterinary medicine** is the branch of medicine that deals with the prevention, diagnosis, and treatment of disease, disorder, and injury in non-human animals. Veterinarians are the medical doctors for all of the Animal Kingdom, minus humans. However, as should be clear from a One Health perspective, the health care veterinarians provide for animals, whether for animals serving humans as food sources, working animals, or companions, or those non-domestic animals important for ecological functions, is imperative for human and environmental health. In fact, a central tenant of the Veterinary Oath as put forth by the American Veterinary Medical Association exemplifies this role for human health. The Oath is:

> Being admitted to the profession of veterinary medicine, I solemnly swear to use my scientific knowledge and skills for the benefit of society through the protection of animal health and welfare, the prevention and relief of animal suffering, the conservation of animal resources, the promotion of public health, and the advancement of medical knowledge. I will practice my profession conscientiously, with dignity, and in keeping with the principles of veterinary medical ethics. I accept as a lifelong obligation the continual improvement of my professional knowledge and competence.

As an academic science, veterinary schools are more recent than human medical schools, with the first College of Veterinary Medicine established in 1762 in Lyon, France. However, prior to this many physicians served as animal doctors across the human to non-human animal spectrum. Even while veterinary colleges were still in their infancy, physicians were often vocal about the close medical relationship of human and animal medicine. The physician and pathologist, Dr. Rudolf Virchow, who was the first person to coin the term zoonoses in 1856, also stated that "between animal and human medicine, there is no dividing line – nor should there be."

Veterinarians are, by definition doctors that may directly diagnose and treat diseases in all animal species except one, *H. sapiens*. Although veterinarians do not have the legal status as doctors for direct human health care, they do in fact contribute to human health in both direct (e.g. ensuring the health of food, working, laboratory, and companion animals) and indirect (e.g. providing health care to free-living animals important for ecosystem function) ways. Within animal health care, there are many disciplines involved beyond the more traditional veterinarian and veterinary technician (animal nurse) roles including **epidemiologists**, behaviorists, animal control specialists, animal keepers, farmers, and others. Additionally, similar to human medicine, veterinarians today may specialize into any number of veterinary specialties, with 22 specialties recognized by the American Veterinary Medical Association, that include surgeons, internists, **theriogenologists**, radiologists, zoological medicine experts, among others.

A growing issue in veterinary medicine is the question of how we decide the type of health care provided to animals that have a diversity of planetary roles and values, at least from a human perspective. One of the more difficult issues confronting animal health care professionals today is the obligation they have to the animal's welfare and the sometime conflicting demands that society places on the animal's role (e.g. for use in research or as food). The veterinarian's role has become more complex with ethical challenges posed by issues such as animal food production that is often on unsustainable scales, increasing economic value of companion animals, experimentation with alternative and complementary medicine, appreciation for the need of non-domestic animals within healthy functioning and resilient ecosystems, and concern for pain management, mental well-being, and welfare of animals. For example, a guinea pig may be a first time pet for a child in North America, but in South America, it may be dinner. How do we determine the health care, and disease risks, for both of these guinea pigs and the persons around them?

## 5.4 Threats to Animal Health on a Changing Planet

The profession of veterinary medicine has become more advanced with specialties and the diversity of health care, at a time that threats challenging animal health have also increased. The threats to animals are more often than not the same health threats to humans and ecosystems. These threats have been covered in Chapters 2 and 3 and include: (i) anthropogenic land use and loss of habitat; (ii) increased exposure to novel pathogens and pollutants; (iii) hunting and poaching; (iv) climate change; (v) emerging infectious diseases; (vi) monetary disparity with the global 1% and the 99% in poverty; (vii) human population explosion; (viii) biodiversity loss; and (ix) the disconnect between timing of animal arrivals and food source availability (e.g. plants emerging from dormancy).

Some of these threats (e.g. hunting and poaching) may seem more relevant as threats to animals; however, it is clear they may also have negative impacts on human health (e.g. zoonotic diseases from eating bushmeat) and ecological health (e.g. loss of mega-vertebrates, such as elephants that alter forest health). Ironically, some of our greatest threats across the One Health Triad are largely due to the production of food animals, as is evident from the role of methane (cow burps and farts!) in climate change. According to the Food and Agricultural Organization (FAO), 37% of human-induced methane comes from livestock and a growing amount of this comes from Concentrated Animal Feeding Operations (CAFO). Although methane warms the atmosphere much more strongly than does $CO_2$, its half-life in the atmosphere is only about eight years, versus at least 100 years for $CO_2$. As a result, a significant reduction in livestock production would reduce greenhouse gases (GHGs) relatively quickly compared with measures involving renewable energy and energy efficiency. This decrease in use of animals as sources of protein would be better for animal health and welfare, environmental health, and for human health since the increase in obesity and cardiovascular disease in humans is often linked to higher animal protein consumption.

## 5.5 Conclusions

Today it is safe to say that we are living on a planet at a time of great change as humans have modified both the planet itself and the animals that share Earth with us. The switch to domestic species, demanding resources and health care on a scale hard to imagine, places costs on planetary and human health. As we strive to feed all 7.6 billion of us, and increasingly by using animal protein to do so, we are often the creators of the many twenty-first-century health challenges.

Being able to feed the human population in a humane way for the animals that provide us food, in a safe way for the humans who consume the food, and in a sustainable way for the Earth without using all the arable land or contaminating environments with pesticides and other chemicals is a true One Health challenge. One need look no further than the loss of bee species from Colony

Collapse Disorder to see how animal health issues result in the loss of food production with significant health and economic impacts on human societies.

How then do we provide health care for, as well as humane treatment of, the billions of domestic animals in such a way that we do not cause more harm than good? For food animals, some people contend that factory farming may cause the least harm to the environment, but the use of antibiotics, growth hormones, and other interventions used to produce animals in these conditions often is far from healthy for the animals themselves or the humans that eat them. Environmental health is also worsening in and around these farms. What of the millions of companion animals that we bring into our homes to share our lives, often to be family members? How do we provide health care for these animals, which allows preventive health for the humans that live with them (think parasite control and vaccination against zoonotic diseases), but without placing too high of a cost to our finite natural resources?

There are many reasons for the One Health movement to strive for animal health if we are to ensure planetary health for *all* life. As noted by many studies in recent years decline in wild animal health in populations as well as population extirpations and even species' extinctions remind us of the **sentinel** roles – the canary in the coalmine so to speak – animals play providing us an indication of declining environmental health and increased disease threats for *all* life. Animal health studies that provide comparative and translational medical advances also have become the cornerstone of so many human health advances. These two human-centric reasons alone – roles as sentinels and translational medicine – are enough reason to care for animal health. We have come to understand that each species may have ecological roles still unimaginable for us to grasp but are of dire significance for planetary health. Animal health is One Health.

# End of Chapter Questions & Activities

A. Thought Questions:
   i) Consider an animal that you interacted with today. This may be as a food source, a companion animal, or a non-domestic bird or other animal you saw when walking to class. How might the health of that animal have an impact on your health?
   ii) How do various physical, social, and economic factors contribute to disease emergence, persistence, and spread in animal and human populations?

B. In-Class/Guided Activities:
   i) Have each student list all the foods they ate in the past 24 hours and then see how many of these had animal products within them.
   ii) Have each student say their favorite animal on the planet. Then give each 15 minutes to look up their current status of endangered or not and if available current estimate of remaining numbers on Earth.

C. At-home Activities:
   i) Take a 15 minute walk near your home. During this time record the species, and numbers, of animals you see during the walk. Then consider the needs of these animals for their health and then the possible health (positive and negative) impacts these animals may have on your health. Bonus points in that the 15 minute walk is good for your health!
   ii) Pick an animal species that is highly endangered (there are lots to choose from) and learn more about it. Determine five things that you can do to help conserve the species.

D. Long-term Action Steps:
   i) As the human population approaches eight billion people, what are some measures you see that may be most

effective to provide animal health in a humane and safe way while providing animal-based protein for the world's people. If you see ways that may help lessen the pressures on the food supply, consider making some of them a part of your lifestyle. Examples might include meat-less Mondays, eating lower on the food web, and buying locally sourced foods.

E. Recommended Reading:

Dunlop, R.H. and Williams, D.J. (1996). *Veterinary Medicine: An Illustrated History*. Mosby.

Fuller Torrey, E. and Yolken, R.H. (2005). *Beasts of the Earth: Animals, Humans and Disease*. Rutgers University Press.

Goodall, J., Maynard, T., and Hudson, G. (2009). *Hope for Animals and Their World: How Endangered Species Are Being Rescued from the Brink*. Grand Central Publishing.

Lewbart, G. (2012). *Invertebrate Medicine*, 2e. Wiley.

Quammen, D. (2012). *Spillover: Animal Infections and the Next Human Pandemic*. W. W. Norton and Company.

## Interview

*An interview with Christine Fiorello, DVM, MS, PhD, Diplomate American College of Zoological Medicine. Dr. Fiorello is a wildlife veterinarian and a conservation biologist. She currently is Staff Veterinarian at the Rio Grande Zoo and Aquarium at the Albuquerque BioPark in New Mexico, USA.*

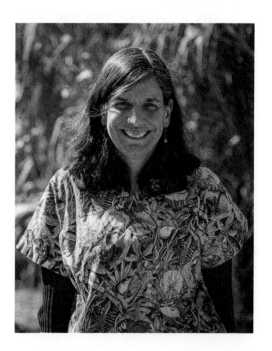

**When did you first hear about One Health?**

It was probably 10 or 12 years ago when it was starting to get more press and veterinary schools were talking about it. Before that, I thought of much of these concepts in terms of conservation medicine and how we help animals and help wildlife populations in the context of health. And that more narrow concept, I think, got sucked into the One Health concept, which is broader.

**How is One Health important to your work?**

Anything that I do that impacts animal health is informed by the concept, I hope. For me, it's internalized and just how I think about things. I am not thinking, "Well, how would I think about this problem?" and then, "Oh, how would I think about this problem using One Health?" It's more holistic than that. As an example, we just worked up an orangutan and I found myself spending a lot of time reading the primary literature in human health, to apply that knowledge to manage this animal's health. I wasn't looking up orangutan health, I was looking up human health, where there's a lot of information about certain diseases, and hoping it would be applicable to the orangutan.

**What can an individual do to make a difference for planetary health?**

I have thought more in the last couple of years about stuff and a little bit less about energy. Energy is huge, obviously but "the stuff" is a massive problem too. We often forget about not just the energy it takes to drive from point A to point B, but the energy it takes to make all the stuff that we buy, and then to recycle all the stuff that we buy and to bring it all to the landfill. One thing people can do is to have less stuff, to use less stuff, to need less stuff. Of course all the corollaries that go along with that, which is to buy used things, buy recycled things, support companies that have those practices that use less packaging, and that use recycled materials. Everybody wants stuff, and yet studies show that people aren't happier with more stuff. The other thing that people can do that's incredibly important is to vote.

**How can we encourage people to care about planetary Health?**

Saying, "Don't buy plastic, it's a pollutant," is not as effective as saying, "Hey, 90% of every single seabird on earth has bits of plastic in it." That plastic does not come from some nebulous factory somewhere that is someone else's problem. That plastic comes from your water bottle, your toys, your packaging, your whatever.

To make these connections that every little bit matters, and that all millions and millions of bits of plastic in the ocean has been contributed by all of us. We need to say, "Hey, we live on this planet, we use stuff. That's okay, but let us use that stuff responsibly. And if we all do it, it might make a difference." In most cases, people do not want their kids to live in a less healthy world than the world they live in, but that's where we are headed as our world gets less healthy.

**How do you feel a One Health approach may differ based on the different subsets of animals?**

It differs because their priorities are different. When it comes to a food animal, the priority is going to be on human health. Whereas in a companion animal, the priority is on that individual animal. When it comes to wildlife, the priority is on that animal and also its ecosystem. We need One Health to keep those approaches, to keep those different roles, from becoming siloed and independent of one another. We need to remind ourselves that, "Hey, there's food animal health that's important for human health, but remember that whatever you do to that animal will impact the environment." To try to make these approaches less different would be an important goal.

---

**Case Study: Rinderpest**

Coauthored by Olivia Hollander & Pascaline Akitani

**Rinderpest** was a highly contagious viral disease of both domestic and non-domestic hoofstook species. The disease is thought to have originated in Asia, spread throughout Asia, Europe, Africa, and Australia, causing devastating losses of cattle for three centuries. Historically, it is believed that rinderpest first spread in the thirteenth century when infected gray oxen of the Central Asian steppe were used to carry baggage of the Mongol armies as they moved through Eurasia, China, and Poland. In the 1700s, the disease then spread rapidly across Asia and Europe, reaching Africa in the late 1800s, where it caused untold losses in domestic and wild ungulates.

The first attempts to control the disease led to innovations such as the first tissue culture produced **vaccine** in 1960. In 1986, the first mass immunization program, Pan African Rinderpest Campaign (PARC), was launched in

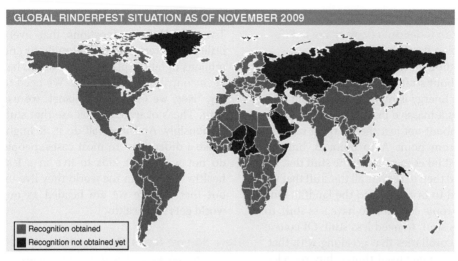

GLOBAL RINDERPEST SITUATION AS OF NOVEMBER 2009

- Recognition obtained
- Recognition not obtained yet

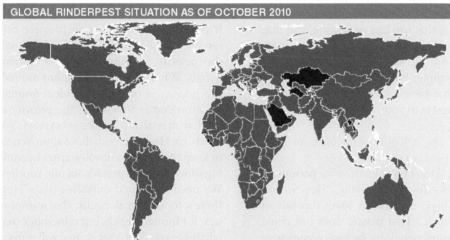

GLOBAL RINDERPEST SITUATION AS OF OCTOBER 2010

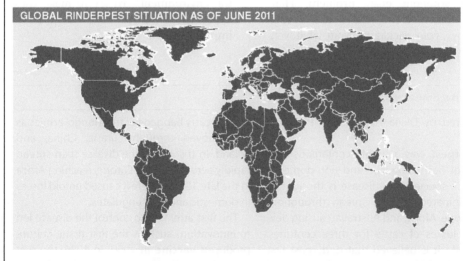

GLOBAL RINDERPEST SITUATION AS OF JUNE 2011

Figure 5.4 Map of countries where Rinderpest was present over time. *Source:* Courtesy of Food and Agriculture Organization of the United Nations, 2011, "Global Rinderest Eradication Programme (November 2009–June 2011)." Reproduced with permission.

an attempt to eradicate the disease. This program covered 34 countries in Africa and was able to vaccinate 300 million animals. However, cost and logistical constraints limited the success of PARC.

In 1994 the World Organization of Animal Health (OIE) and the FAO came together to form the Global Rinderpest Eradication Program (GREP); a program designed to eradicate rinderpest by 2010. The GREP incorporated many of the same approaches that PARC had used. However, the approaches were implemented on a global scale, and included three key measures. The first was to have a large network of laboratory scientists. Through the network, scientists were able to monitor the disease with a global perspective. The second was the use of a thermostable vaccine. One of the limiting factors for PARC was the inability to keep vaccines cold during distribution across Africa. Therefore, thermostable vaccines, with a shelf life of eight months, were viable even if unrefrigerated for up to 30 days, thus allowing access to the remotest areas. The third part of the program was the use of community based animal health workers (CAHWs). These CAHWs traveled on foot to deliver and administer the thermostable vaccines to livestock throughout the world. As community members, the CAHWs had knowledge of local herd sizes, their locations, and seasonal movement patterns, which was instrumental in choosing the optimum time to vaccinate cattle.

Community vaccination programs lead by GREP achieved **herd immunity** levels of 80%, a necessary level for a virus, such as rinderpest, in the Family Paramyxoviridae. The last known outbreak of rinderpest occurred in Kenya in 2001. Rinderpest was officially declared globally eradicated at the FAO Conference in 2011 (Figure 5.4). In the final assessment, rinderpest caused the death of millions of cattle and other animals, both domestic and wild, with associated economic costs and human hunger issues in Africa, Asia, and Europe. The eradication of rinderpest brought much relief to people in Africa, the last stronghold of the disease. For example, Chad credits a 3% increase in its GDP to the absence of rinderpest and household income across Ethiopia rose by $45.1 million as a result of rinderpest control and eradication. Additionally, the cost–benefit ratio of the costs of the eradication program to post-eradication range from 11% in Ivory Coast to 118% in Burkina Faso.

Rinderpest is the first eradicated animal disease. It is only the second viral disease to have been eradicated with human small pox virus the first one and officially declared eradicated by the World Health Organization in 1980. The eradication of infectious agents is a difficult undertaking that requires collaboration from many sectors. The One Health benefits of the eradication of rinderpest is both a human health benefit from ensuring livestock is available for human protein and the cessation of the devastating wildlife losses that also occurred when rinderpest was in a region.

## Works Cited

AVMA° Our Passion. Our Profession. (2017) Veterinarian's Oath. https://www.avma.org/KB/Policies/Pages/veterinarians-oath.aspx (accessed December 12, 2017).

Blake, S., Deem, S.L., Strindberg, S. et al. (2008). Roadless wilderness area determines forest elephant movements in the Congo Basin. *PLoS One* 3 (10): e3546. http://dx.plos.org/10.1371/journal.pone.0003546 (accessed December 12, 2017.

Camerona, S.A., Loziera, J.D., Strangeb, J.P. et al. (2011). Patterns of widespread decline in North American bumble bees. *Proceedings of the National Academy of Sciences of the United States of America* 108 (2): 662–666. doi: 10.1073/pnas.1014743108.

Collen, B., Böhm, M., Kemp, R. et al. (2012). *Spineless: Status and Trends of the World's Invertebrates*. United Kingdom: Zoological

Society of London https://www.researchgate.net/publication/259820252_Marine_Invertebrate_Life_in_Spineless_Status_and_Trends_of_the_World%27s_Invertebrates_Eds_Collen_B_Bohm_M_Kemp_R_Baillie_JEM (accessed December 12, 2017.

Cuthbert, R.J., Dave, R., Sunder Chakraborty, S. et al. (2011). Assessing the ongoing threat from veterinary non-steroidal anti-inflammatory drugs to critically endangered gyps vultures in India. *Oryx* 45: 420–426.

Deem, S.L. (2007). Role of the zoo veterinarian in the conservation of captive and free-ranging wildlife. *International Zoo Yearbook* 41: 3–11.

Delgado, C., Rosegrant, M., Steinfeld, H. et al. (2001). Livestock to 2020: the next food revolution. *Outlook on Agriculture* 30: 27–29.

Hallmann, C.A., Sorg, M., Jongejans, E. et al. (2017). More than 75 percent decline over 27 years in total flying insect biomass in protected areas. *PLoS One* 12: e0185809. https://doi.org/10.1371/journal.pone.0185809 (accessed December 12, 2017.

Hoff, B. (1982). *The Tao of Pooh*. New York, NY: E.P. Dutton & Co., Inc.

Margalida, A., Bogliani, G., Bowden, C.G.R. et al. (2014). One Health approach to use of veterinary pharmaceuticals. *Science* 346 (6215): 1296–1298.

Markandya, A., Taylor, T., Longo, A. et al. (2008). Counting the cost of vulture decline – an appraisal of the human health and other benefits of vultures in India. *Ecological Economics* 67: 194–204.

Naidoo, V., Wolter, K., Cuthbert, R. et al. (2009). Veterinary diclofenac threatens Africa's endangered vulture species. *Regulatory Toxicology and Pharmacology* 53 (3): 205–208.

Oaks, J.L., Gilbert, M., Virani, M.Z. et al. (2004). Diclofenac residues as the cause of vulture population decline in Pakistan. *Nature* 427: 630–633.

Rabinowitz, P.M. and Conti, L.A. (2010). Foodborne Illness. In: *Human-Animal Medicine: Clinical Approaches to Zoonoses, Toxicants, and Other Shared Health Risks* (ed. P.M. Rabinowitz and L.A. Conti), 331–342. Maryland Heights, MO: Saunders.

Stanwell-Smith, R., Bloomfield, S.F., and Rook, G.A. (2012) The hygiene hypothesis and its implications for home hygiene, lifestyle, and public health. International Scientific Forum on Home Hygiene. http://www.ifh-homehygiene.org (accessed December 12, 2017).

The Global Rinderpest Eradication Programme: Progress Report on rinderpest eradication: Success stories and actions leading to the June 2011 Global Declaration. http://www.fao.org/ag/againfo/resources/documents/AH/GREP_flyer.pdf (accessed December 12, 2017).

# 6

# Human Health as One Health

In 1844, an epidemic began somewhere in the Americas and then traveled to Belgium. From there it spread quickly across Europe to the British Isles where it found its most vulnerable victims in Ireland. Over one million Irish died and up to two million more were displaced. The population of Ireland has still not returned to pre-epidemic numbers. This scourge, however, was not caused by a virus or bacterium, and it could not be transmitted from person to person. Instead, the primary host of this outbreak was the potato, in particular, the Irish Lumper (*Solanum tuberosum* cultivar: Irish Lumper), we now know that the causative agent was the oomycete *Phytophthora infestans*, a fungus.

The Irish Lumper is not a particularly appealing potato, but it grew well in unproductive soil and was the primary source of calories for the poor in Ireland in 1844. The Irish dependence on this crop put them at risk. Any crop grown as a monoculture, no matter how perfectly suited to its environment, is vulnerable. The right pathogen can wipe out the entire species, as *P. infestans* did in 1844–1845, instigating the Great Irish Famine, the desperation of which is captured in Figure 6.1.

There were socioeconomic and political factors underlying this story as well. The United Kingdom of Great Britain and Ireland in the mid-1800s marginalized Ireland's poor. This was largely because of political control by unengaged English landholders and a set of laws, the British Corn Laws, which restricted the import of grain products by placing exorbitant excise taxes on them. These laws forced citizens to buy only British-grown foods, and when the potato crop failed, the Irish were left with two choices: emigrate or starve. These were certainly not the first **ecorefugees**, but they were a large enough group that their displacement has had a notable effect on the social, political, and genetic structures of not just Ireland but also many non-Irish countries.

Today an estimated 70 million people worldwide claim Irish heritage, while the island itself is home to a population of only six million. As the Irish dispersed around the globe, they carried with them a genetic uniqueness, the "Celtic Curse." Rather than a curse, it was an altered version of the C282Y gene involved in iron storage. It is likely that the Irish, over thousands of years of evolution, have experienced **heterozygote advantage** for this gene. For those in whom only one of the two gene copies, or **alleles**, is mutated, the extra storage of iron gives them a survival advantage when faced with an environmental **selective pressure** unique to Ireland. Several hypotheses have been put forward as to what that pressure might be: the iron-poor diet that results from foods grown in iron-depleted soil, Celiac Disease (also common among the Irish), or perhaps the response to a parasite. Unfortunately, those who inherit two mutated alleles (i.e. coming from *both* parents) store so much iron that it becomes toxic, a potentially fatal

*Introduction to One Health: An Interdisciplinary Approach to Planetary Health*, First Edition.
Sharon L. Deem, Kelly E. Lane-deGraaf and Elizabeth A. Rayhel.
© 2019 John Wiley & Sons, Inc. Published 2019 by John Wiley & Sons, Inc.
Companion website: www.wiley.com/go/deem/health

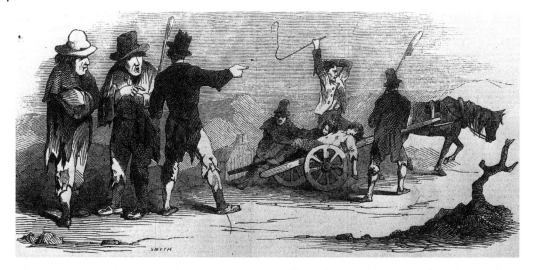

Figure 6.1 La Grande Famine, *Illustrated London News* par *Smyth*, 1847. The sketch, *A Funeral at Skibbereen*, shows the body of a young Irish man on a cart to be carried, coffin-less, to a pauper's grave. Stories carried in the *Illustrated London News* were meant to shock Victorian England into an understanding of the death and despair in Ireland. *Source:* Samuel Austin, https://fr.wikipedia.org/wiki/Fichier:Patate_famine.jpg. CC BY-SA 3.0.

condition known as **hemochromatosis.** Similar relationships between genetic makeup and ancestral geographic origins occur between people of African descent and sickle-cell anemia and Tay-Sachs disease and the Ashkenazi Jewish population. In preceding chapters, we have shown how humans are shaping the environment and the health of animals, but animals and the environment have shaped us as well.

Like most species, humans embody a diversity of traits and backgrounds that make us different from one another. At the same time, all humans share 99.9% of their DNA, unifying us into one cohesive species with essentially the same health needs. We – and all animals – need clean air to breathe, clean water to drink, nutritious food to eat, and a hospitable environment in which to thrive. **Life expectancy** at birth is a measure of overall health for a population in a given region, and better medicines and nutrition are increasing life expectancy overall. However, Figure 6.2 shows the past and projected life expectancies for people by region, and the data shown speak to a stunning inequality in life expectancy for those born in

different parts of the globe, with clear distinctions between the northern and southern hemispheres. Many of the causes of this inequality have a place in the One Health perspective on human health.

## 6.1 Human Health as One Health

The definition of **health** is open to debate. However, the World Health Organization (WHO) defines human health as "a state of complete physical, mental, and social well-being and not merely the absence of disease or infirmity." This definition describes the health *goal* and not just the minimum acceptable standard. In that spirit, the following discussion of human health in the context of One Health begins with the ways in which animals and the environment enrich us and enhance our well-being.

Plants, algae, and other microscopic photosynthetic lifeforms are the only lifeforms able to fix the carbon and nitrogen that animals need to make proteins, and they alone can harness the sun's energy to produce

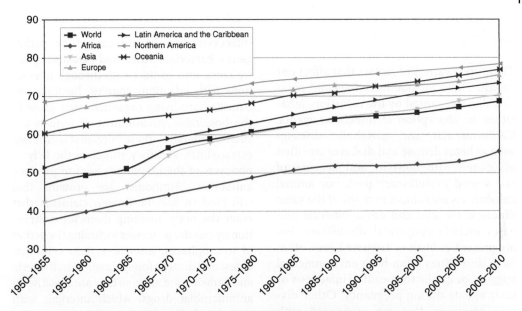

**Figure 6.2** Life expectancy at birth by region. Future projections are based on continuation of current trends, such as further reductions in deaths due to HIV/AIDS in Africa. Data from the UN World Population Prospects, 2012 Revision: Key Findings and Advance Tables, by Department of Economic and Social Affairs Population. *Source:* R Cragun, https://commons.wikimedia.org/wiki/File:Life_Expectancy_at_Birth_by_Region_1950-2050. png. CC BY 3.0.

oxygen and fuel. These processes are crucial to human life, but there is more. In addition to establishing terrestrial food chains, plant products have given us shelter, warmth, fuel, medicines, and other beneficial compounds. The bark of the White Willow tree (*Salix alba*) has been used as a painkiller since roughly 1500 BCE. We now know that it contains salicylic acid, the active ingredient in aspirin. However, the discoveries of bioactive compounds are not only tales from history; the widely used anticancer drug taxol was first isolated in the 1970s from the Pacific Yew tree. Today an estimated 40% of our medications came originally from plants, and continued deforestation and plummeting biodiversity will remove an unknown number of yet to be discovered drugs and cures.

Animals are just as crucial to our survival as plants. They provide us with ecological services such as the pollination of roughly 35% of our food crops, seed dispersal, soil aeration, and decomposition of the dead (with help from fungi and bacteria). In addition to the crucial work of sustaining the environment, animals have also enhanced our health. As omnivores, most of us eat them, but most people see animals as more than just meat. Our shared ability to move about and interact is the basis of a powerful bond that has formed between humans and animals. We use them to pull loads, we watch in awe as they fly overhead, and we play chase with them in our yards. They also make us healthier. Studies have shown a variety of health benefits provided by pets to their owners, including reductions in stress, blood pressure, and depression, and increases in lung function and immunity in children. Animals also provide companionship that has been useful in therapy and rehabilitation settings for humans as well as service to people with disabilities. They have been reliable teammates in the hunting of animal food (e.g. horses, raptors, and dogs), and they are integral to several human sports. Finally, many animals have skills that humans utilize in dangerous situations, like bomb- and drug-sniffing dogs. Some animals have even shown the capacity to smell diseases in humans.

## 6.2 Human Disease in the Context of One Health

There are a variety of factors that affect our health. These include infectious and parasitic disease, caused by the ingestion, inhalation, or absorption of infectious agents. Cardiovascular and metabolic diseases such as heart disease and diabetes are often associated with lifestyle, and because of our shared evolutionary past, our animal cohabitants are subject to many of the same illnesses. Genetic and developmental diseases include congenital disabilities that are present at birth or triggered soon after. Such disabilities often have environmental triggers, or can be the result of infectious or toxic agents during pregnancy. Other disease processes that are associated with environmental exposures include cancers, auto-immune dysfunctions, neurological and mental diseases, and endocrine disruptions. Traumatic injuries caused by accidents or disasters are part of the health equation as well. The psychological problems that we experience include depression, anxiety, addictions, Post-Traumatic Stress Disorder, eating disorders, and more. Many of these are made worse by adding the stress of displacement, fear, and malnourishment to the mix. Problems that can arise during pregnancy and childbirth finish out the list. Pediatric, obstetric, and gynecological health are One Health concerns on several fronts: exposure to toxins is particularly damaging to developing tissue; putting fetuses and children at increased peril. Additionally, access to gynecological and prenatal care is sparse in many parts of the world, and where it is available, women are often restricted in their family-planning options. Finally, genital mutilations, physical abuse, and pregnancy affect women's health far more significantly than their male counterparts. Several human diseases that are included in the One Health triad are introduced in the following sections.

### 6.2.1 Infectious Diseases

Infectious diseases are caused by pathogens – bacteria, viruses, and parasites – that we come into contact with through interactions with infectious sources. Bacteria and parasites are living organisms that grow in the hospitable environment of human tissues. Generally, these organisms remain extracellular, and they stimulate the B lymphocytes of the immune system to produce antibodies. Antibodies are proteins that will bind to specific foreign elements that enter the body, marking them for destruction by cellular processes including the action of macrophages, immune-system cells that ingest and destroy foreign materials. Bacteria and parasites are alive, so they are sensitive to antimicrobial drugs, which interfere with their metabolism. Antimicrobials are powerful tools in fighting bacterial infections, however, with repeated exposure to these drugs, bacteria that can withstand the effect of antimicrobials will prevail, leading to strains of bacteria that are antimicrobial resistant. Viruses enter a person's tissues and then insert into the cells themselves. This intracellular location makes them harder to destroy. Eliminating a virus, as well as some intracellular bacteria (e.g. *Mycobacterium* spp.), requires eliminating the cell in which it exists, which is the job of a variety of T lymphocytes.

Once an infectious agent enters a person, it is usually recognized and neutralized by cells of the immune system. This process takes time, and in the interim, the person will experience the symptoms of the disease. However, in many cases, the immune system retains a memory of the encounter, and subsequent encounters are handled more efficiently. The person has developed immunity to that organism and is protected. This process is utilized when vaccines are used to immunize an individual. Vaccines contain **antigens**, molecular bits of an infectious agent that cannot make a person ill. They do, however, initiate the lymphocytic processes described above, which results in immunity. Vaccines are another powerful tool in fighting infectious diseases. However, finding just the right antigenic variant can be difficult. As an example, in the three decades since HIV was recognized internationally, no suitable vaccine has been marketed because of the speed at which HIV **evolves**.

The environmental drivers of emerging and re-emerging infectious diseases are described in Chapter 3. These infectious diseases are more than twice as likely to be zoonotic, putting people who routinely interact with animals in harm's way. This includes livestock handlers, hunters, farmers, those living in the midst of vectors such as mosquitoes, individuals who share family-living spaces with animals, and those who eat animals. A 2002 study of poultry workers in Thailand assessed zoonotic exposure following the 1997–1998 outbreak of **H5N1** flu and found a significant, positive relationship between H5 seropositivity – an indicator that the person was exposed to the virus and retains **immunological memory** – and the number of poultry-related tasks performed by an individual. Examples of emerging and re-emerging zoonoses include Zika, Dengue, Sudden Acute Respiratory Syndrome, Avian Influenza, Tuberculosis (TB), Malaria, and Lyme Disease.

### 6.2.2  Disruption of Embryonic and Fetal Development

Human health begins with proper embryonic development, a process in which stem cells divide, mobilize, and specialize to form tissues and organs. Getting the proper cell type to the correct position in the growing body is a highly coordinated process that depends upon unperturbed chemical communication between cells and between cells and the matrix upon which they sit. As the process proceeds, there are critical developmental periods during which faulty genes or the actions of pathogens and chemicals can alter the process. The majority of these sensitive periods occur early, making the first eight weeks of development particularly vulnerable to disruption. **Teratogens** are substances extrinsic to the embryo that can result in abnormal development and include substances found in our environment, infectious agents, radiation, and mechanical forces. Environmental teratogens may originate in plant, animal, viral, and protozoan organisms.

As the environment absorbs the wastes of human industry, the rate of congenital disabilities has climbed accordingly. Chapter 4 details the mechanisms by which a variety of these substances enter the environment, including lead, mercury, endocrine-disrupting agents, and pesticides. All of these, if present during this early developmental period, impact neural development and subsequent IQ potential. Endocrine-disrupting chemicals are particularly troubling as they are both ubiquitous in the environment and have been revealed to alter sexual development in animals, with evidence suggesting that human development may be similarly vulnerable.

Infectious agents can also interfere with the developmental process. The US rubella (German measles) epidemic of 1963–1965 resulted in as many as 20 000 fetal deaths, and of those exposed during the first five weeks *in utero*, as many as 30 000 more infants were born with heart, eye, and ear defects. More recently we have seen the effects of Zika, a viral zoonosis most commonly transmitted by mosquito vectors (*Aedes aegypti* and *Aedes albopictus*). A woman infected during pregnancy can pass the virus to her fetus with potentially devastating effects, including microcephaly, or failure of the brain to develop properly. Other viruses of risk to developing fetuses include HIV, the herpes viruses, Cytomegalovirus, and Varicella Zoster (chickenpox). Less frequently, developmental disruption occurs as a result of bacteria or protozoan infection. However, one commonly encountered protozoan is *Toxoplasma gondii* (*T. gondii*), a protozoan parasite carried by cats, making the litter box perilous for any pregnant woman who has not previously been exposed to the parasite. *T. gondii* during pregnancy can result in preterm birth or even **congenital** toxoplasmosis which is associated with disruption of brain and eye development, and less frequently heart, kidneys, blood, liver, or spleen. An estimated 400–4000 cases of congenital Toxoplasmosis occur in the USA each year. You will see in Chapter 8 that *T. gondii* is a problem for other animals as well.

The process of development continues through childhood, adulthood, and into **senescence**. However growing tissues are particularly vulnerable to the effects of toxicants, pollutants, and other agents that disrupt normal growth. Therefore, children are at far greater risk of environmentally induced death and disease than adults. Reducing the number of total deaths in children under the age of five was one of the UN's **Millennium Development Goals** (MDGs), and, after a significant effort, this number has dropped from roughly 12.6 million in 1990 to 5.6 million in 2016. While that is progress, many of the remaining deaths are preventable and fall into One Health categories. Figure 6.3 shows the major causes of death for **neonates** and children under five, with pneumonia, malaria, diarrhea, and injury topping the list.

### 6.2.3 Diseases of Nourishment

The vast majority of nutrients enter the human body through the digestive tract: the mouth, esophagus, stomach, and the small and large intestines. This continuous, muscular tube that propels its contents from entry to exit has points along the way where water and nutrients are absorbed across its walls and into the bloodstream. Due to this absorptive capacity and direct exposure to

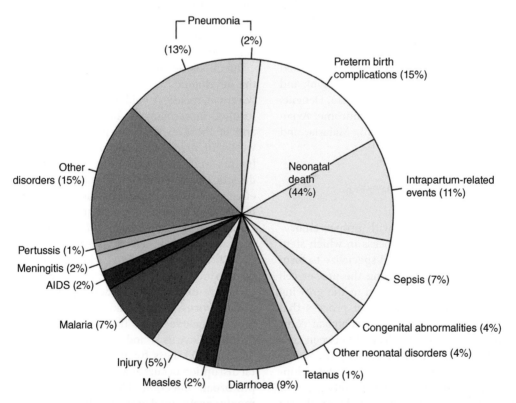

**Figure 6.3** Global causes of children under-five deaths in 2015. Forty-four percent of deaths in this age group occur in the first year (in yellow shades above). The remaining 56% of deaths occur between ages 1 and 5. *Source:* Reprinted from: Liu et al. (2015) with permission from Elsevier.

external sources of infection, the digestive tract is one of the major portals of entry for foreign substances into our bodies. The walls of the digestive tract are lined with cells of the immune system, ready to identify and destroy any infectious agents that enter. Ingested toxins and toxicants generally enter the body this way as well. The digestive tract is also home to million of bacteria and other microscopic life forms, collectively known as the **microbiome**.

Undernutrition is a global problem. The World Food Programme estimates that one-in-nine people experience hunger on a daily basis, and even more, one-in-three, suffer from some form of malnutrition. Undernutrition occurs in all countries, though it is significantly more prevalent in the developing world than the developed, with less than one-in-twenty experiencing malnutrition in the USA. Deficient overall caloric intake leads to suffering and disease; however, a diet with sufficient calories but inadequate intake of any specific nutrient is problematic as well. For example, lack of protein in the diet can result in **kwashior-kor**, a condition in which low amounts of protein upset the body's osmotic balance, which results in swelling and the buildup of abdominal fluids. This lack of protein undermines the immune system as well, interfering with the production of antibody proteins, making the underfed even more vulnerable to infection and disease. Frustratingly, part of the problem associated with getting food to people has to do with distribution and resource allocation rather than the absence of food. In parts of the world where infrastructure is lacking, or greed and corruption have undermined governance, undernutrition is a problem of society rather than science.

Overnutrition, a form of malnutrition, is significantly more prevalent in developed countries where food is readily available. Easy access to food provides people with the option of making poor choices in food consumption and overconsumption of calories. In developed countries, the metabolic syndrome of increased blood pressure, high blood sugar, excess body fat around the waist, and abnormal cholesterol or triglyceride levels, increases the risk of heart disease, stroke, and diabetes, adding billions of dollars to national healthcare expenses. The choice of protein source in the developed world has One Health-associated ramifications as well. Meat and other animal products (e.g. cheese, milk, eggs) are resource-intensive to produce. When your food eats food, the overall amount of food consumed is more. As discussed in Chapter 3, the cost of global meat consumption includes continued habitat destruction and greenhouse gas emissions as more land is turned into pasture or farms.

Unsafe Water can expose human populations to infectious agents as well. Water-borne diseases, long associated with unsanitary water, are well-documented and include diarrheal diseases, like cholera and shigella, helminthic diseases like Guinea worm and schistosomiasis, typhoid fever, paratyphoid fever, and other gastrointestinal and respiratory maladies. According to the United Nations Children's Fund (UNICEF),

> about 4 billion cases of diarrhoea per year cause 1.8 million deaths, over 90 per cent of them (1.6 million) among children under five. Repeated episodes of diarrhoeal disease makes children more vulnerable to other diseases and malnutrition. Diarrhoea is the most important public health problem directly related to water and sanitation. The simple act of washing hands with soap and water can cut diarrhoeal disease by one-third. Next to providing adequate sanitation facilities, it is the key to preventing waterborne diseases.

Access to clean drinking water was another of the high-priority MDGs and education efforts by UNICEF and the WHO resulting in a 60% decrease in the number of children worldwide that died of diarrheal disease between the years of 1990 and 2012. There are still those without safe water, predominantly in rural areas of Central Africa and Southeastern Asia, but it is clear that workable solutions to the problem exist. The remaining One Health challenge is making these solutions available to all who need them.

Ingestible toxins also enter the body through the digestive tract. An estimated 5.2 billion pounds of pesticides are applied to farms globally each year, the bulk of which are transformed into agricultural runoff once it rains. Contaminated water then finds its way into nearby streams, waterways, and drinking water. The main two pesticide types, **organophosphates** and neonicotinoids, work similarly by modulating the actions of acetylcholine, the neurotransmitter required to control nerve transmissions at synapses. These neurotoxins affect all animals, including humans. In the summer of 2013, organophosphate poisoning caused the death of at least 25 children aged four to twelve who had eaten a tainted lunch at their school in Mashrakh, India. The neonicotinoids have been implicated in exacerbating the deterioration of bee colonies experiencing Colony Collapse Disorder, yet another indirect threat to human health, by the rapid decline in pollinator numbers. A 2017 report in Science Magazine showed significant levels of neonicotinoids in honey samples worldwide.

**Glyphosate** (a.k.a. Roundup˚) is a popular herbicide, and while it is technically an organophosphate, it works quite differently from the pesticides mentioned above. It is not a neurotoxin, in fact, it works by interfering with an enzyme that only occurs in plants and thus, should be safe for animal consumption. However, conflicting data from occupational exposures regarding glyphosate's ability to cause human lymphomas led the WHO, in 2015, to designate it as "probably carcinogenic." Studies in mice suggest that it may disrupt endocrine pathways, as well. To make matters even worse, pest plants are beginning to show resistance to the chemical, leading to massive overuse of the product and levels in agricultural runoff that have not been approved by regulatory agencies.

### 6.2.4 Respiratory Disease

The mammalian respiratory system is well conserved, making the process of inhalation similar across species. Muscles pull air into the mouth or nose and down a long flexible tube, or trachea, which divides to deliver air to each lung. As the air continues along its path, it enters the smaller but more muscular bronchioles, before finally reaching its destination: tiny, bubble-like alveoli. Alveolar walls are so thin that substances are easily shared between alveolar air and the blood, which flows through adjacent vessels. Air can also carry pathogens and toxicants deep into the lungs, and as a result of this exchange, the lungs are another portal of entry. Like the digestive system, the respiratory tract is equipped with tools to evade infection, including immune cells and mucus to entrap would-be pathogens. Inhaled foreign objects or substances can also affect health by irritating and inflaming airways, making it harder to breathe. The One Health concerns that we focus on in this section include asthma, infectious diseases like pneumonia and TB, and air pollutants.

Asthma occurs when the airways overrespond to irritating or allergy-inducing substances in the air. These can be naturally occurring, such as pollen and mold, or air pollutants like fine particulates, ozone, and carbon monoxide. During an asthma attack, the muscles in the bronchiole walls contract and restrict airflow. Inflammation in the cells of the airway causes them to swell and produce extra mucus, further reducing the diameter of the tube. According to the WHO, asthma is the leading chronic disease in children, and an estimated 235 million people globally have asthma. Asthma rates are increasing worldwide, particularly in urban areas, likely because of the levels of pollution. A recent study showed that children who live near busy streets were more likely to have decreased lung function due to car exhaust and exposure to fine particulates in the air. Other risk factors associated with asthma include exposure to cockroach remains, and interestingly, infant exposure to *Pichia pastoris*, a fungal member of the gut microbiome. This further emphasizes the role of the microbiome and its potential importance to human health.

Globally, pneumonia is the leading cause of death for children under five (Figure 6.3). The two most common causes of pneumonia are *Streptococcus pneumoniae* and *Haemophilus influenzae type b*. Mortality from the disease is linked to poor nutrition, indoor air pollutants, and restricted access to healthcare. Notably, there are vaccines to protect against both of the common causative agents, but as with the distribution of food, these life-saving vaccines are often not available to those most vulnerable.

Tuberculosis is an infectious, respiratory disease most often caused in humans by the bacterium *Mycobacterium tuberculosis*. Currently, one-third of the world's population is thought to be infected with TB, but not all of these people are actively sick. TB **bacilli** first enter the lungs as tiny, infectious droplets. Once inside, the bacteria are engulfed by **macrophages**; however many mycobacterial cells can survive the environment inside the cells that are trying to digest them. Something akin to a stalemate begins, during which the bacteria and immune cells are contained inside a capsule-like structure called a **granuloma**. As long as the bacteria are held in check, the infection is considered **latent**, and the infected person remains symptom-free. However, a variety of factors including concurrent HIV infection, undernutrition, diabetes, smoking, and alcohol consumption can tip the balance in favor of the bacteria, allowing them to overpower the immune cells and escape into open lung spaces and beyond. At that point, the person has active TB, which occurs in about 10% of TB-infected persons. Extrapulmonary TB can develop in many locations, including the covering of the brain, the lymphatic system, the genitourinary tract, or even bone. In the active state, the bacteria can also be transmitted to another person through sneezing or coughing.

Humans are not the only animals that can get TB. Bovine tuberculosis (bTB, caused by *Mycobacterium bovis* rather than *M. tuberculosis*) infected cows can subsequently infect humans through direct contact or ingestion of contaminated meat, cheese, and milk. In developed countries the pasteurization of milk products has lowered the human risk of disease, although it remains a problem in developing countries. bTB frequently results in the loss of cattle, however, and in the UK, the discovery of a dead badger on a cattle farm in Gloucestershire, England, in 1971 stirred up a firestorm that still rages today. The dead badger tested positively for bTB, and it was soon found that there was a high prevalence of bTB in the English badger population. The resulting skirmish focused on two concerns: how to accurately assess the risks of transmission between wild and domestic animals, and how to determine the proper response to this zoonosis. Despite science that suggests the ineffectiveness of culling to address this problem, the UK has undertaken several waves of mass culling of badgers that test positively for bTB, much to the dismay of a growing number of British badger activists. In September 2017, in response to escalating costs to British farmers, the British government announced an increase in badger culling from $10,000$ in 2016 to up to $33\,500$ in 2017, prompting Rosie Woodroffe, disease ecologist at the Zoological Society of London to say,

> It's depressing that the government is pursuing badger culling over such huge areas when the benefits remain so uncertain. Data published today suggest that, after three years of culling, cattle TB in the first cull zones was still no lower than that in unculled areas.

This story emphasizes the need for improved communication of science, particularly One Health science, which addresses best approaches to complex health situations, and increased inclusion of science by those who govern.

Finally, pollution is responsible for one in six deaths globally each year, with air pollution being the greatest killer by far. Comparative data indicate that air pollution is roughly threefold deadlier than water pollution, and sixfold more deadly than occupational and soil-borne pollutants (Figure 6.4). Aerosols, as discussed in Chapter 4, are the most dangerous of the air pollutants, particularly the smallest particulates which are generally reported as **PM$_{2.5}$**. Air pollution is implicated in stroke, heart disease, lung cancer, and respiratory diseases including asthma. Unexpectedly, there is the growing list of associations between air pollution and non-respiratory diseases such as non-lung cancers, diabetes, osteoporosis, and obesity. Recent studies in mice show that these pollutants also affect the brain, either indirectly through the production of inflammatory molecules, or directly by traveling along the olfactory nerves to gain access to brain tissue. Either way, particulates can cause damage, which may result in dementia.

### 6.2.5 Cancer

Cancer, or unchecked cell growth, can form in any tissue, although it is more likely in tissues that are routinely prolific, like blood, skin, and reproductive cells. Any tissues that are exposed to high levels of **carcinogens**, like tobacco smoke or UV radiation, are prone to cancers, as well as tissues that are infected by cancer-inducing viruses like Human Papilloma Virus. Usually, cells become cancerous as a result of a mutation in genes, and most often it is a sequence of mutations rather than one single genetic alteration that allows cells to become immortal and invasive. These may be mutations that silence cancer-suppressing genes or mutations that activate cancer-promoting genes. Environmental oncology is a growing field of modern medicine because many carcinogens are found in the air and water. Indeed, the toxic pollutants discussed in Chapter 4 are so prevalent in our environment that cancer biologists and toxicologists are beginning to speak of the **exposome**, the catalog of

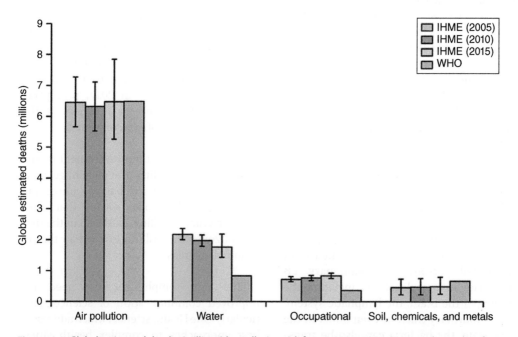

**Figure 6.4** Global estimated deaths (millions) by pollution risk factor, 2005–2015. Data used are taken from the Global Burden of Disease report produced by the Institute for Health Metrics and Evaluation (IHME) (2015 data) and by WHO (2012). *Source:* Reprinted from: Landrigan et al. (2017) with permission from Elsevier.

chemicals and toxins that humans encounter over a lifetime. These are substances that can have immediate ill effects, or may even influence future generations by generating epigenetic modifications as discussed in Chapter 4.

Translational medicine is one area where cancer provides opportunities for productive One Health collaboration. Human and animal physiologies are similar enough that generations of laboratory animals have served as invaluable substitutes for humans in the study of disease and development of drugs and treatments. Recently, however, the observation that the mechanisms and progression of certain diseases in animals and humans are similar has prompted human and veterinary oncologists to pool their knowledge and work in tandem to develop treatment protocols for patients in both species. As an example, a team including veterinarians from the University of Missouri – Columbia, College of Veterinary Medicine are working with human cancer researchers from Washington University's School of Medicine to develop a **viroimmunotherapy** procedure in dogs with malignant melanoma that will be readily applicable to human disease.

## 6.3 Climate Change and Human Health

The drivers of climate change are discussed in Chapter 3, and nearly all of the human health threats mentioned here are made worse by climate change. Figure 6.5 shows how increases in greenhouse gases and the resultant increase in temperature impact our nutritional status, mental health, and cardiovascular and respiratory diseases. Additionally, it leads to algal blooms and the expanded ranges of vector-borne diseases, with interconnecting and synergistic effects. The Lancet Commission concludes that the following four climate-mitigating steps must be taken to reduce this threat to human health: (i) a rapid phase-out of coal-fired plants to protect cardiovascular and respiratory health; (ii) a transition to cities that support and promote healthy lifestyles; (iii) investment in research, monitoring, and surveillance; and (iv) scaled-up financing for climate-ready health systems.

Further, anthropogenic changes to the environment increase the number and frequency of storms, floods, droughts, and fires. Rising sea levels will devastate coastal communities, and fracking activities increase earthquake frequency. These are natural disasters with unnatural accelerants. In most disaster scenarios, there is first a wave of death and injury from the disaster itself, followed by continued health risks associated with the destruction of infrastructure necessary for access to clean water, food, medicines, and other needed resources. In the days and weeks following the arrival of 2017's Hurricane Maria in Puerto Rico people died for a host of reasons, many of which were not officially attributed to the storm. When clean water is scarce, people will turn to whatever water is available, making secondary infectious diseases inevitable. In Puerto Rico, there was an outbreak of Legionnaire's disease, a respiratory illness associated with ill-managed water. In addition, the rate of death by heart attack rose, as did the suicide rate, and sepsis was a problem for people in disabled hospitals. Similarly, the 2010 earthquake in Haiti was followed by 9000 deaths from cholera (*Vibrio cholerae*).

As areas are made uninhabitable by such natural disasters, there will be those who can flee, and those who are left to live in intolerable conditions. It falls upon the WHO to coordinate responses to these disasters, and there have been mixed results in the WHO's ability to mobilize and move quickly. The WHO response to disease outbreaks is discussed further in Chapter 13.

## 6.4 Going Forward

Most human physicians do not encounter the concept of One Health in their medical training, although this is beginning to change.

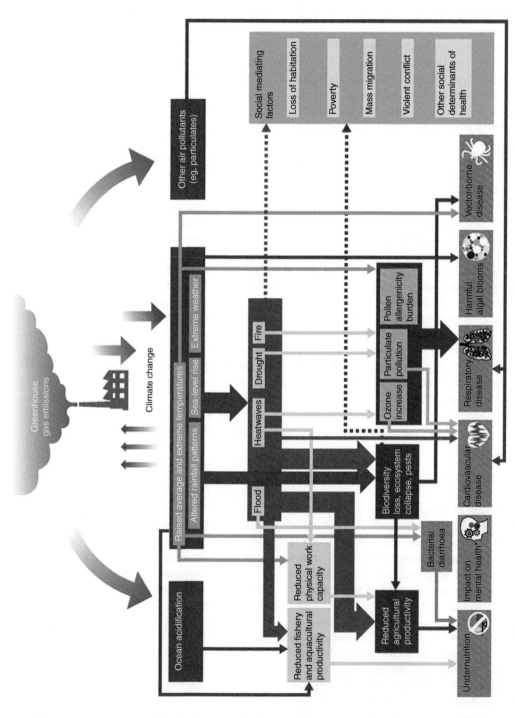

**Figure 6.5** The Interconnected Health Effects of Climate Change. The direct and indirect impacts that climate change can have on various aspects of human health are shown. *Source:* Reprinted from: Watts et al. (2017) with permission from Elsevier.

In Chapter 9, we will address the inclusion of One Health in medical training programs, a high-priority goal of the One Health movement. This will improve the overall understanding within the medical community of how the interconnections play out for their patients. Doctors and veterinarians are ubiquitous in US society. Most people routinely encounter medical doctors, and pet owners and livestock farmers frequently visit with their veterinarians. The recruitment of these medical professionals as One Health trainers will have far-reaching benefits because their sphere of influence is vast. The human physician has a patient who lives in the environment and is surrounded by animals, they are part of that patient's medical history, and we will all benefit when this is incorporated into the point of view of all medical professionals.

## End of Chapter Questions & Activities

A. Thought Questions:
   i) What health issues have you or members of your family experienced? Do any of them have an environmental component?
   ii) When you visit your physician with an illness, does the physician ever ask about your exposure to animals, such as asking if you have pets at home? Do you think the physician should do so and why or why not?
B. In-Class/Guided Activities-In small groups:
   i) Discuss 10 ways in which your health is impacted by animals every day.

   ii) Discuss 10 ways in which your health is impacted by plants every day.
   iii) Discuss 10 things that you do every day to improve the welfare of the environment or animals. Brainstorm 10 more and make a plan to do them.
C. At-home Activities:
   i) Try cutting your daily spending in half. Make a list of the things that you had to do without.
   ii) Consider your family, friends, and neighbors. Do any of them have health needs that you could meet? If anyone is ill, does their dog need walking? Does their cat need its box emptied? Think of ways that you can be useful.
D. Long-term Action Steps:
   i) Research volunteer organizations that you could help with donations of time or money.
E. Recommended Reading:
   Buckman, R. (2002). *Human Wildlife: The Life That Lives On Us*. Key Porter Books.
   Natterson-Horowitz, B. and Bowers, K. (2013). *Zoobiquity*. Vintage Books.
   Plotkin, M.J. (1993). *Tales of a Shaman's Apprentice*. Penguin.
   Rabinowitz, P.M. and Conti, L.A. (2010). *Human-Animal Medicine: Clinical Approaches to Zoonoses, Toxicants and Other Shared Health Risks*. Saunders.
   Reader, J. (2009). *Potato: A History of the Propitious Esculent*. Yale University Press.
   Wasik, B. and Murphy, M. (2012). *Rabid: A Cultural History of the World's Most Diabolical Virus*. Viking.

## Interview

*An Interview with Barbara Natterson-Horowitz, MD: Professor of Medicine in the Division of Cardiology at the David Geffen School of Medicine at UCLA and* *the co-director of the Evolutionary Medicine Program at UCLA. Dr. Natterson-Horowitz is also the author of the book* **Zoobiquity.**

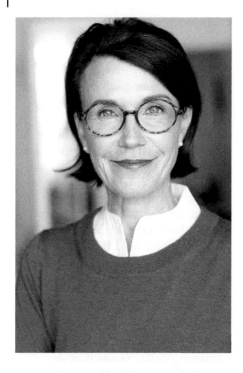

**When did you first hear about One Health?**

I began providing cardiovascular consultation for great apes at the Los Angeles Zoo. Through that exposure to the veterinarians at the zoo, I became intrigued by the many connections between human and animal health, particularly those connections that are non-infectious. I began exploring the overlaps between spontaneous occurring diseases of human and non-human animals. That led to the publication of *Zoobiquity*, and the creation of Zoobiquity conferences which bring veterinarians and physicians together to share knowledge and information.

**How is One Health important to your work?**

Once awakened to the overlap in human and animal pathology my entire career took a 90° turn. My academic work now focuses on the common origin of disease across animal species – namely evolutionary explanations for vulnerability. In my research and teaching I emphasize the need for physicians to considering environmental factors and comparative factors when learning about human disease.

**Do you see yourself as a One Health practitioner?**

I see One Health as a series of lenses and a collection of tools that we can use to better understanding some of the most complex and seemingly intractable problems in human and veterinary medicine.

**What can an individual do to make a difference for planetary health?**

Health care providers of all kinds should always bear in mind that the patient in front of you may be your *primary* responsibility, but the ecosystem in which that patient lives is also a responsibility. Of course, remaining mindful of both of these responsibilities simultaneously can be challenging, and may create tension, and conflict, and difficulty. But one of the responsibilities linked to the privilege of being a healthcare provider in the modern era is the importance of living in an interconnected world. Thinking outside of our individual silos will make all patients (human or animal) healthier.

**What motivated you to write** *Zoobiquity*?

Once I started consulting at the LA Zoo and attending rounds with the veterinarians, I was struck that their discussions of the management of breast cancer, diabetes, hypothyroidism, etc. were so similar to the conversations that I had participated in for many years in human hospitals. I realized how under-informed I was about the connections between animal and human health and became convinced that my profession (human medicine) could benefit from looking to our veterinary colleagues for insights. That there was a gap in the literature.

I thought writing a book about this would contribute to the medical literature.

**What would you like to share with students interested in One Health?**

For veterinarians, I would probably point them in the direction of public health. Public health veterinarians engage with human medical communities a great deal, and there is so much need in this area. To physicians, or to medical students, I would encourage them to begin thinking comparatively through their medical education and to consider engaging in scholarship and collaborations with animal-health experts in medical school, in post-graduate training. We are at the beginning of a new era of collaboration, and any medical student who is interested and works to advance this, will find herself or himself as a leader in the years to come.

---

### Case Study: Loss of Biodiversity Effects on Human Health

Co-authored by Zachary Carel

The effects of human activity on the environment are undeniable. From greenhouse gas production to deforestation, the spectrum of human behavior that damages the environment is vast. It is remarkable how little the planet is prioritized in everyday life. Most people are at least somewhat familiar with environmental struggles that result from their everyday behavior; however, what people seem to ignore is the effect that human activity has on wildlife, including biodiversity loss, and more importantly, the secondary effects that biodiversity loss has on human health. Some areas where biodiversity loss affects people are nutrition, infectious disease, and the effectiveness of modern medicine.

The high rate of deforestation in Africa has resulted in biodiversity loss across the continent, and many species have suffered the consequences, including loss of genetic diversity within populations. Although controversial, the dilution effect suggests that the less diverse a disease source population is, the more likely they are to have been targeted by disease vectors. Though this might seem unimportant, primates are the animals that are the most genetically similar to humans, and they are a major source of food in Africa. Therefore, any human that hunts or handles primate products (bushmeat) is more likely to be exposed to a variety of genetically divergent viruses if the population of primates experiences declining diversity.

Another harmful anthropogenic practice is pesticide use to improve the rates of plant growth. Such practices have become very common in today's society as they are very effective in eliminating insects from destroying plant growth; however, one common side effect is that they can also be fatal to non-target species. For example, many commonly used pesticides can prove fatal to amphibians with which they come into contact. Once again, this does not seem like something that is particularly relevant to humans, but frog skin has become an important ingredient in new types of antibiotics. It has been recognized since 2010 that frog skin contains chemicals that have the power to combat drug-resistant infections. Hundreds of antibiotic substances have been isolated from frog skin secretions, including one that is effective against Methicillin-Resistant *Staphylococcus aureus* (MRSA). Unfortunately, that substance was isolated from the Foothill Yellow-Legged Frog (*Rana boylii*), which is now facing extinction.

If these patterns and rates of biodiversity loss continue, it is inevitable that human health will ultimately be harmed.

## Works Cited

Alderete, T.L., Habre, R., Toledo-Corral, C.M. et al. (2017). Longitudinal associations between ambient air pollution with insulin sensitivity, β-cell function, and adiposity in Los Angeles Latino children. *Diabetes* 66 (7): 1789–1796. doi: 10.2337/db16-1416.

Borgobello, B. (2010) Frog skin could thwart antibiotic-resistant germs. https://newatlas.com/frog-skin-antibiotic-resistant-germs/16164 (accessed December 29, 2017).

Bosch, F.X. and de Sanjosé, S. (2007). The epidemiology of human papillomavirus infection and cervical cancer. *Disease Markers* 23 (4): 213–227.

Bousquet, J. and Khaltaev, N. (eds.) (2007). *Global Surveillance, Prevention and Control of Chronic Respiratory Diseases: A Comprehensive Approach*. Switzerland: WHO Press, Geneva.

Bryan, J.N., Curiel, D., Dmitriev, I. et al. (2016) Viroimmunotherapy for malignant melanoma in the companion dog model. In: Stroud, C. A.). One health overview, facilitating advances in comparative medicine and translational research. *Clinical and Translational Medicine* 5 (Suppl 1): 26.

Carrington, D. (2017) Huge Increase in Badger Culling Will See up to 33,500 Animals Shot. *The Guardian*, 11 September 2017. https://www.theguardian.com/environment/2017/sep/11/huge-increase-badger-culling-see-up-to-33500-animals-shot (accessed July 11, 2018).

Carrington, D. (2018) What is biodiversity and why does it matter to us? The Guardian, 12 March 2018. https://www.theguardian.com/news/2018/mar/12/what-is-biodiversity-and-why-does-it-matter-to-us (accessed July 11, 2018).

Cassidy, L.M., Martiniano, R., Murphy, E.M. et al. (2016). Neolithic and Bronze Age migration to Ireland and establishment of the insular Atlantic genome. *Proceedings of the National Academy of Sciences of the United States of America* 113 (2): 368–373.

Christianson, A., Howson, C.P., and Modell, B. (2005). *March of Dimes: Global Report on Birth Defects, the Hidden Toll of Dying and Disabled Children*. White Plains, NY: March of Dimes Birth Defects Foundation.

Costanzo, L.S. (2014). *Physiology*. Philadelphia, PA: Saunders.

Finlay, B.B. (2017) The Role of the Microbiome in Early Childhood. *Presented at the AAAS 2017 Annual Meeting*. Boston, MA.

Gauderman, W.J., Avol, E., Gilliland, F.M. et al. (2004). The effect of air pollution on lung development from 10 to 18 years of age. *New England Journal of Medicine* 351: 1057–1067.

Gilbert, S.F. and Barresi, M.J.F. (2016). *Developmental Biology*. Sunderland (MA): Sinauer.

Graham, J.P., Leibler, J.H., Price, L.B. et al. (2008). The animal-human interface and infectious disease in industrial food animal production: rethinking biosecurity and biocontainment. *Public Health Reports* 123: 282–299.

Haynie, D. (2016) *10 Countries With the Most Irish Emigrants* https://www.usnews.com/news/best-countries/articles/2016-03-17/10-countries-with-the-most-irish-emigrants (accessed December 29, 2017).

International Agency for Research on Cancer of the World Health Organization (2016) Questions and Answers on Glyphosate. https://www.iarc.fr/en/media-centre/iarcnews/pdf/Q&A_Glyphosate.pdf (accessed December 29, 2017).

Kaur, J. (2014). A comprehensive review on metabolic syndrome. *Cardiology Research and Practice* 2014: 943162. doi: 10.1155/2014/943162.

Landrigan, P.J., Fuller, R., Nereus, B.E. et al. (2017). The Lancet commission on pollution and health. *The Lancet* 391: 462–512. doi: 10.1016/S0140-6736(17)32345-0.

Liu, L., Oza, S., Hogan, D. et al. (2015). Global, regional, and national causes of child mortality in 2000–13, with projections to inform post-2015 priorities: an updated systematic analysis. *The Lancet* 385 (9966): 430–440.

Mitchell, E.A.D., Mulhauser, B., Mulot, M. et al. (2017). Worldwide survey of neonicotinoids in honey. *Science* 358 (6359): 109–111.

Nunes-Alves, C., Booty, M.G., Carpenter, S.M. et al. (2014). In search of a new paradigm for protective immunity to TB. *Nature Reviews in Microbiology* 12: 289–299. doi: 10.1038/nrmicro3230.

O'Haire, M. (2010). Companion animals and human health: benefits, challenges, and the road ahead. *Journal of Veterinary Behavior* 5 (5): 226–234.

Ostfeld, R.S. (2009). Biodiversity loss and the rise of zoonotic pathogens. *Clinical Microbiology and Infection: The Official Publication of the European Society of Clinical Microbiology and Infectious Diseases* 15 (Suppl. 1): 40–43.

Peeters, M., Courgnaud, V., Abela, B. et al. (2002). Risk to human health from a plethora of simian immunodeficiency viruses in primate Bushmeat. *Emerging Infectious Diseases* 8 (5): 451–457. http://wwwnc.cdc.gov/eid/article/8/5/01-0522_article (accessed April 9, 2016).

Philpott, T. (2013) New Study: Common Pesticides Kill Frogs on Contact. http://www.motherjones.com/tom-philpott/2013/01/new-study-common-pesticides-kill-frogs-contact (accessed April 9, 2016).

Plotkin, S.A. (2006). The history of rubella and rubella vaccination leading to elimination. *Clinical Infectious Diseases* 43: S164–S168.

Prada, D., Zhong, J., Colicino, E. et al. (2017). Association of air particulate pollution with bone loss over time and bone fracture risk: analysis of data from two independent studies. *Lancet Planetary Health* 1: e337–e347.

Quigley, F. Haiti's Earthquake was Devastating, the Cholera Epidemic was Worse. *The Nation (online)* 15 October 2016. https://www.thenation.com/article/haitis-earthquake-was-devastating-the-cholera-epidemic-was-worse (accessed May 17, 2018).

Reece, J., Urry, L.A., Cain, M.L. et al. (2014). *Campbell's Biology*. Boston: Pearson.

Sam, D.C. (2017). Congenital toxoplasmosis: time for a new treatment approach. *Global Journal of Intellectual and Developmental Disabilities* 2 (1): 555579.

Siddiqui, A.A. (18 July 2013). *Autopsies on Indian School Children Confirm 22 Died from Poisoning Caused by Insecticide in Lunch*. Associated Press.

Sutter, J.D., Santiago, L., and Khusubu, S. Maria's Uncounted Dead. *CNN (online)*, 20 November 2017. http://www.cnn.com/2017/11/20/health/hurricane-maria-uncounted-deaths-invs/index.html (accessed December 29, 2017).

Tantibanchachai, C. (2014) Teratogens: The Human Embryo Project. https://embryo.asu.edu/pages/teratogens (accessed July 11, 2018).

United Nations, Department of Economic and Social Affairs, Population Division (2017) World Population Prospects: The 2017 Revision, Key Findings and Advance Tables. Working Paper No. ESA/P/WP/248.

United Nations Inter-agency Group for Child Mortality Estimation (UN IGME), *Levels & Trends in Child Mortality:* Report 2017, Estimates Developed by the UN Inter-agency Group for Child Mortality Estimation, United Nations Children's Fund, New York, 2017.

Underwood, E. (2017). The polluted brain. *Science* 355 (6323): 342–345.

Veersham, C. (2012). Natural products derived from plants as a source of drugs. *Journal of Advanced Pharmaceutical Technology & Research* 3 (4): 200–201. doi: 10.4103/2231-4040.104709.

Vrijheid, M., Slama, R., Robinson, O. et al. (2014). The Human Early-Life Exposome (HELIX): project rationale and design. *Environmental Health Perspectives* 122: 535–544. doi: 10.1289/ehp.1307204.

Watts, N., Adger, W.N., Ayeb-Karlsson, S. et al. (2017). The Lancet Countdown: tracking progress on health and climate change. *The Lancet* 389 (10074): 1151–1164. doi: 10.1016/S0140-6736(16)32124-9.

World Food Programme (2016) The Year in Review. http://www1.wfp.org/zero-hunger (accessed December 29, 2017).

World Health Organization (1948) Constitution of the World Health Organization. http://www.who.int/governance/eb/who_constitution_en.pdf (accessed December 26, 2017).

Yoshida, K., Schuenemann, V.J., Cano, L.M. et al. (2013). The rise and fall of the Phytophthora infestans lineage that triggered the Irish potato famine. *eLife* 2: e00731. doi: 10.7554/eLife.00731.

**Part III**

**Practitioners and Their Tools**

7

# The One Health Practitioner

On December 2, 2013, a two-year-old boy became ill. His name was Emile, and he lived in the village of Meliandou in Southern Guinea. Earlier that day, Emile and several other children from the village had been playing in a hollow tree just outside of their town. Scientists would soon discover that the tree housed a large colony of insectivorous bats, but that night, when Emile developed a fever and headache, no one paid much attention. His parents assumed that he had picked up an ordinary bug.

Four days later, Emile was dead. Emile is presumably patient zero of the 2014–2015 Zaire Ebola (EBOV) epidemic, which eventually spanned three continents and killed over 11 000 people. Emile's sister, mother, and grandmother succumbed to the virus as patients two, three, and four, after which the virus spread to friends and relatives who had tended to the family and attended their funerals. Emile's great aunt had traveled from her nearby village of Dawa to help prepare her sister for burial, and then unknowingly carried the virus back home with her. That same week a midwife traveled from Meliandou to Dandou Pombo Village, where she and several family members became ill and died. By New Year's Day, stories of the mysterious, deadly illness had spread throughout the area, prompting the afflicted to seek skilled help at the only nearby clinic, a malaria clinic in the town of Guéckédou. The clinic was run by Médecins sans Frontières (MSF) (also known as Doctors

without Borders), an internationally recognized, medical aid organization that had been battling endemic malaria in the region for decades. But this outbreak was different, and the following week, despite taking all proper precautions, a clinic worker and a doctor fell ill. The clinic worker and her mother died, and there was a large family gathering in Guéckédou for their burials. The doctor also died, but his brothers transported his body to yet another village, Kissidougou, for burial. At least seven mourners at that funeral contracted the disease and died. Throughout the winter, the mysterious illness spread death throughout the remote region, village-to-village, and across porous borders, largely unnoticed by the rest of the world. By February, the death toll was rising in the three countries that converged at ground zero of the outbreak: Guinea, Sierra Leone, and Liberia. On March 10, medics on the ground alerted the Ministry of Health of Guinea and MSF headquarters in Geneva that there was an outbreak of something with a troublingly high mortality rate. MSF testing identified it as Ebola Virus (EBOV) (Figure 7.1).

Ebola was not new to Africa in 2014, but it was new, and unanticipated, in West Africa. The assumption by healthcare workers that they were dealing with the usual and the expected allowed EBOV to get a head start of several months on the epidemiologists who would now need to contain it. As Ebola spread across Western Africa, it exposed weaknesses

*Introduction to One Health: An Interdisciplinary Approach to Planetary Health*, First Edition.
Sharon L. Deem, Kelly E. Lane-deGraaf and Elizabeth A. Rayhel.
© 2019 John Wiley & Sons, Inc. Published 2019 by John Wiley & Sons, Inc.
Companion website: www.wiley.com/go/deem/health

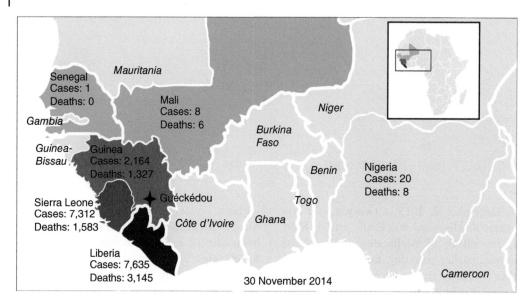

Figure 7.1 Map of the area effected by Ebola dated November 30, 2014. The number of cases per country are shown. The epicenter of the outbreak is the village of Guéckédou. *Source:* Art by Mikael Häggström, updated by Brian Groen (CC0 1.0 Public Domain).

in the systems that were supposed to protect the people of the area. All three governments struggled with a lack of resources and the inability to ramp up a response. Before Ebola, Sierra Leone's medical system provided two nurses for every ten thousand people, and the other two countries were only slightly better prepared. None of the involved countries had isolation-ward capabilities, and when the weight of an EBOV epidemic hit, it quickly overwhelmed the failing medical infrastructures that were in place.

By June, only a handful of international aid organizations were still willing to work in the West-African region. Those groups were severely overextended, and their staffs were exhausted. MSF reported dealing with active Ebola in more than 60 locations in all three countries. In Liberia, two American aid organizations, Samaritan's Purse and Serving in Mission, tried to expand their facilities to meet the need but each day they could only admit the number of new patients that would replace those that had died the night before. The rest were sent home.

Social forces were at work as well, which made this outbreak even more volatile.

A history of political instability, corruption, and devastating poverty had engendered among the people a distrust of government and foreigners. The fact that the arrival of foreigners wearing head-to-toe biohazard suits coincided with the outbreak of a devastating disease only validated people's distrust. Worse still, the foreign doctors insisted on removing the dead in sealed bags, before families could say their goodbyes. In Liberia, many believed that their own government was using the hospitals to poison them in a government-led slaughter. Rumors spread, and in July, thousands marched on the Ebola treatment unit in Kenema, Sierra Leone, after a former nurse at the facility suggested that the virus was a hoax to conceal cannibalism at the hospital. Communication and trust were required, but late to the stage, in the fight to contain Ebola in 2014.

We now know the last pieces of the puzzle regarding how this virus got so far out of control so quickly. This was no ordinary EBOV. In any zoonotic event, one of the first questions for epidemiologists is: how is the pathogen spreading? In one scenario there is an animal source, and people come into repeated contact with the infectious animals. In another, the virus jumps to the human population but then begins person-to-person transmission. The first study to come out of this outbreak was ready for print by August 2014, which is lightning fast in scientific circles, but it had been costly; five of the authors succumbed to the disease before the results could be published, including Sierra Leone's top epidemiologist, Dr. S. Humarr Khan. Their work was critical to the Ebola response, however, as it gave vital information about transmission of the disease. Working with the Kenema Government Hospital in Sierra Leone, the group discovered evidence of person-to-person transmission associated with the funeral of a popular local healer, an event that they could link to over three hundred EBOV cases.

At the height of the outbreak, people in affected areas were desperate, mistrustful, and unconvinced of the risks. They treated their dead as they always had, which included a lot of washing and touching of the body. In rural areas, the education of imams, pastors, and chiefs of the risks resulted in behavioral changes associated with caring for the ill, and burial. Such trusted voices were not available in the cities, where there were riots against the healthcare workers, ambulance drivers, and burial personnel. It was frustrating and demoralizing for the volunteers on the ground, who were trying to help a terrified and distrustful public without the necessary resources to save lives. MSF staff were braced for a continued struggle when in the fall of 2014, the outbreak began to subside. No one knows exactly why, but hypotheses include greater availability of beds, increased efforts to control infection, and a general agreement by the public to change their burial practices.

## 7.1 Who Is a One Health Practitioner?

An analysis of the successes and failures of the Ebola outbreak response allows the identification of the professionals who were, or

would have been, crucial to dealing with this notable One Health challenge. On the front lines of the outbreak, doctors, nurses, allied health professionals, public health professionals, ambulance drivers, and volunteers who cared for the ill were critical One Health practitioners. However, they were quickly overwhelmed and lacking was a team of backup personnel trained to handle a highly infectious disease as well as additional healthcare workers to absorb the non-crisis medical needs of the community. This support materialized once the WHO proclaimed the status of Public Health Emergencies of International Concern, but the process of communicating the seriousness of the situation delayed that proclamation. From the wildlife perspective, initial reactions to the disease were devastating. Because Ebola is a zoonotic disease, fear caused people to respond with indiscriminant and uninformed violence toward wildlife, leading to a little-reported biodiversity crisis in the region. Also, gorillas and other great ape species are susceptible to Ebola and over a third of their global population has fallen victim to the virus, many during the 2014–2015 episode. Backup support for the conservationists and public-health veterinarians who could monitor the status of wildlife and educate the people at risk would have helped tremendously. Thus it makes sense that a One Health team approach to future zoonotic outbreaks should include professionals with wildlife experience from the start.

Community needs are another area where a One Health approach will be beneficial in future outbreaks. During the Ebola outbreak a specific social behavior, the treatment of the dead with hands-on interactions, put people at risk of infection. Eventually, WHO anthropologists convinced community and religious leaders to approve of safe burial methods, and that was critical to the eventual containment of the outbreak. A One Health team should include professionals who focus on the social, historical, and political atmosphere of the region, in order to

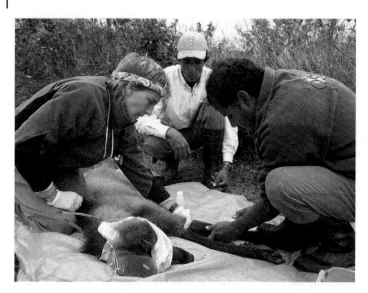

Figure 7.2 Monitoring the health of Maned Wolves of Noel Kempff Mercado National Park. A team of veterinarians take blood from a Maned Wolf (*Chrysocyon brachyurus*), an International Union for Conservation of Nature near threatened species. Monitoring the health status of wildlife is one area where One Health practitioners can make a significant contribution to planetary health.

coordinate the most effective approach. Also, the social and animal welfare organizations were swamped by the unexpected enormity of the crisis, resulting in problems ranging from the inability to handle the sudden onslaught of orphans to the dead leaving untended farms and the resultant drop in food production. Animals were abandoned, homes left empty, and there were not enough gravediggers to meet demand. All of these issues point to the need for organized, quickly mobilizing response teams that can work within, and supplement, the local emergency-response organizations.

Regarding leadership, the governments involved in the 2014 outbreak were understandably reluctant to announce a health crisis within their borders, leading to a delay in response that ultimately cost lives. A plan for global response to an emergency that does not financially penalize the country of impact would minimize the fear of financial loss. Business is inevitably disrupted during a major health crisis. One Health logisticians, businesspeople, and service coordinators, with experience in arranging for infrastructure repairs, redirecting tourists to unaffected parts of the country, and rerouting product and supply routes, would be valuable indeed.

One Health, however, expands far beyond zoonoses and epidemics. When the professionals needed to address the One Health issues documented throughout this text are included, the true scope of the need for One Health practitioners is revealed. But, who is a One Health practitioner? One Health relies on a team approach, but most of those involved think of themselves in terms of what it is they bring to the group: such as public health professionals, educators, veterinarians, social workers, politicians, or a diverse collection of other professional identities (Figure 7.2). In the end, however, anyone with something to offer to the solution of a complex One Health issue *is* a One Health professional.

In the remainder of this chapter, we identify some of the key professional and educational components of a One Health practitioner, beginning with the foundational skills of interdisciplinary, team-based, problem solving.

## 7.2 The Beauty of an Interdisciplinary, Team-Based Approach

Valuing diverse input is one of the keys to successful teamwork. For instance, if a team that includes an insect biologist is designing a One Health-based city, they do not need to bring in more insect biologists, since that point-of-view is covered. The team would need skilled architects, transportation specialists, and perhaps some engineers. Thus, diversity on a team can prevent knowledge gaps. However, the benefit of diversity in a team goes beyond an expanded knowledge and perspective base. Research published in 2010 suggests that participation in diverse teams transforms the participants, by prompting them to prepare more thoroughly and to perform better, than when participating in a homogenous team. A different study was published in 2014, in which investigators used the surnames of the authors of 2.5 million articles published in peer-reviewed journals based in the USA, to make two interesting observations. First, like everyone else, scientists tend to collaborate with colleagues of their own ethnicity, as there was not much diversity among the authors of a paper, and second, papers with more diversity in authorship tended to be published in higher-impact journals.

Team approaches consider the points of view of all contributing voices, and bring a diverse set of skills to the table. The greatest challenges of the Anthropocene are complex, and as with the Ebola outbreak, solutions and responses will need coordinated input from many sectors. The chapter case study deals with the association between tuberculosis (TB, a disease caused by *Mycobacterium tuberculosis*) and poverty. That topic can provide one potential example of the benefit of the coordinated approach of One Health. A traditionally trained scientist might see a TB outbreak from a purely microbial perspective, in which getting the proper antibiotics to the patient is of paramount importance. However, poverty and homelessness are factors in the spread of TB, and a social-services provider might see patient housing solutions as equally important to containing the outbreak. These are not mutually exclusive actions, and with a team-based One Health approach, members of a response team will respect other points of view, valuing inclusivity and creativity in opinion for problem solving. Even among closely aligned professionals, there can be a need for bridge-building, as scientists and medical professionals often have a siloed and isolated educational background.

### 7.2.1 Problem Solving

Problem solving is a life skill that everyone uses every day, but when confronted with large, complicated, and socio-politically charged problems, the process can be daunting. Support in the face of challenge is another reason why a team is beneficial, but problem-solving also calls for creativity. Albert Einstein said, "If I had an hour to solve a problem I'd spend fifty-five minutes defining the problem, and then five minutes looking for solutions." In many cases, people fail to understand the true source of a problem and spend valuable time chipping away at symptoms rather than causes. Practice in problem solving helps develop analytical skills that allow people to cut right to the heart of a problem. Interestingly, Einstein also quipped, "We cannot solve our problems with the same thinking we used to create them." The approach to such problems as climate change, global income inequality, the increase in human–wildlife interactions, food insecurity, and others will require creative thought. The One Health approach is itself one such creative solution. However, within One Health, for each concern that arises, we will need people who think outside the box. Inventors, engineers, and technological entrepreneurs are needed to imagine a future with floating cities, biodegradable cars, and other such preposterous but potentially world-changing ideas.

## 7.2.2 One Health Is Anticipatory

One of the major premises of One Health is that it will be far cheaper to prevent catastrophe than to deal with one that has occurred. This was the conclusion of the 2010 meeting of the Energy, Environment and Development Programme and the Centre on Global Health Security at Chatham House, a think tank of experts in animal, human, and environmental health. Determining the actual cost of a catastrophe can be a complicated and unsatisfactory practice, as discussed in Chapter 12. The need for these data opens the door to opportunities for economy-minded personnel in One Health. Understanding costs, values, and economic behavior, and framing arguments and policies in those terms, is important to convincing people, municipalities, and governments to invest in preventive strategies.

Prevention requires an ability to predict the outcomes of current events. Global climate change is a notable example where the multitude of variables results in predictions and models that can vary slightly from model to model. The World Climate Research Programme coordinates the Coupled Model Intercomparison Project (CMIP). It is a massive effort to normalize and integrate the models and predictions of over 30 modeling groups annually to increase the predictive power of the models.

In addition to climate change, the Chatham House report mentioned earlier includes two other notable health concerns that have potential interventions "upstream" of disease transmission: land use change and global trade practices, which opens the door to farming and food production as One Health-associated sectors.

## 7.3 Occupational Opportunities in One Health

This text presents six over-arching themes or areas in which there are roles for One Health practitioners. Part I, *An Introduction and Impetus for One Health*, gives an understanding of how planetary health has come to need a new approach. In Part II, *The One Health Triad*, introduces the health concerns that stem from the interconnected wellbeing of the environment, animals, and humans. The current Part, *Practitioners and Their Tools*, explores the opportunities and necessary skills for One Health practitioners, and Part IV, *How to Start a Movement*, addresses the challenges involved in advocacy and education concerning science, risk, and the need to change. Part V explores the *Humanities of One Health*, and the interdisciplinary points of view that are critical to producing coherent and effective One Health strategies.

### 7.3.1 The One Health Triad

Almost any human-medicine professional, such as doctors, nurses, osteopaths, dentists, nurse practitioners, and physician assistants, can be One Health practitioners if they choose to do so. Some specialties in which One Health opportunities exist are oncology, infectious disease, emergency medicine, allergy and immunology, obstetrics and gynecology, ophthalmology, pediatrics, dentistry, preventative medicine, and toxicology. As an example, an oncologist might focus on the environmental triggers of cancers. Similarly, the allied-health specialties have options in One Health. These include medical laboratory specialists with expertise in pathogen identification, nutritionists, and therapists with experience in occupational, physical, or mental health therapy.

Similarly, the veterinary specialties of oncology, infectious disease, and emergency medicine are potential areas for One Health practice, but within the animal domain, there are other pertinent fields as well. These include wildlife care and management, zoological practice, food-animal management, preventive practice, toxicology, laboratory-animal, and translational medicine in which animals are active participants in disease research and drug development. Professionals in this area include veterinarians, veterinary assistants, and disease ecologists.

While the medical specialists for animals and humans are easy to identify, those who mitigate diseases or imbalances in nature are less clear. In a sense, anyone who works with habitat protection, animal conservation, ecology, water and air management, or many of the other One Health specialties listed here, works to repair small pieces of the ecosystem. Some examples of professions in environmental protection are botanists, conservation biologists, environmental engineers, and plant pathologists.

Treatment of disease often involves medications and preventatives, which opens up another field within One Health. However costs for therapeutic drugs and preventative vaccines can be prohibitive, making the development of cheap and effective therapies a goal, for both human patients and animals. Because drug discovery is an expensive undertaking, this is an area where public-private partnerships can be useful, as well. Examples of occupations in this area include pharmacologists and drug or vaccine-production specialists.

Public health practitioners are a crucial piece of the One Health picture. Dealing with public health crises is part of the mandate in public health, making these practitioners well aligned with the goals and objectives of One Health. Examples of occupations and activities within the field of public health include epidemiologists, health educators, and field investigators.

The basic sciences are where the mechanisms and characteristics of diseases are discovered and, as with medicine, almost any of the basic sciences can take on a One Health perspective. Some examples of potential One Health occupations from the biological sciences include developmental biologists, geneticists, toxicologists, biochemists, ecologists, and disease ecologists. From within the environmental sciences, examples include bioclimatologists, botanists, conservation biologists, environmentalists, environmental engineers, and wildlife management specialists.

Finally, food safety is a significant sector for One Health. At any point along the path from the wild, the ocean, or pasture, meat may be infected with disease causing agents. Meat handlers from hunters to small-farmers to large meat processing factories must take care to properly handle and inspect meat quality. In addition, the resources needed to produce meat, especially beef, are burdensome enough that it is unsustainable as the only protein source for a growing human population. Additionally, as the demand for food increases, farmers are faced with One Health decisions as they weigh the need to feed their families against the use of damaging pesticides and fertilizers. Such things as organic and intensified farming, hydroponics, and water-conserving vertical farming are just a few farming innovations. Similarly, water must be managed and monitored for access and safety. One Health occupations in food safety include farmers, ranchers, butchers, policy makers, watershed managers, and more.

### 7.3.2 One Health Practitioners and Their Tools

One Health tool development includes some areas of basic science, certainly, but new tools for One Health are also invented in corporate labs, software firms, or possibly a basement workshop. Computer programming and device development are essential to the science of One Health, with possible areas of focus including biodiversity tracking, disease tracking and projections, climate change modeling for proactive attention, and modeling for conservation and human public-health needs, as land and water use changes occur. Developing technologies that can be applied to One Health include cellular phone systems, the internet, and devices that allow remote information gathering such as drone reconnaissance, and monitors for data collection on everything from animal movements to the weather. Examples of occupations in tool development include computer programmers, bioinformaticists, GIS specialists, meteorologists, and humanitarian engineers.

### 7.3.3 How to Start a Movement

This part of the book focuses on reaching out to the public to inform, convince, and inspire them to adopt an attitude of awareness. It includes a discussion of the state of science education, and the communication skills needed to influence people. Science education at all levels can and should include a One Health perspective. Teaching children about the interconnectedness of life will allow the next generation to develop One Health perspectives early, which, hopefully, will persist into adulthood. Teachers and specialists in schools and the informal educational venues such as zoos, aquariums, museums, and such are instrumental in engaging the general public. Similarly, communication with the general public is critical to promoting responsible behavior and advancing One Health informed decision making. While some scientists are good communicators, there is a concerted effort within the science community to improve communication skills. Examples of occupations from this area include teachers, journalists, novelists, storytellers, and the photographers who bring One Health to life.

### 7.3.4 The Humanity of Science

Understanding One Health in the context of daily life is the focus of this section. The social services play a vital role in managing human need during a crisis. Even if only the moderately dire predictions of climate change come to pass, a significant amount of currently inhabited land will become uninhabitable, initiating predictable refugee problems for both humans and animals, wild and domestic. Also, as shown in the Ebola story, meaningful outreach to an impacted community must begin with an understanding of the culture, behavior, and attitudes of those affected. Communication during a crisis must acknowledge the humanity and values that underpin any society. Examples of occupations in this area include social

workers, anthropologists, historians, linguists, ethicists, religious leaders, crisis volunteer coordinators and humanitarian engineers, and wildlife conservationists.

Governments, generally, provide for the wellbeing of their citizens. To that end, the One Health community must develop local, regional, federal, and international leaders in justice, law, and policy. The need for globally understood and respected human rights has never been greater. This will inevitably worsen if the human population increases to the point of overwhelming its resources, while climate change and pollution reduce access to air, water, and food. Local governments also manage urban development. As the majority of the human population now live in cities, the functionality of cities becomes pivotal. Local-resource management and conservation, environmental, resource, and transportation engineers will be critical in developing cities that work. Crisis management also comes under governmental oversight, and includes the ability to respond locally, regionally, and even internationally to infectious and environmental crises. These predictably require temporary housing, animal, family and orphan fostering, food and water delivery, emergency, medical and funeral service management, and infrastructure management, because natural disasters often disrupt water, communications, and electricity.

Providing for the security of its people is a role of government, and there are several security-related areas in One Health. The military often handles large-scale security threats, which can include war. Wars are inevitable; thus for military One Health advocates, the goal is to conduct war in the midst of people, animals, and the environment, while protecting the health of as many as possible. Also, with bioterrorism as a continuing threat, the ability to determine the cause of any infectious outbreak is of immediate concern. In an intentionally produced infectious crisis, the military and law enforcement personnel would need to increase vigilance for secondary attacks. Further, climate change puts our food and future at risk, and many consider this to be a national security concern. Examples of occupations in these areas include lawyers, politicians, diplomats, judges, city planners, resource managers, landscape and greenspace artists, first responders, military strategists, and bioterrorism experts.

Finally, from the economics and business perspective, the success of One Health will depend on whether it is financially feasible. It is assumed that it is more efficient to be proactive than reactive and to combine services and reduce expenses, but that will need to be shown. It is difficult to ascertain the exact cost of any disaster, and impossible to calculate the savings realized by avoiding one. Economists model these complicated scenarios and will be instrumental in determining the bottom-line, as well as best approaches, for future One Health issues. Business leaders understand the complexity of maintaining productivity in the face of challenge. When an area is impacted by disease, drought, or other, the local businesses must be able to thrive, and resources must continue to flow. Logistics experts, global trade organizations, and such can help support local economies in the face of crisis.

Business innovation is also an area for One Health. Figure 7.3 shows vertically produced lettuce, just one of the agri-business innovations that could change the way we produce food. Moreover, we are moving toward a One Health / green economy that prioritizes people, animals, and the environment while maintaining profitability.

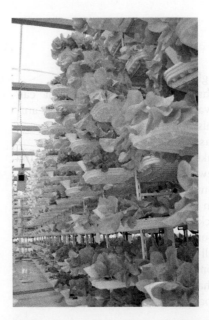

Figure 7.3 Vertical Farming. Vertical farming is just one innovative idea for reducing water and land needed to feed the growing human population. Here lettuce is grown in an indoor, controlled environment. *Source:* Valcenteu, https://commons.wikimedia.org/wiki/File:VertiCrop.jpg. CC BY-SA 3.0.

## 7.4 The Citizen Practitioner

Ultimately, we all make decisions every day that have an impact on health within the One Health Triad. Should we use chemicals on our lawns? What textiles were used to make the clothes we buy? What dyes? Do we eat locally produced foods, or import them from half a world away? Do our choices have an impact on orangutans? It is not realistic to think that the general public has the time or interest in corralling all of the details required to live a completely health-positive life, but when there is a pervasive culture of One Health, the choices will be clearer. This approach should start with children, who can learn good habits rather than have to break old, bad ones. Parent educators can have an enormous impact on the future. Truly, anyone who models a One Health-conscious lifestyle is also a non-professional practitioner: the avid recycler or the person who gives to One Health causes. When people start making their daily decisions based on the common good of life on the planet, One Health thinking will have taken hold.

## End of Chapter Questions & Activities

A. Thought Questions:
  i) What skills do you have that can advance the health of humans, animals, and the environment?
B. In-Class/Guided Activities:
  i) Take almost any headline from the newspaper and look for One Health connections.
  ii) On paper, build a fantasy team to tackle a complicated health issues in your community, like where to build a ball-field.
C. At-home Activities:
  i) Whatever your level of training, try to expand your circle of influence. Model One Health for classmates, clients, family, students.
D. Long-term Action Steps:
  i) Develop a list of One Health occupations or specialties that interest you and explore the requirements and steps needed to enter the field.
E. Recommended Reading:
  Baron, N. (2010). *Escape from the Ivory Tower: A Guide to Making Your Science Matter*. Island Press.
  Feinsinger, P. (2001). *Designing Field Studies for Biodiversity Conservation*. Island Press.
  Gibbs, J.P., Hunter, M.L. Jr., and Sterling, E.J. (1998). *Problem-Solving in Conservation Biology and Wildlife Management: Exercises for Class, Field, and Laboratory*. Blackwell Science, Ltd.

## Interview

*An Interview with Lise Saffran, MPH, MFA: the Director of the Master of Public Health Program at the University of Missouri, Columbia*

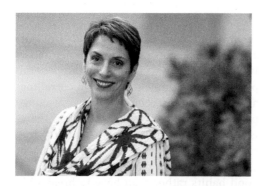

**How is One Health important to your work?**

Public health, with its focus on populations, is really about taking a step back and looking at the evidence for patterns in health outcomes, and for opportunities for prevention. One Health, since it focuses on the connections between humans, animals, and ecosystems, is another way to explore these patterns. It pushes us, as public health practitioners, to ask additional questions: not just how will human health be impacted, but what are these relationships?

**Do you see yourself as a One Health practitioner?**

I do. Public health is impacted by and impacts everything, and I think you could argue the same for One Health. So, the challenge is: how to focus? You have to understand that health requires a cross-cutting approach, but you also have to do something somewhere, and you cannot do all things. I do consider myself a One Health practitioner because I have learned to ask those questions. If I focus on human health, or on educating graduate students who are going to make human health their focus, I keep those One-Health connections in mind. Because if you have those connections and patterns and relationships in your mind, it will make you approach the work differently.

**What can an individual do to make a difference for planetary health?**

I do think that the greatest impacts are made on the policy level, and by that I mean the internal policies and laws of each nation participating, as well as international efforts and policies. So individuals need to be asking about, and paying attention to, policy. So anything from laws and regulations that protect air and water. Are these being strengthened? Or are they being disregarded? Who are the people in the agencies who are taking climate change seriously and what policy plans do they propose?

And fortunately, individuals, especially in this country (USA) can impact policy. We have mechanisms to impact policy in our country, and they do make a difference. So that's primarily where change is going to happen if it's going to happen. However, obviously, individuals can take other measures, conservation measures, conserving energy and recycling, and buying less new stuff. I do not think those things are mutually exclusive though.

**How can we encourage people to care about planetary health?**

One of the reasons that I teach my storytelling classes is there's a lot of research evidence that supports the idea that people become engaged in issues and persuaded by evidence when it is accompanied by contextual information. Stories and anecdotes, and things that involve them emotionally make them care about the issue. It's not just focused on sort of a dry representation of the data, even though the data is really important. And I am often surprised at how unprepared scientists and academics are to convey how important issues are that they are working on and the work they do to the general public. There are exceptions, of course, folks that are very good storytellers. And by stories, I do not mean making things up. I just mean making things vivid. And so I am surprised by the fact that not only are people who have important information to share not very good at that sometimes, but they are also sometimes kind of suspicious of the whole enterprise. "Why should I have to make these data compelling? Why should I have to pretty it up with a story? People should just look at the numbers and act." But of course, human beings do not respond that way to anything, people are not generally motivated by charts. And they are not going to be just because they ought to be. And so, I think that's an important skill. And the other thing that I have learned from teaching for a couple of years now is that you can learn. Anyone can do better at communicating and making your science information compelling. It's not rocket science.

**What are the aspects of public health that are essential for a One Health professional?**

Some of the core components of public health include the social and behavioral science in public health, epidemiology, and biostatistics. And thinking of human behavior and why people behave as they do, what kinds of things actually can get people to change their behavior. I think that's a really important aspect that all of the participants should be familiar with because humans are at the center of driving these changes that affect all the three domains. So, what to do about humans is the central question. And that's a lot more mysterious in some ways, I think, than some questions of biology that are interesting, but in terms of mystifying, and puzzling, and challenging, human behavior can be really key.

I also think that public health is good at illuminating the fact that it's never just about the science, it's also about values; about what to do. So, do you restrict freedoms or not, do you distribute resources or not? Those are all values-questions that are informed by the science, and one of the things I think that public health can contribute to this conversation is to understand that the tension around values needs to be acknowledged in our communication efforts and our intervention designs.

### Parting Thoughts?

I guess I would just say that this whole idea of interdisciplinary work is really at the core of One Health, as it is at the core of many of the most important things that we are doing. You don't have to understand everyone else's discipline as well as you understand your own, but you should get a sense of what your discipline brings to the conversation, what is the unique perspective that your approach or your data brings to the overall conversation?

---

### Case Study: Poverty and TB

Coauthored by Elizabeth Rechtien

According to a report published in October 2016 by the World Health Organization, TB has surpassed HIV/AIDS as the most deadly infectious disease. In 2015, over ten million people fell ill with TB, and nearly two million died from the disease. The bacteria that causes TB (*M. tuberculosis*) is widespread across the globe, but infection is much more common in impoverished areas. It is recognized that the poorer a community is, the greater the likelihood of its population becoming infected with the TB bacteria and developing clinical disease. Over 95% of TB deaths occur in low- and middle-income countries, and six countries – India, Indonesia, China, Nigeria, Pakistan, and South Africa – account for nearly 60% of the total number of new cases of TB each year.

One of the reasons TB is so common in these countries is that many people who live in absolute poverty are also homeless. People experiencing homelessness are subject to conditions that increase the risk of TB, such as substance abuse, HIV infection, and crowded shelters. A study conducted in India in 2012 sought to investigate the mechanisms by which poverty increases the risk of TB. After analyzing self-reported cases of TB throughout the poorest communities in India, the results indicated that indoor air pollution is one of the key determinants of disease. The TB bacteria persists in the air and spreads more easily in dark, poorly ventilated places.

Poor nutrition is another factor associated with poverty that increases the risk of TB. Malnutrition weakens the immune system, which makes people more vulnerable and prone to infection. Consequently, if an infection does occur, the body has a reduced chance of fighting it off. Studies have shown that "60% of adults with a healthy immune system can completely kill tuberculosis bacteria." The 2012 study also showed that low Body Mass Index (BMI) is the strongest mediator of the association between TB and poverty and that for those who share the two factors of low BMI and poor indoor air, the risk of clinical TB increased almost fivefold over those who had neither risk factor.

Finally, the lack of access to healthcare, which is common in impoverished nations, also contributes to the spread of TB. It is extremely difficult for people in low- and middle-income countries to be treated for anything related to their health, but serious infectious diseases present an even bigger challenge. "Of the nine million people who develop tuberculosis each year, around three million never reach a qualified doctor." For people living in impoverished nations, lack of ready access to medical care means it is virtually impossible for them to acquire an early diagnosis of TB. With no health services to diagnose or treat patients, there is a longer delay between the onset of disease and a cure. Further, the cost of traveling to a clinic can also be expensive, so many people living in poverty are unable to afford to make the journey to receive treatment, even if the treatment itself is free.

The complicated set of variables that link TB and poverty are daunting. However, if health is a human right then poverty is clearly jeopardizing that right for millions of people.

# Works Cited

Blaize, S., Pannetier, D., Oestereich, L. et al. (2014). Emergence of Zaire Ebola virus disease in Guinea. *New England Journal of Medicine* 371: 1418–1425. doi: 10.1056/NEJMoa1404505.

Bousquet, J. and Khaltaev, N. (eds.) (2007). *Global Surveillance, Prevention and Control of Chronic Respiratory Diseases: A Comprehensive Approach*. Geneva, Switzerland: WHO Press.

Brovkin, V., Boysen, L., Arora, V.K. et al. (2013). Effect of anthropogenic land-use and land-cover changes on climate and land carbon storage in CMIP5 projections for the twenty-first century. *Journal of Climate* 26: 6859–6881. doi: 10.1175/JCLI-D-12-00623.1 (accessed December 29, 2017).

Chatham House Centre on Global Health Security (2010) Meeting Report: Shifting from Emergency Response to Prevention of Pandemic Disease Threats at Source. https://www.chathamhouse.org/sites/files/chathamhouse/public/Research/Energy%2C%20Environment%20and%20Development/0410mtg_report.pdf (accessed December 19, 2017).

Deem, S.L., Bronson, E., Angulo, S. et al. (2012). Morbidity and Mortality. In: *The Maned Wolves of Noel Kempff Mercado National Park*, Smithsonian Contributions to Zoology 639 (ed. L.H. Emmons), 77–89. Washington, DC: Smithsonian Institution Scholarly Press.

Deem, S.L., Parker, P.G., and Miller, R.E. (2008). Building bridges: connecting the health and conservation professions. *Biotropica* 40 (6): 662–665.

Freeman, R.B. and Huang, W.J. (2014). Strength in diversity. *Nature* 513: 305.

Gire, S.K., Goba, A., Andersen, K.G. et al. (2014). Genomic surveillance elucidates Ebola virus origin and transmission during the 2014 outbreak. *Science* 345 (6202): 1369–1372. doi: 10.1126/science.1259657.

Halliday, J.E.B., Hampson, K., Hanley, N. et al. (2017). Driving improvements in emerging disease surveillance through locally relevant capacity strengthening. *Science* 357: 146–148.

Médecins sans Frontiéres (2015) Ebola: Pushed to the limit and beyond. http://www.msf.org/en/article/ebola-pushed-limit-and-beyond (accessed December 29, 2017).

Oxlade, O. and Murray, M. (2012). Tuberculosis and poverty: why are the poor at greater risk in India? *PLoS One* 7 (11): e47533. doi: 10.1371/journal.pone.0047533.

Phillips, K.W. (2014). How diversity makes us smarter. *Scientific American* 311 (4): 42–47. https://www.scientificamerican.com/article/how-diversity-makes-us-smarter (accessed December 29, 2017).

Saéz, A.M., Weiss, S., Nowak, K. et al. (2014). Investigating the zoonotic origin of the West African ebola epidemic. *European Molecular Biology Organization Molecular Medicine* doi: 10.15252/emmm.201404792.

Stephen, C. and Stemshorn, B. (2016). Leadership, governance and partnerships are essential One Health competencies. *One Health* 2: 161–163.

World Health Organization. Global tuberculosis report 2017. Geneva, Switzerland. License: CC BY-NC-SA 3.0 IGO.

# 8

## Essential Tools for One Health Practitioners

*"All the tools, techniques and technology in the world are nothing without the head, heart and hands to use them wisely, kindly and mindfully."*

Rasheed Ogunlaru

Using a real world challenge involving water – one of the most vital elements binding the health of all life – we may see in action both the discipline-specific tools, as well as the need for the core competencies important across all One Health disciplines. This example involves a single-celled parasite (*Toxoplasma gondii*), domestic cats (*Felis catus*), water, and the endangered California sea otter (*Enhydra lutris*) (Figure 8.1). Medical and veterinary professionals are both well-versed in *T. gondii*. *T. gondii* is a protozoan parasite that causes serious and sometimes fatal, human health complications, particularly in pregnant women; and cats are the **definitive host**. Domestic cats are commonly subclinical carriers of *T. gondii*, meaning they do not have clinical signs, but they may shed thousands of eggs in to the environment. They are the only taxa that can shed viable eggs. Once in the environment, humans and other animals may consume the eggs in contaminated food, water, or soil.

Less understood, until recently, was the environmentally resistant nature of *T. gondii* eggs, and specifically their ability to survive and remain infectious, in fresh and salt water. Both indoor (especially when people

flush cat feces down the toilet) and outdoor cats contribute to environmental contamination with *T. gondii* eggs. These eggs are in soils and wash into water systems and rivers which eventually lead to the ocean. Once in the ocean, *T. gondii* eggs may survive for months and may infect sea otters through the bivalve animals they eat (Figure 8.2). And, unfortunately sea otters are highly susceptible to disease caused by this terrestrial cat parasite.

Determining the link between a parasite of domestic cats (a terrestrial animal) and the sea otter (a marine mammal) mortalities involved a diverse One Health team, from pathologists and veterinary clinicians to ecologists, biologists, and epidemiologists. Understanding water flow and the movement of *T. gondii* eggs within these systems benefited from hydrologists and landscape ecologists. Public awareness campaigns on how to prevent domestic cats from spreading this parasite, and ultimately, causing deaths of sea otters required strong communication skills. These campaigns included messages such as not flushing kitty litter and cat poop down the toilet but rather placing indoor cat's poop in sealed containers and in the trash to prevent eggs from leaching into the environment (Figure 8.3). This sea otter conservation challenge also benefited from having human health professionals involved, which was easily accomplished due to the fact that *T. gondii* is a zoonotic pathogen that can, and does, cause devastating human

*Introduction to One Health: An Interdisciplinary Approach to Planetary Health*, First Edition.
Sharon L. Deem, Kelly E. Lane-deGraaf and Elizabeth A. Rayhel.
© 2019 John Wiley & Sons, Inc. Published 2019 by John Wiley & Sons, Inc.
Companion website: www.wiley.com/go/deem/health

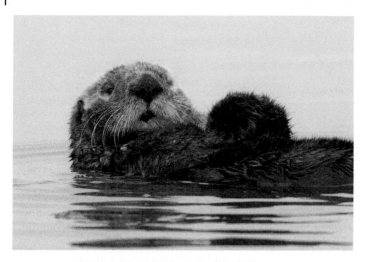

Figure 8.1 California sea otter (*Enhydra lutris*). *Source:* Mike Baird, https://commons.wikimedia.org/wiki/File:Sea_otter_cropped.jpg. CC BY 2.0.

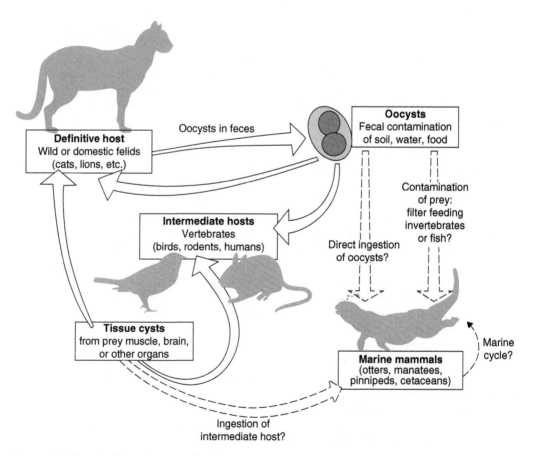

Figure 8.2 Lifecycle of *Toxoplasma gondii* – from terrestrial cats to marine sea otters. *Source:* Courtesy of Frontiers in Public Health.

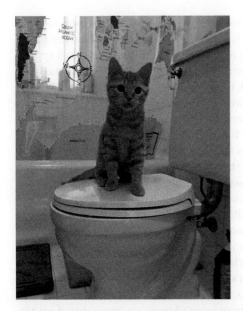

Figure 8.3 Be #1 with your cats #2; trash it, don't flush it.

health issues. Solving the mystery of sea otter deaths and working to prevent *T. gondii* environmental contamination is a win-win for conservation and public health.

Considering this One Health challenge we see there are many disciplines, each providing their academic knowledge and skills that were valuable in finding answers and solutions to this species-spanning health concern. This collaborative team determined the problem of sea otter deaths (the what, where, why, how, when) and then developed solutions to minimize impacts, such as the control of cats and cat feces to limit *T. gondii* run-off and sea otter *T. gondii* prevention and therapeutic strategies. The diverse range of stakeholders demanded a respectful and effective communication across these groups. This example demonstrates how a love of domestic animals and the animal-human bond that companion animals bring to so many people may have additional, and unwanted, health costs to environments, humans, and threatened wildlife species. This example illustrates a One Health challenge, and the possible solutions, from disease issues with water at the center. It is far from the only example.

Water systems globally are under pressure with over 1.5 million people, mostly children, dying of diarrheal diseases associated with poor quality water, worldwide each year. In the USA, *Cryptosporidia* spp. outbreaks in people, with the vast majority of cases from chlorinated water sources, have caused significant morbidity and mortality and have led to a number of economic challenges for cities. The ecology of water-borne diseases represents a critical area of future study to better understand and prevent water-borne human and other animal health threats. In addition to infectious agents, there are growing issues of water supplies contaminated with chemicals, toxins, and by-products of drugs and hormones, such as endocrine disruptor chemicals (see Chapter 3). Each of these substances may pose significant health challenges. These, like the story of sea otters and *T. gondii*, demand a One Health approach with tools that will help us solve the health challenges of today.

## 8.1 Why We Need One Health Tools

As a classically trained veterinary epidemiologist, whenever I evaluate a health challenge I consider the what, where, when, who, why, and how of the issue. Now that we have presented the what of One Health (Chapter 1), the where, when, and why of One Health (Chapters 2 and 3), and the who of One Health (Chapters 4–7), we may look at the how of One Health. How do we as One Health practitioners accomplish all the tasks that must be performed if we are to understand the health challenges of today and more importantly find the solutions to solve these challenges?

In this chapter, we will consider the tools – both tangible and intangible – of One Health. The tools used in a One Health approach are many and varied. These tools include those that all One Health practitioners should possess as well as those tools that are more specific for individuals within a specific discipline. Tools may be the physical items (e.g. medical supplies) or the harder to quantify, but just as important, skills of individuals (e.g. communication and leadership). To be most effective, One Health practitioners must have the tools necessary to collaborate, to cross disciplines, and to solve the complex problems of global health. In this chapter, we will explore what these tools include and how One Health practitioners might develop or acquire these tools.

The transdisciplinary nature of the One Health approach may feel intuitive to those of us working in the health fields for even the shortest of time. The **multifactorial** nature of the serious health challenges confronting people, plants, and animals demands a holistic – One Health – approach. However, having these diverse disciplines with professionals, who each may view the world through different educational and experiential lenses, suggests that One Health teams require an almost infinite number of tools. In this chapter, we will present the tools we believe to be key to One Health. We will not present all the tangible "hard" tools for each of the One Health disciplines as that is beyond the scope of this book. The reader is encouraged to go further into their chosen discipline, or area of expertise, so they may more fully understand what the core tools are for practitioners in the discipline (e.g. ecology, sociology, economics, statistics, human or veterinary medicine, agriculture, politics). There are however a number of core tools that *all* One Health practitioners should have in their individual toolbox if they are to be successful working in this complex and interconnected world.

## 8.2 The Tools of One Health

Often when thinking about tools we think of, well… "tools." The materials we can reach for to help with some task-at-hand. Tools such as the hammer or saw, and more commonly in the health fields, the needle, scalpel, or stethoscope. The tools we need to perform a function. A common definition of a tool is any device or implement, especially one held in the hand, used to carry out a particular function or to accomplish a task. We can all appreciate this definition of a tool. "Please pass me that tool, the screwdriver sitting over there." However, the word tool may also take on a far different meaning. For example, "she has all the tools to succeed as a great actress." This calls to mind her natural abilities, or tools of her trade. Other tools might include the books on a scholar's shelf that she reaches for to answer a difficult question or a software application that an IT specialist utilizes to accomplish some virtual task. In the first example, tools are inherent qualities (competencies) people possess. The other two examples are external materials that we reach for to help us in our endeavors. In One Health, both of these types of tools are imperative if we are to be successful in One Health activities.

To obtain these tools, One Health practitioners may have inherent talents to contribute or they may require advanced education or training to develop the tools. Alternatively, it may require that we have access to materials (devices) that allow us to do the work needed for understanding and solving today's health challenges. Each of these tools are part of a "One Health Toolbox." This toolbox must contain all the tools, from human competencies to the more concrete devices constructed from natural resources, in order for the One Health practitioner to be most successful.

As might be expected in an approach as holistic as One Health, and one with so many disciplines, these tools are many. Here we cover what we believe are the core tools that even if not being used by every individual, will more than likely be a tool that some member of your One Health team may bring to the table.

### 8.2.1 The Tangible: Hard Tools of One Health

All disciplines have tools of the trade. Doctors, nurses, veterinarians, and veterinary technicians have their stethoscopes, landscape ecologists their maps, and molecular biologists their polymerase chain reaction (PCR) machines. We might think of these as the "hard tools" of One Health; the tools that help us in most everything we do as professionals. Interestingly, from a One Health angle, it was believed that tool use was one of the things that separated humans from other animals. Now we know that tool use occurs across taxa, from sea otters to chimpanzees to finches; again reminding us of our shared evolution and membership in the animal kingdom.

The diversity of One Health disciplines (Chapter 7) and scope of the challenges that occupy the practitioner's time are broad and almost limitless (Table 8.1). Therefore, as you might imagine the tangible tools of One Health are also nearly limitless. What tools does the wildlife veterinarian need to safely remove a snare from an elephant's leg (Figure 8.4)? We may appreciate that the veterinary skills and training needed include knowledge of elephant anatomy (e.g. 70% of air exchange occurs through the trunk), but what of the equipment? A darting gun to deliver the anesthetics, the anesthetics themselves, monitoring devices, cutters and pliers to remove the snare, medicines to treat the wound, and prevent tetanus and infection at the wound site. What tools are needed by the public health nurses working in Vietnam to advance preventive measures that will improve hygiene in a village? They may need tools for mosquito control (e.g. mosquito nets), safe toilets, and water purification kits. Or, we may think of the needs for the medical doctor working in Central Africa at a hospital that has just diagnosed the **index case** of Marburg virus at the start of yet another hemorrhagic fever outbreak. This doctor will need **personal protective equipment** (PPE) and medicines to treat the symptoms of hemorrhagic disease while ensuring his own protection as well as the other persons caring for the patient. Or what tools will the landscape ecologist or epidemiologist, solicited to map the spatial distribution of an ongoing *Campylobacter jejuni* outbreak in the USA, require to perform their work. The hard tools

**Table 8.1**  Scope of One Health.

Agro- and bio-terrorism

Animal agriculture and animal sciences

Antimicrobial resistance

Basic and translational medicine

Biomedical research

Clinical medicine

Combating existing and emerging diseases and zoonoses

Comparative medicine

Conservation medicine

Consumer support

Diagnosis, surveillance, control, response, and recovery directed at natural or intentional threats that are chemical, toxicological, or radiological in nature

Entomology

Ethics

Food safety and security

Global food and water systems

Global trade and commerce

Health communications

Health of the environment and environmental preservation

Implications of climate change

Infectious disease ecology

Integrated systems for detection

Land use and production systems and practice

Mental health

Microbiology education

Occupational health

Public awareness and public communications

Public health and public policy

Regulatory enforcement

Scientific discovery and knowledge creation

Support of biodiversity

Training

Veterinary and environment health professionals and organizations

Wildlife promotion and protection

*Source:* https://www.avma.org/KB/Resources/Reports/Documents/onehealth_final.pdf

needed by these professionals, working to make sense of this zoonotic epidemic in an ecological context, may include global positioning system (GPS) equipment and geographic information system (GIS) packages, maps and cartography equipment, normalized

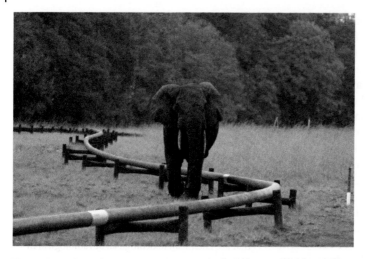

**Figure 8.4** African forest elephant (*Loxodonta cyclotis*) with snare around its leg, walking in an oil field.

difference vegetation index (NDVI) assessment tools, climatic monitors, and software and hardware to allow for all the databases required to collate these data.

### 8.2.2 People Power: The Intangible Tools of One Health

We all know that even the best hammer is all but useless if the person holding it has never seen one before. The same is true for most all of the tangible tools we have at our disposable to advance One Health. The stethoscope is mostly useless to the untrained ear as is the PCR machine to the researcher who knows nothing of molecular biology. The skills necessary to utilize these tools are often developed through formal educational opportunities and/or apprentice training. There are however, other tools of the trade that One Health practitioners should be cognizant of, if not proficient in (Table 8.2).

One Health practitioners must be proficient in the knowledge, skills, behaviors, and attitudes that go beyond their discipline-specific academic training. These are the intangible "soft tools" that are just as important, but harder to quantify, as the hard tools and include such things as the ability to communicate across cultures or the ability to give a stimulating presentation on One Health to a lecture hall full of people. For example, we all know that language barriers exist when we do not know the language of local peoples. This barrier may be overcome by learning multiple languages, or at the least the language of the region where you are working. However, less appreciated may be the fact that language barriers occur even when people speak the same language, since words maybe perceived differently by different people. The botanist delivering his One Health lecture to a room full of medical doctors must be cognizant that his use of a word, such as detritus, may have a very different meaning or no meaning at all for the audience that hears it.

Education, discussed further in Chapter 9, may be key for acquiring many of these core tools. Fortunately, there are a growing number of One Health courses and degrees, at the undergraduate and graduate levels, in universities across the world, helping to advance the One Health approach (Table 8.3). These academic courses have much to provide while training professionals in the core One Health competencies. Additionally, there are a number of less formal ways to acquire these soft tools through real world educational and experiential pathways.

We all have a certain set of skills, and any practitioner brings these discipline-specific

Table 8.2 Core competencies for One Health practitioners.

| Source | Management | Communication and informatics | Values and ethics | Leadership | Team and collaboration | Roles and responsibilities | Systems thinking |
|---|---|---|---|---|---|---|---|
| | | | | **Major domains** | | | |
| Bellagio working group | Working across boundaries | Communication | Ways of being[a] | Visionary and strategic | Influence | Change makers/ achieving results | Working across boundaries |
| Stone Mountain Meeting Group | Human capital management, resource management | Communicates lessons learned, communication | Integrity | Vision integration | Collaboration; diplomacy; builds diverse teams; interpersonal skills | Problem solving; flexibility; self-development | External awareness; strategic thinking |
| USAID/ RESPOND | Planning and management; analysis and assessment | Applied informatics; communication, and collaboration | Ethics and professionalism | Leadership and systems thinking | Communication and collaboration | Leadership | Leadership and systems thinking; cultural competence; policy and regulation |
| Rome synthesis | Leadership and management | Communication | Values and ethics | Leadership and management, conflict resolution | Teamwork | | Systems analysis/thinking (external awareness and big picture); creating an enabling environment and advocating change |
| Example competencies proposed during the Rome synthesis | Able to manage cross disciplinary teams-understands roles and responsibilities of team and its individual members – holds team accountable | Utilizes diplomacy – able to negotiate – able to resolve conflicts – achieves collaboration | Values honesty – possesses strong knowledge of self-possesses integrity | Advocates for change – fosters a change environment – understands individual and shared leadership models – possesses an external awareness (social, political, legal, and cultural) | Able to identify shared values and goals – values diversity of discipline, culture, ideas, background, and experience – establishes trust – thinks strategically | | Awareness of big picture and interdependent of stakeholders – understands and embraces a One Health approach – able to identify problem and its impact on the system |

[a] Used to describe a portfolio of value-driven personal attributes: confidence, courage, credibility, emotional intelligence, empathy, ethics, passion, self-awareness, spirituality, and wisdom.

Table 8.3 One Health Programs at the Undergraduate or Higher Level.

| University | Country | Program | URL |
|---|---|---|---|
| Murdoch University | Australia | Masters of Veterinary Studies in Conservation Medicine | www.murdoch.edu.au/study/courses/course-details/Master-of-Veterinary-Studies-(Conservation-Medicine)-(MVS) |
| | | Postgraduate Certificate in Veterinary Conservation Medicine | www.murdoch.edu.au/School-of-Veterinary-and-Life-Sciences |
| Universitat Bonn | Germany | Doctoral Program in One Health and Urban Transformation | https://www.zef.de/onehealth.html |
| Kerala Veterinary and Animal Sciences University | India | Post Graduate Certificate in One Health Post Graduate Diploma in One Health | www.coheart.ac.in/index |
| Massey University | New Zealand | One Health Epidemiology Fellowship | http://www.onehealthnetwork.asia/ohefp |
| Ross University of Veterinary Medicine | St. Kitts | Masters of Science in One Health | http://veterinary.rossu.edu/postgraduate/msc-one-health.html |
| University Of Basel and Swiss Tropical and Public Health Institute | Switzerland | One Health Certificate – Online | https://www.futurelearn.com/courses/one-health |
| University of Liverpool | UK | Veterinary Conservation Medicine (BVSc) | www.liverpool.ac.uk/study/undergraduate/courses/veterinary-conservation-medicine-intercalated-honours-bsc |
| University of Edinburgh | UK | One Health (Online Distance Learning) (MSc, PgDip, PgCert, PgProfDev) | www.ed.ac.uk/studying/postgraduate/degrees/index.php?r=site/view&id=814 |
| Royal Veterinary College London with London School of Hygiene and Tropical Medicine | UK | Masters of Science in One Health | www.lshtm.ac.uk/study/masters/one-health |
| Berry College | USA | Undergraduate Minor in One Health | http://www.berry.edu/academics/majors/onehealth |
| Columbia University | USA | Conservation Biology Certificate with course in "Conservation Medicine" Disease Ecology" | http://sfs.columbia.edu/content/certificate-conservation-biology-and-environmental-sustainability-1 |
| Cornell University | USA | Master of Public Health / College of Veterinary Medicine – One Health approach | https://www2.vet.cornell.edu/departments/population-medicine-and-diagnostic-sciences/public-health-and-international-programs |
| Duke University | USA | One Health Training Program | https://globalhealth.duke.edu/projects/one-health-training-program |
| Fontbonne University | USA | One Health Minor (undergraduates) One Health Certification (post-baccalaureates) | https://www.fontbonne.edu/academics/departments/biological-and-physical-sciences-department/center-for-one-health |

Table 8.3 (Continued)

| University | Country | Program | URL |
|---|---|---|---|
| Michigan State University | USA | Masters, PhD Specialization in Fish & Wildlife Disease Ecology and Conservation Medicine | https://reg.msu.edu/AcademicPrograms/ProgramDetail.aspx?Program=5256 |
| Ohio State University | USA | Masters of Public Health – Veterinary Public Health | http://vet.osu.edu/education/veterinary-public-health-program |
| Tufts Cummings School of Veterinary Medicine | USA | Masters in Conservation Medicine | https://grad.vet.tufts.edu/ms-conservation-medicine/ |
| University of Arizona | USA | Masters of Public Health in One Health | https://publichealth.arizona.edu/departments/epi-bio/one-health-program |
| University of California – Davis | USA | Masters of Preventive Veterinary Medicine (MPVM) with electives in One Health and Wildlife Disease & Ecology | http://www.vetmed.ucdavis.edu/mpvm |
| University of Florida | USA | Masters Health Sciences in One Health | http://egh.phhp.ufl.edu/degree-programs/masters-programs/mhs-one-health/ |
| | | PhD in One Health | http://egh.phhp.ufl.edu/degree-programs/phd-programs/phd-in-one-health/ |
| | | Graduate Certificate in Wildlife Forensic Sciences and Conservation | https://wildlife.forensics.med.ufl.edu/programs/courses/conservation-medicine |
| University of Illinois | USA | Dual DVM/ Masters of Public Health | http://vetmed.illinois.edu/education/doctor-veterinary-medicine-degree/dvm-master-public-health-degree |
| University of Minnesota | USA | Dual DVM/ Masters of Public Health | http://www.sph.umn.edu/academics/dual-joint-degrees/veterinary-medicine |
| University of Missouri – Columbia | USA | Masters of Public Health – Veterinary emphasis (MVPH) | https://healthprofessions.missouri.edu/mph/mph-degree/competencies |
| | | Dual DVM/ Masters of Public Health | https://healthprofessions.missouri.edu/mph/mph-degree/dual-degrees/mphdvm-doctor-veterinary-medicine |
| University of Washington School of Public Health | USA | Graduate Certificate in One Health | http://deohs.washington.edu/cohr/graduate-certificate-one-health |
| Westminster College | USA | Undergraduate Major in One Health | http://www.westminster-mo.edu/academics/degree-requirements/major-minor-summary-sheets/Documents/Majors/Majors_PDF/One%20Health%20Major.pdf |

skills and knowledge to a One Health team. Furthermore, many of these skills, behaviors, and approaches, including cross-sectional collaboration, communication, and respect, are necessary for all One Health practitioners to possess. Soft tools may be categorized under seven core competency domains, as has been suggested by a number of authors. The seven core competency domains include: (i) Management; (ii) Communication; (iii) Values and Ethics; (iv) Leadership; (v) Teams and Collaboration; (vi) Roles and Responsibilities; and (vii) Systems Thinking. Some of the most important tools for any One Health team to possess are listening skills, collaborating skills, and the ability to appreciate differences (Table 8.2).

The soft tools of One Health are in many ways intangible, since most do not have a clear metric for assessment. For example, how does one measure an individual's listening skills? We each have a vision of someone that we think of as a good listener, but is there a "listen-o-meter" that allows us to fully measure this ability? Probably not. This is true for the other intangible tools, which although just as important as the hard tools are often difficult to measure. Here we briefly cover these competencies.

To be effective One Health practitioners we must have management skills, including the ability to manage our own actions. Management requires that we set goals, divide these goals into manageable tasks, and measure targets we set forth when developing the manageable tasks. Additionally, in this fast-paced world of today, good management requires that we work to continually develop people; both our own development as well as others on our team. We also must be able to communicate if we are to advance the work. Communication requires that we are able to convey our thoughts to others and that we do so with the intended meaning (see Chapter 10). Communication requires that we have mutually agreed upon definitions of words. This may in fact be a challenge for One Health teams, since our various disciplines may use words in slightly different ways.

The values and ethics we each bring to One Health should be the anchor that centers our efforts. These values and ethics ensure that we do tasks with integrity and honesty. Core to the mission of One Health is the drive for providing health benefits across the One Health Triad, and this requires of us to work with integrity and to consider all stakeholders. Additionally, by definition, One Health requires that we are able to work collaboratively and within teams. This requires that we have skills to influence as well as skills to operate with diplomacy while striving for shared values and goals. Within any One Health team we each have roles and responsibilities that must be understood and performed to achieve the goals set out at the beginning of the work. We each must know our roles and responsibilities and then be able to achieve them. We should also operate with an appreciation of systems thinking, and the ability to have an external awareness of the big picture is key for One Health. We must be able to identify a problem and its impact on the system and then work to address it.

Lastly, within the seven core competencies that have been suggested is leadership. Leadership differs somewhat from management while sharing many of the same qualities. Leadership is the ability to lead and guide a group. This may be accomplished through both words and actions. Whether we wish to be "the leader of the group" or not, we are all leaders. By definition, leadership is the use of our words and actions to lead others (to influence) to do something we wish them to do. Each of us should have this as a goal within our professional careers. In One Health, there is both room for, and a need of, many leaders if we are to solve the twenty-first century health challenges.

### 8.2.3 Disease Risk Analyses: Linking the Tangible with the Intangible Tools of One Health

It should be evident that tools are necessary to perform all One Health actions, with some tools being imperative and others extremely useful and varied depending on the situation. These tools allow us to acquire data, work across disciplines, and develop solutions. Again, each of us, as we find our passion and our role in One Health, will learn about the "nuts and bolt tools" that are necessary for working within our disciplines. The less tangible tools may be harder to acquire in the traditional training programs within our disciplines. However, this may be changing as all these disciplines are realizing the necessity for practitioners to have communication and other people skills. Fortunately, there are tools that allow us to link these tangible tools with the intangible ones. These are often the tools that are developed to bring the data collected using hard tools (e.g. prevalence data collected of Zika **antigen** from blood samples collected and tested using PCR) so that we may use these data to effect change. One such method for linking tangible and intangible tools is **Disease Risk Analysis**.

Disease Risk Analysis is a multidisciplinary process used to evaluate existing knowledge in order to prioritize risks associated with the spread or occurrence of diseases. A disease risk analysis consists of four interconnected phases: (i) hazard identification; (ii) risk assessment; (iii) risk management; and, (iv) risk communication (Figure 8.5). All the phases are interactive with the others as the process should not simply flow in a one to four chronological order. Hazard identification is the identification of what may go wrong. We must identify what diseases have potential effects harmful enough to warrant inclusion in the risk analysis. Some criteria used for ranking infectious disease hazards include prevalence and incidence data, infectivity, pathogenicity (e.g. morbidity, mortality, fitness costs, reproductive costs), transmissibility (e.g. routes, rates, competent vectors), susceptibility (e.g. species), and economic impacts associated with the disease (e.g. for wildlife species, domestic animals, humans, and the ecosystem). Risk assessment is the range of calculations required to estimate release, exposure, and consequence parameters for infectious dis-

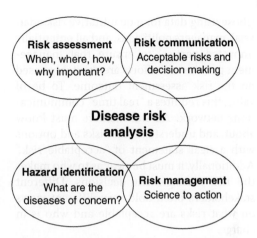

**Figure 8.5** A Disease Risk Analysis consists of four interconnected phases: (i) hazard identification; (ii) risk assessment; (iii) risk management; and, (iv) risk communication. *Source:* Photo credit to Jamie L. Palmer, Saint Louis Zoo.

eases of concern. The process of assessing the risk will help to understand the when, where, how, and why of a potential disease risk. A subsequent estimate of the "total" risk may then be calculated based on the above parameters for each of the identified hazards. Hazard identification and risk assessment are sometimes grouped together as they are clearly inter-related. They also may be applied to noninfectious diseases with slight variations on the types of data used to rank the hazard and risks associated with it.

Risk management focuses on responses that may decrease the likelihood of an adverse outcome and reduce the consequences if such an outcome occurs. This element of risk analysis may best be viewed as the reason for performing the analysis so that science may move into action. Risk management may be the single most important component, as it translates the identification of diseases and assessment of associated risks into management actions that may mitigate these risks. Risk communication is a continuous process, necessitating respectful communication among the multiple stakeholders throughout the risk analysis. Risk communication should occur between field staff (those on the ground collecting data), modelers (those using data for a quantitative risk analysis), managers politicians, and all potentially impacted parties, to ensure that management policies and efforts are equitably based on the risk assessment outcome. To be of value, this requires a "real time" communications network. All stakeholders must know about, and understand, the risks and options with a clear statement of "acceptable risk." Additionally, it must be clear as to who makes the risk management decisions. Different stakeholders often hold very different views on what risks are acceptable and who is in charge.

The criteria used to identify diseases of concern may also be used to assess the level of their associated risks. In many risk analyses, hazard identification and risk assessment are performed based solely on expert opinion or literature review. In fact, one of the most valuable products of disease risk analysis is the identification of missing data points which if obtained would enhance a broader understanding of disease risks for a population or project. In order for a disease risk analysis to provide the highest quality outputs, hazard identification and risk assessments should be based on scientific data collected from the field and pertinent to the analysis in question. Providing these necessary data points for disease risk analysis is best performed by implementing standardized disease surveillance and monitoring systems.

Several databases exist to provide One Health practitioners the data that will help in disease risk analyses. These databases, created from the application of hard tools, provide the data to use in risk assessment, management, and communication. One example is the Enhanced Infectious Disease Database (EID2), a comprehensive and open-access "big data" record of over 60 million scientific papers, electronic sources, and textbooks associated with infectious diseases. The integration of data from disease surveillance programs has been accomplished in recent years to include human, animal, and environmental surveillance in a One Health approach. Examples include

an integrated surveillance program based out of Accra, Ghana; the United States Agency for International Development (USAID) funded pandemic preparedness program that has databases available from these programs (Predict, Respond); the World Health Organization (WHO) databases; and a USA specific surveillance program through the US Geological Survey (USGS).

## 8.3 Tools to Help Start a One Health Movement

The tangible and intangible tools mentioned earlier may be used in countless ways to help in all One Health initiatives. One increasingly common mode of use for these tools is to start a movement that addresses a concern. In some cases these movements have remained local, but for a growing number of movements there has been global reach. These movements have been able to advance some aspect of One Health, and the drivers of these movements have been able to influence others with their words and actions.

The steps to starting a movement may be helped by taking a disease risk analysis approach as presented earlier. We must first identify the problem that we wish to tackle. Health challenges today are for the most part interconnected and multifactorial. This first step in starting a movement may require the identification of a number of stakeholders that will play important roles in the movement. Once the problem and the stakeholders are identified, the transdisciplinary team necessary to work on the problem must be built. This occurs alongside, and as a result of, data gathering as well as while the solutions that are the impetus of our movement unfold. The movement's team will get the most bang for its buck if communicators and politicians help to move the findings into the public domain, facilitating changes at the political table. We may look at the USA at the time of writing, and the war on science, and realize that the task of developing an effective public awareness campaign and gaining an elected seat at the political table is vital for any movement's success. Having a collaborative team in place is only the start of the work. The final step is to work respectfully to maximize the core competencies held by various members of the team and work so that you may effect change (see Chapter Case Study).

## 8.4 Conclusions

Tools used to perform the tasks necessary to approach health challenges across the six degrees of One Health are varied and many. A One Health approach, by nature of the complex, interconnected health challenges on which it focuses, requires a diversity of tools, both tangible and intangible, if we are to succeed in our efforts. Many of these tools are the "traditional tools" of the individual disciplines which make up any One Health team. Other tools, however, are the intangible competencies that a One Health practitioner should possess to successfully work as part of a collaborative team.

It may seem daunting for any one of us to consider how we might possess all the core tools suggested as beneficial for One Health. Still, we should strive to obtain as many as possible. Just as importantly, we must be able to accept when we do not have a core competency. Knowing individual strengths and weaknesses can help a team be as effective as possible. The One Health toolbox should include all the tangible devices we use in our studies and the core competencies that the team possesses from language skills and communication to shared responsibilities and management styles. However, we are not in this alone, and one of the biggest tools of One Health is the growing number of practitioners that may each bring to the team their own tools.

We began this chapter with water – one of the most important substances connecting the health of all life from environments to human and non-human animals. This example highlighted how connected we truly are as we explored the add-on costs that may result from the human-companion animal bond. In this case, conservation concerns for a beloved wildlife species and public health concerns for humans factored in to a response that benefited both human and non-human animals alike. It also exemplified the complexity of these connections and the need for a transdisciplinary approach and the many tools used by the persons within these disciplines. There is an increasing number of stories, similar to the *T. gondii* challenge, and each demands a One Health approach and the tools necessary to perform such an approach. Acquiring and developing the tools of One Health is imperative if we are to combat these challenges.

## End of Chapter Questions & Activities

A. Thought Questions:

   i) Essential tools for One Health practitioners may have a number of uses. Provide a list of tools that you think are important for One Health and indicate if they are tangible or intangible? Do they differ from those presented in the chapter?

   ii) We start the chapter using a One Health challenge of today, *T. gondii*. Can you think of another challenge that includes domestic and wild animals, environmental contamination, and human health? If so, write it out and then list the tools (tangible and intangible) that you feel are necessary to handle the challenge.

   iii) Understanding that it is not possible for any One Health practitioner to possess all the tools in a One Health toolbox, provide a strategy, using your example in question (ii), for how a One Health team might have the tools necessary for accomplishing the goal at hand.

B. In-Class/Guided Activities:

   i) Visit the websites for the integrated surveillance programs mentioned in the text and think of how you might use these data. They include Accra, Ghana http://www.indepth-network.org); USAID funded pandemic preparedness program that has databases available from these programs (Predict, Respond) (http://data.predict.global); WHO databases (http://www.who.int/csr/resources/databases/en); USGS map https://catalog.data.gov/dataset/usgs-national-geologic-map-database-collection

C. At-home Activities:

   i) Find a program on TV that you feel has a One Health quality to it. There are many to choice from – a human health drama, nature show, anything on animal planet – and then see if during the hour long program you can find examples of where they missed an opportunity to present the topic through a One Health lens. Alternatively, determine if they did in fact present the show using a One Health approach.

D. Long-term Action Steps:

   i) As you move through your studies as an undergraduate or graduate student, consider if you are receiving training in the seven core, intangible, tools discussed in this chapter. If you are not receiving this training, figure ways to do so either through independent study or by electives that you had not previously considered.

   ii) Take any one of the seven core intangible tools discussed in the chapter and during the coming year, find ways to advance your skills in this competency (e.g. take a language, a leadership course, storytelling course).

E. Recommended Reading:

Beck, B. (2013). *Guidelines for Reintroductions and Other Conservation Translocations*. IUCN.

Covey, S. (1989). *The Seven Habits of Highly Effective People: Powerful Lessons in Personal Change*. Simon & Schuster.

Gallo, C. (2014). *Talk Like Ted: The 9 Public Speaking Secrets of the World's Top Minds*. St. Martin's Press.

## Interview

*An interview with Ekaette Mbong, PhD. Dr. Mbong is a science policy expert, trained in both Virology and Neuroendocrinology.*

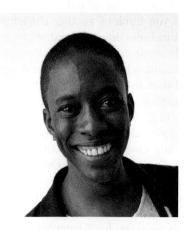

**Tell us a little about yourself**

I am a scientist. I found my way to science by taking biology classes. I was heading to medical school but then changed paths and decided graduate school fit. I completed a PhD in Biological Sciences with a focus in Virology. I switched gears for my postdoc and went on to study something completely different. I did Neuroendocrinology and studied the effects of obesity on fertility. However, I always had this itch for policy. I am interested in how we translate research into policy. During a two-year fellowship, I was able to look at science policy as it relates to education. Specifically I considered, "How do we ensure that we have a diverse pool of scientists when it comes to the workforce?" I now do consulting on the science policy front.

### How is One Health important to your work?

As scientists, we may do a good job of research. However, in order to get our messaging out to lay people, we have to meet them on their level. Often this means we should "speak to them like speaking to your grandmother who knows nothing about what you do." My research to policy reach through effective communication is core to my work and it embodies One Health. It is going to take voices of scientists speaking up, coming out into their communities, be it the library, their churches, or synagogues or elsewhere. We need to tell people what is going on.

### Do you see yourself as a One Health practitioner?

Yes. As a person, a scientist, and a global citizen, I embody One Health. I saw a problem in science leadership and I am working to change that. I joined 500 Women Scientists in order to make sure that we are able to address the problem of white male domination across all sciences and look for ways to get women into these fields.

### How do your actions reflect One Health, personally or professionally?

We as scientists need to move away from just doing research and move into roles of leadership. For me, that looks like eventually running for public office. How am I doing this? I am still doing my research and still consulting; still doing all the things that keep me a well-respected scientist. However, I also go to community meetings, see what is going on in my community, where there is need. By getting more scientists into public-facing roles, it will help us make informed decisions to make effective policies, for our climate, for earth, for the animals, and so forth.

### How can we encourage people to care about planetary health?

The biggest thing people can do is start at home. It is like when you throw a pebble into a lake. There is a little ripple and then the ripple is across the lake, and you can see it expanding. Do you think about the electricity that you use unnecessarily? Do you recycle? Do you compost? Then you expand even further. Once you have a solid grasp on your household, then you can share tips with friends so they are involved. Then they tell their friends. You note a little thing, and you run with it, and get other people onboard. One and one and one and one – they add up very quickly.

### Where is One Health headed?

We are in a unique situation right now. People are being galvanized to do things that they never did before. That's not necessarily a bad thing. Sometimes you need a little fire in order for people to come out of their houses and start fighting back. We are starting to have conversations. If there is anything One Health is doing, it is promoting this idea of a conversation. A conversation goes a long way. It allows you to find common ground for moving forward.

### How do you suggest that students keep pace with technological advances?

Do not be afraid to learn something new. That is how you keep up. When new technologies come out, be excited about it. Try to figure out how it works, because you are not going to be able to make progress by staying in the technology you already know. It is always changing, and you can choose to be upset that it changes and it's not moving at the pace that you like, or you can take a different approach – "How can I improve on this and be the next groundbreaker for a technology down the road?"

Parting Thoughts?

Be reflective in all that you do. It's easy to run with a degree, if you are a biology major, naturally the next step would be to choose a master's degree or a PhD program, or immediately go into work. Slow down. None of us has the answers as to what the future holds. We can only make predictions. I still have no idea what I want to do in my life. But, I am moving in a direction that I really like. Be okay with where you are now and move forward at a pace that allows you to enjoy the moment while picking up new knowledge along the way.

---

### Case Study – Starting a Movement: Sea Turtles and Clean Beaches

Co-authored by Christopher Graham

If you wish to start a movement – any movement – it is vital that you start with a plan. There have been all types of movements throughout history, from the Environmental Movement to the American Revolution. No matter how different the movement, they all follow a similar pattern in development. When considering a One Health challenge you wish to tackle, consider taking the steps necessary as you work to gather an army of people to help with your efforts. Applying these steps, many organizations have worked tirelessly during the past few decades to tackle the global problem of marine debris that liters beaches throughout the world. Considering the efforts of one organization, Sea Life Trust, their movement relied on using sea turtles as the hook that ignited people to care. Since all seven sea turtle species rely on beaches for reproductive success, any work to clean beaches also helps sea turtle conservation.

Most successful movements follow five basic steps to be effective. These include to (i) find a way to connect people; (ii) find actions that can take place to push your movement forward; (iii) set targets; (iv) recruit people; and (v) measure progress. These steps at first glance may seem basic, but they are necessary for effectively starting a movement. When we look at the movement to clean beaches and help conserve sea turtle populations, the steps along the way were key to the success of the movement.

The first step was to find a connection that would make people care about clean beaches. This was achieved by using sea turtles as the poster animal for beach cleanup efforts. The sea turtle offers a tangible image to portray the necessity to perform beach cleanups. The public was made aware of the challenges that face female sea turtles and their eggs and hatchlings when the beaches where sea turtles come to lay and incubate eggs are littered with garbage. Although the beach cleanup efforts benefit more species other than just sea turtles, the sea turtle gave the public justification for why these actions were important.

The second step was to recognize that there were two major actions that would aid in pushing the movement forward. The first action was to clean the beaches. Bringing the public together to clean beaches builds a strong purpose for the cause and as importantly provides a tangible product that people could feel proud of – clean beaches. The second action that the cleanup needed was for the public to be able to witness hatchling turtles safely moving from nests on the beach to the oceans. The third step was to set targets. This was done by selecting areas in need of cleanup, and setting up activities in these areas for the community to assist. This allowed for an extremely large-scale issue to be broken down into smaller more achievable goals. The fourth step was to recruit people. As the cleanup efforts became more popular it was easier to appeal to more people. People from across the community were involved through outreach programs in schools, funding drives with businesses, and activities that attracted all members of the community. The final step was to measure progress. With beach cleanup efforts, it is easy to measure progress. You may quantify pre- and post-cleanup garbage to see if there is a reduction. And, you may monitor overall wildlife presence and health. Sea turtle monitoring that provides data on number of nests, number of successful hatchings per nest, and hatchling survival are all important measures pre- and post-cleanup efforts.

This example shows how one group followed easy steps to start a movement. If the base of the movement is built correctly, it will then continue to build on itself. It is important to address all the necessary steps in order to make the movement effective. If one of the steps is lacking, the movement may not move forward successfully.

## Works Cited

Barrett, M. and Bouley, T.A. (2015). Need for enhanced environmental representation in the implementation of One Health. *EcoHealth* 12: 212–219.

Davis, M.F., Rankin, S.C., Schurer, J.M. et al. (2017). Checklist for one health epidemiological reporting of evidence (COHERE). *One Health* 4: 14–21.

Deem, S.L. (2008). Tracking a snared elephant. In: *The Rhino with Glue-On Shoes* (ed. L.H. Spelman and T.Y. Mashima), 138–147. New York, NY: Bantam Dell Publishers.

Deem, S.L. (2012). Disease risk analysis in wildlife health field studies. In: *Fowler's Zoo and Wild Animal Medicine: Current Therapy 7* (ed. R.E. Miller and M.E. Fowler), 2–7. Saint Louis, MO: Saunders Elsevier.

Deem, S.L., Karesh, W.B., and Weisman, W. (2001). Putting theory into practice: wildlife health in conservation. *Conservation Biology* 15: 1224–1233.

Deem, S.L., Parker, P.G., and Miller, R.E. (2008a). Building bridges: connecting the health and conservation professions. *Biotropica* 40: 662–665.

Deem, S.L., Ezenwa, V.O., Ward, J.R. et al. (2008b). Research frontiers in ecological systems: evaluating the impacts of infectious disease on ecosystems. In: *Infectious Disease Ecology: Effects of Ecosystems on Disease and of Disease on Ecosystems Princeton University Press* (ed. R.S. Ostfeld, V.T. Eviner and F. Keesing), 304–318. NJ: Princeton.

ENHanCEd Infectious Diseases (EID2) database. (2017) https://eid2.liverpool.ac.uk/ (accessed November 15, 2017).

Frankson, R., Hueston, W., Christian, K. et al. (2016). One Health core competency domains. *Frontiers in Public Health* 4: 192. doi: 10.3389/fpubh.2016.00192.

INDEPTH Network. (2017). http://www.indepth-network.org (accessed November 15, 2017).

Kim, Jim Y. (2012). 5 Tips on Starting a Social Movement. The World Bank. http://blogs.worldbank.org/voices/5-tips-on-starting-a-social-movement (accessed November 15, 2017).

King, L.J., Anderson, L.R., Blackmore, C.G. et al. (2008). Special report: executive summary of the AVMA One Health initiative task force report. *Journal of the American Veterinary Medical Association* 233 (2): 259–261.

Lebov, J., Grieger, K., Womack, D. et al. (2017). A framework for One Health research. *One Health* 3: 44–50.

Miller, M.A. (2008). Tissue cyst-forming Coccidia of marine mammals. In: *Zoo and Wild Animal Medicine: Current Therapy* (ed. M.E. Fowler and R.E. Miller), 319–340. Saint Louis, MO: Saunders Elsevier.

Office of International Epizootics (2004). Import risk analysis. In: *Terrestrial Animal Health Code, 13the*, 872. Paris: Office of International Epizootics.

One Health: A New Professional Imperative. (2008) American Veterinary Medicine Association One Health Initiative Task Force: Final Report. https://www.avma.org/KB/Resources/Reports/Documents/

onehealth_final.pdf 76 pp. (accessed September 12, 2017).

Sea Life Trust. (n.d.) Clean-Up for Hatchlings. http://www.sealifetrust.org.au/news/latest/clean-hatchlings (accessed July 9, 2018).

Thrusfield, M. (2007). Appendix XXIV: risk analysis. In: *Veterinary Epidemiology*, thirde (ed. M. Thrusfield), 482–502. Oxford, UK: Blackwell Publishing.

US Geological Survey. (2016) USGS National Geologic Map Database Collection. https://catalog.data.gov/dataset/usgs-national-geologic-map-database-collection (accessed December 15, 2017).

USAID – FROM THE AMERICAN PEOPLE. (2017) http://data.predict.global/ (accessed November 14, 2017).

World Health Organization (2017) Emergencies preparedness, response. http://www.who.int/csr/resources/databases/en (accessed December 15, 2017).

Zinsstag, J., Schelling, E., Bonfoh, B. et al. (2009). Towards a "One Health" research and application toolbox. *Veterinaria Italiana* 45: 121–133.

Zinsstag, J., Schelling, E., and Waltner-Toews, D. et al. (2011). From "one medicine" to "one health" and systemic approaches to health and well-being. *Preventive Veterinary Medicine* 101: 148–156.

Part IV

How to Start a Movement

# 9

# Education and Critical Thinking in One Health

On August 22, 1999, the New York Times ran a story in its regional section entitled "NEIGHBORHOOD REPORT: BAYSIDE; At Fort Totten and Elsewhere, Crows Dying Mysteriously." The reporter, Corey Kilgannon, noted that for two weeks bird watchers had seen a growing number of dead birds, particularly crows, strewn around the base of feeders. Concurrently, a veterinarian in Bayside, New York, had treated and released several crows suffering from a neurological disease of unknown origin. Robert Lieblein, a spokesman for the state's Department of Environmental Conservation (DEC), told Kilgannon that he had been getting reports of dead birds for weeks from neighborhoods in and around Queens. He had sent bird corpses to the Department's laboratory for testing and awaited the results. Kilgannon also spoke to Jill Weiss, the assistant director of environmental education at the Alley Pond Environmental Center, a nonprofit group, who suspected a toxic food source in the neighborhood. The story closes with this quote from Ms. Weiss, "It doesn't draw attention because people don't really value crows for some reason, and don't see where they fit." Meanwhile, at the Wildlife Conservation Society's Bronx Zoo/Wildlife Conservation Park, the head pathologist, Dr. Tracey McNamara, was also taking notice of the dead crows. Necropsies that she had performed showed evidence of extensive brain and spinal cord inflammation. Dr. McNamara had also sent samples to the state

DEC lab, which reported negative results for aspergillosis, poison, and bacteria. The DEC pathologist then requested that the New York State Department of Health test the bird samples for viruses, and was redirected to the Cornell University Veterinary laboratory. They redirected the pathologist to the National Veterinary Services Laboratory in Ames, Iowa. That same week, the third week of August, three flamingos (*Phoenicopterus chilensis*), a pheasant (genus *Lophura*, species unknown), a golden eagle (*Aquila chrysaetos*), and a cormorant (*Phalacrocorax bougainvillea*) died at the zoo.

Across town, at the Flushing Hospital, the Chief of Infectious Diseases noticed that there had been an uptick in spinal taps and reviewed the files for five elderly patients admitted with meningoencephalitis. He brought this to the attention of the New York City Department of Health, who quickly discovered three more cases in Queens and nearby Brooklyn. The following week, two of the elderly patients died, and their brain tissues were submitted for testing by the New York State Health Department lab. The samples were positive for the mosquito-borne flavivirus group, and mosquito-control measures began across the city. The state health department also sent patient samples to the US Centers for Disease Control (CDC) along with an email stating that polymerase chain reaction (PCR) results for the St. Louis Encephalitis-type flavivirus (SLEV) were negative. Two days later the CDC announced

*Introduction to One Health: An Interdisciplinary Approach to Planetary Health*, First Edition.
Sharon L. Deem, Kelly E. Lane-deGraaf and Elizabeth A. Rayhel.

positive enzyme-linked immunoabsorbent assay (ELISA) results for SLEV. The press released an announcement of the outbreak, and a hotline was established for those who thought they might be ill. By then, on September 2, there were up to 40 suspected human cases.

Dr. McNamara considered the possibility that the two diseases, bird and human, were linked, but the pattern did not fit. SLEV would not kill the species of birds that had died, and birds that should be sick with SLEV were fine. Wanting a definite diagnosis for her animals, she called the DEC pathologist again, who had by then examined over 400 dead birds. They decided to send samples to the National Wildlife Health Center in Wisconsin, which caused a delay of approximately five days due to shipping and transit constraints. Dr. McNamara contacted the CDC in Atlanta and was redirected to the CDC Division of Vector-borne Infectious Diseases in Fort Collins, Colorado. They suggested that her exotic bird samples would be more appropriately sent to the National Veterinary Services Laboratory in Ames. Simultaneously, but unknown to Dr. McNamara, a CDC vertebrate ecologist was traveling to New York to collect samples from live zoo birds at the request of the NYC health department. By September 12, three human patients and unknown hundreds of birds had died, and the New York State Health Department lab had rerun their PCR test for SLEV numerous times, all with negative results.

In mid-September, the National Veterinary Services Lab announced that the bird virus was a flavivirus, but not any type they had ever seen, including SLEV. At that point, there was a convergence in the study of the human and animal samples, and on September 23, the CDC Division of Vector-Borne Diseases announced positive results for a virus not seen before in the Western Hemisphere: West Nile (WNV).

As the disease spread from New York to neighboring states, Dr. McNamara helped to initiate a collaborative effort between zoos and public health officials to monitor the spread of WNV, but the main question from this story was, "why weren't these professionals sharing their information and results in the first place?" In a paper describing the outbreak, Dr. McNamara suggests the following:

> Confusion resulting from the antigenic similarities between West Nile and St. Louis encephalitis viruses, combined with the unexpected nature of the introduction of WNV into the United States, resulted in a delay in the identification of the etiologic agent responsible for this outbreak. Also serving to delay the identification was a failure to recognize an association between extensive mortality among wild avian species, which had been observed earlier.

That there are connections between human and animal health has been understood since the domestication of dogs brought with it the first human cases of rabies, and historically the study of medicine and science have been one and the same. Human dissection has been frowned upon throughout most of our history, meaning that the majority of pre-twentieth-century physicians used animals to learn anatomy, physiology, and surgical procedure. Further, animals have served as models of human disease since the eighteenth century, motivating Rudolf Virchow (1821–1902), a human pathologist and the man who coined the term "zoonosis," to say, "Between animal and human medicine there are no dividing lines – nor should there be. The object is different, but the experience obtained constitutes the basis of all medicine."

Recently, however, the educational and professional spheres of veterinarians, physicians, and basic scientists have diverged. The genetics and biotechnology revolutions of the twentieth century significantly expanded the knowledge bases of human and animal medicine. The study of disease on both sides of the aisle became focused on mechanisms of pathology at their most fundamental, cellular, and genetic levels. The depth of specialized knowledge required for this level of understanding is not conducive to broad-based points of view. This siloing of knowledge helped to create the isolation of medical professionals evident in the WNV story.

At the same time, globalization in the twentieth century along with human overpopulation and ecosystem destabilization ushered in complex and entangled health problems that required experts with broad and interdisciplinary approaches. And while there have been calls for cooperation and collaboration by leaders in both human and veterinary medicine throughout the twentieth century, it has only been in the last few decades that events such as the WNV outbreak have brought One Health to the forefront. That focus has grown in the two decades since WNV, and in July 2017, Dr. Tedros Adhanom, a man who has proclaimed himself a "champion of the One Health approach at all levels" was named the Director General of the World Health Organization.

In this chapter, we explore several ways in which education and One Health intersect. One Health is interdisciplinary by nature and represents a rich opportunity for undergraduate liberal arts programs and cross-discipline majors and minors. In addition, comprehensive pre-medical and pre-veterinary programs would benefit from the inclusion of One Health concepts in studies of conservation biology and disease transmission as well as a solid foundation in problem-solving and critical thinking. The post-baccalaureate setting in which professionals are trained is an important One Health consideration as well, given that narrowly focused and exclusive human and animal medical-education systems are how the siloing of fields occurred in the first place. One Health-based programs offer the opportunity for doctors, veterinarians, public health officials, and researchers-in-training to communicate and collaborate with colleagues from other disciplines to avoid forming silos of knowledge. Further, practicing health professionals

need a path to One Health credentialing that provides a foundation in the One Health perspective and the language needed to communicate with professionals from other fields.

However, formal training is not the only intersection of One Health and education. Public outreach is a component of many One Health careers, and this requires an understanding of how to connect and communicate with diverse, non-science audiences. The science-related interests and behaviors of the general public are discussed later in the chapter as well as a brief review of formal and informal science education. This is important because increasing the science and health interest and literacy levels of the public is crucial to promoting a universal culture of One Health. Finally, we discuss the recent phenomenon of science/health denial. Worldwide, but notably within the USA, a sector of the population disregards many of the scientific conclusions that inform One Health, despite overwhelming evidence and the consensus of scientists globally. The denial of science has spawned a good deal of study and debate, which is summarized at the chapter's end.

## 9.1 Higher Education and One Health

One Health is interdisciplinary in nature and well suited to the undergraduate environment. It involves anticipating, understanding, and either mitigating or effectively managing risks that occur within the triad, and this requires teams with knowledge of science as well as many non-science subjects such as law, policy, management, social services, communication, and more. In fact, it is difficult to name a discipline that cannot be included in a One Health framework. Historians on a One Health team offer a broad perspective of the geopolitical atmosphere. Sociologists can help with an understanding of the culture, traditions, and motivation of the people impacted by the risk. Social workers and those within the public health infrastructure have an understanding of the societal pressures, politics, and policies involved, and those with theological knowledge can help interpret any religious issues that might arise. The list includes engineering, urban planning, marketing, education, nursing, and on and on. The perspective of One Health is far reaching, and as such, One Health can sit at the center of any well-structured liberal arts program that encourages problem solving, critical thinking, and team work.

Undergraduate science and health programs, such as pre-medical, pre-veterinary, and pre-public-health would also benefit from exposure to the One Health environment. Students interested in entering these fields usually begin with a major in biology or chemistry, with curricula that may or may not include coursework in immunology, conservation biology, or ecology. Prerequisite coursework for entry into human medical-training programs vary widely, but few specify the elective science courses taken for the major. Most medical schools require a year of introductory biology, a year of introductory physics, and two years of chemistry that include general and organic chemistry. The Medical College Admissions Test covers biology, including evolution, but according to the Association for American Medical Colleges, there are no questions on conservation or ecology on the test. Veterinary school entrance requirements are similar to human medical programs although there are lists of recommended elective courses that vary widely from school to school. Most do not mention humanities beyond the courses needed for the bachelor's degree nor are conservation or ecology generally recommended electives. Admission to graduate programs in biology or public health requires bachelor's degrees with outstanding GPAs, but again, they are inconsistent and often do not specify required science or non-science coursework.

At the time of this writing, there exist a handful of undergraduate One Health programs. These include a major available at Westminster College in Fulton, MO, a minor available at Fontbonne University in St. Louis, MO, a minor at Berry College in Mount Berry, GA, and a learning community experience for freshman and sophomore students at Texas A & M in College Station, TX. This number will almost certainly increase, a trend that will require personnel to provide introductory One Health training for faculty in both science and non-science departments.

Another area where undergraduate One Health programs can find acceptance is in the education of future teachers. One Health should be incorporated into the elementary curriculum, as the interconnectedness of life is something that captures most children and can engage them in science. However, before One Health can show up in K-12, teachers must be trained in the content. The One Health Commission produced a report in 2016 advancing several strategies for incorporating One Health into elementary education, including grants for teacher training in One Health, potential online collaborations, and a presumptive K-12 curriculum.

There is a clear opportunity for One Health experiences at the graduate level, including medical, veterinary, basic research, and public health programs. As detailed in previous chapters, some of the greatest threats to our health future include the environmental impacts of climate change, zoonoses, and food-borne illnesses. These complex threats cannot be meaningfully disentangled to consider only their human, animal, ecosystem, or basic science implications nor does approaching them from isolated perspectives go very far toward finding solutions. The WNV story that opened the chapter revealed the critical nature of cross-discipline collaboration and the need for it has only increased as the tools have advanced to include highly specialized genetics and genomics. Additionally, there are points of mutual interest between disciplines, such as the pathophysiology, evolution, and treatment of cross-species diseases like cancer and heart disease. Too often, the response to a health crisis is, "How do I approach this?" rather than, "What team do I need to call together?" Working together, medical, veterinary, and other scientists should learn to value a team approach from the outset, increase the efficiency with which disease mechanisms are studied by pooling efforts, and better value the role that animals play in the research arena. While these connections are easier to accomplish on large campuses that house human and animal medicine, and a variety of other graduate programs, it is certainly possible to connect remotely. In some cases, students have taken the lead on making these connections. One Health student groups have formed on medical, veterinary, public health campuses; and as the faculty in these programs become increasingly aware of One Health, the connections of research opportunities, collaborative summer programs, and internships are bound to increase.

However, the One Health perspective could be valuable to allied health and even non-health graduate programs as well. As examples, lawyers interested in environmental law or policy would need to know the best science for species involved, and the impacts to businesses and financial partners in any conservation effort are important to consider. Those seeking a Master's in Business Administration would benefit from an understanding of the environmental costs and benefits that their companies control. Graduate-level social workers will certainly face families and communities impacted by crises that arise within the triad, and the allied health professionals, particularly physician assistants, nurses, and nurse practitioners, will likely play an increasingly important role in community health, especially in the neighborhoods most vulnerable to disaster.

For students in allied health and graduate research programs, as well as for professionals in a variety of fields, there is a need for focused and efficient credentialing programs in One Health. These programs must equip health professionals with the knowledge needed to communicate across boundaries, as well as inform the work of politicians and policy makers, those in social and behavioral fields,

businesspersons, and the educators of our next generation from elementary to undergraduate classrooms. Professional certification programs are suited to meet this need. The basic requirement of such a program is to provide an introduction to One Health, experience with the tools and language used by professionals across the range of One Health, and networking and access to resources available to One Health professionals. One such program is the One Health Practitioner Certification Program at the Center for One Health at Fontbonne University.

## 9.2 One Health Practitioners as Educators

Several of the organizations that oversee health and wellbeing of the planet have included education as a critical part of enduring a healthy future. The closest thing Earth has to a planetary governing body is the United Nations (UN), and many One Health organizations point to the 2030 Sustainable Development Goals, adopted by the UN in 2015, as an authoritative document. It calls for global action on many One Health concerns, including poverty, health, clean water, responsible energy, climate action, and more. Goal four of the Agenda seeks to ensure "inclusive and equitable quality education and promote lifelong learning opportunities for all," suggesting that the skills acquired through education are what make people successful and resilient in their professional and personal lives. Additionally, the UN Educational, Scientific and Cultural Organization, states that "education is the most effective means that society possesses for confronting the challenges of the future." Education is also a priority of the Organization for Economic Cooperation and Development (OECD), a governmental think tank dedicated to communication between governments seeking solutions for commonly faced problems. The OECD's mission is to promote policies that will improve the economic and social wellbeing of people around the world. Beginning in 2000, the OECD, through their Program for International Student Assessment has sponsored triennial, global testing of 15-year-old-students from 72 countries in an effort to understand the issues involved in educational success in order to inform education policy.

Given the importance of education to the future health and well-being of planet Earth, it must also be a priority for One Health. And if One Health is active at the interface between human, animal, and the environment, then the people who live or work at that interface are the people that we, as a One Health practitioners, might need to educate. They may be families whose children play in an urban back yard, or they may be families whose children are malnourished survivors in a war zone. The One Health environment can be local, including issues like wildlife-encounter protocols or the passage of ani-mal- and environmentally-friendly business policies, or it can be global, as in developing a response plan to emerging viruses. But in most cases, the bottom-line consumer of One Health information is a non-scientist

member of the general public. It is they who must be taught, and in some cases persuaded, how to interact with nature in ways that are best for all involved.

The ability to communicate with the public about health and science is not innate. As discussed in Chapter 10, the weight of evidence does not always win the day with a non-science audience, and the ability to connect with people where they and their interests are is a valuable tool to have on hand. Considering American attitudes, a survey sponsored by the American National Science Board (NSB), focused on public attitudes and behavior concerning science and engineering. This report includes survey information gathered by the NSB's own researchers, by groups such as Gallup and Pew. Considerations of the comparative value of such data, as well as the caveats that go along with survey results, apply here, but still, the report provides insights into the mindset of the general audience. In most cases, the surveys gave respondents the response options of "very interested," "somewhat interested," "not at all interested," and

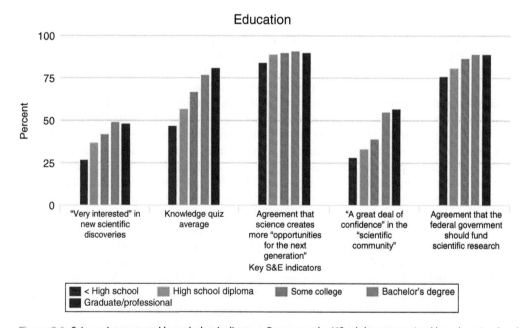

Figure 9.1 Science interest and knowledge indicators; Responses by US adults, categorized by education level attained. *Source:* Reprinted from the National Science Board. 2016. Science and Engineering Indicators 2016. Arlington, VA: National Science Foundation (NSB-2016-1).

"I don't know." Figure 9.1 shows the answers of US adults from five educational demographics to questions regarding four key science indicators as well as their basic science knowledge as determined by a quiz. From these data, it is clear that we need to do more to spark interest in science, but encouragingly, all demographics surveyed agree that science holds great opportunities for future generations and that the government should continue to fund it. Additionally, while the results *appear* to show a lack of confidence in leaders within the science community, the report states that only leaders in the military routinely score higher on this scale, which speaks to a place for science and engineering professionals in politics and public service.

Concerning the aspects of science that US adults find interesting, Figure 9.2 shows that 41% of the US population are "very inter-

ested" in new scientific discoveries, a number that goes up to 59% when the discoveries are medical in nature. Concerning controversial topics, only 40% were "very interested" in environmental pollution, a number that has dropped from its high of 60% in 1990. Similarly, fewer than 40% feel that climate change poses a serious threat to their way of life (Figure 9.3). This is in sharp contrast to global attitudes, where a 2016 Ipsos poll found that 84% of respondents from 27 countries found climate change to be a serious problem. This declining interest among the US public may reflect confidence stemming from the approval of the Paris Accord to combat climate change. It will be interesting to see if this nonchalance about the climate continues in the current (2017) political atmosphere. With respect to energy, most (60%) of US adults said that they would choose con-

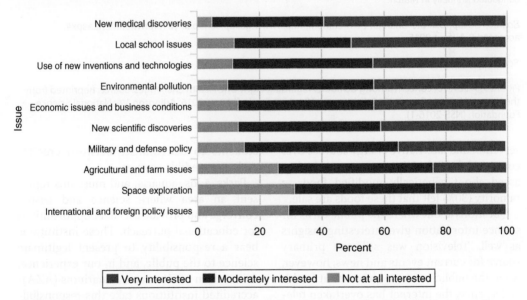

*Notes:* Responses to *There are a lot of issues in the news, and it is hard to keep up with every area. I'm going to read you a short list of issues, and for each one I would like you to tell me if you are very interested, moderately interested, or not at all interested.* Responses of "don't know" are not shown.

*Source:* University of Chicago, National Opinion Research Center, General Social Survey (2014). See appendix table 7-1.

*Science and Engineering Indicators 2016*

Figure 9.2 Interest level of US adults in a variety of science areas. *Source:* Reprinted from the National Science Board. 2016. Science and Engineering Indicators 2016. Arlington, VA: National Science Foundation (NSB-2016-1).

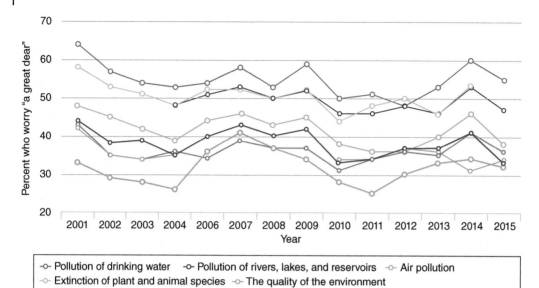

Figure 9.3 Level of concern among US adults regarding eight One Health challenges. *Source:* Reprinted from the National Science Board. 2016. Science and Engineering Indicators 2016. Arlington, VA: National Science Foundation (NSB-2016-1).

servation and alternative energy sources over continued fossil-fuel development, and when asked about genetically modified foods, a minority (30%) felt that these foods are safe.

Questions about where the public turns for science information give interesting insights as well. Television was still the primary source for current events and news; however, when the public wants to know about health and science, the internet has overtaken television as the first stop. This suggests opportunities for internet-based communication for One Health practitioners. Increasing the presence of One Health on the internet must become a priority, particularly on sites that are attractive to the public, such as zoo and animal-issue sites. However, the expansion of use of the internet as a science resource must be accompanied by sustained efforts to teach

students to discriminate between credible and non-credible sources.

Parks, zoos, aquaria, and museums represent an area where science and leisure converge and provide excellent opportunities for educational outreach. These institutions bear a responsibility to present legitimate science to the public, and in our experience, Association of Zoos and Aquariums (AZA)-accredited institutions take this responsibility quite seriously and do an outstanding job of displaying science in a way that interests and engages children while exposing their parents to the underlying evidence. However, these institutions must continually be careful not to discourage, overwhelm, or enrage their volunteer audience. This is an incredibly tight line to walk, and many compromises must be made. For more on this, read the chapter interview with Ms. Louise Bradshaw, Director of Education for the Saint Louis Zoo. Ms. Bradshaw suggests that finding common interests with an audience is a good beginning. An as example, our chapter case study explores the global decline of a beloved group of animals: the amphibians.

Public **skepticism** of scientific conclusions is an area of concern for One Health. From climate denial and anti-vaccination campaigns to the consumption of products that medical science has deemed unhealthy, health professionals stand in awe as warnings go unheeded. While many in the science community blame a lack of science literacy in the general population, which could be overcome by improved education in elementary and secondary schools, recent studies do not support this conclusion. Using the US relationship to climate change as an example, if this hypothesis of "science-deficit" were supported, one would expect that US scores in basic science understanding would correlate with the degree to which the US population disregards climate science. They do not. Only 66% of US respondents view climate change as a serious threat, yet according to the 2015 Programme for International Student Assessment (PISA) results, US 15-year-olds score in the top 30 of the 70 OECD countries on science understanding. Additionally, the NSB report shows that adult understanding of scientific inquiry, probability, and experimental design, and their ability to correctly interpret scientific information has increased by 14, 2, 19, and 5 percentage points, respectively, in the period between 1999 and 2014. Importantly, a study from 2012 found that science denial has more to do with differences in world view than science knowledge. In fact, a greater percentage of climate deniers scored *higher* in science literacy and numeracy than most non-deniers.

Why do knowledgeable people ignore science? There are several possible reasons for this, but the first is that trained scientists think and communicate differently than most people. Scientific studies use inductive reasoning (the type of reasoning that draws general conclusions from limited samples),

and as such, always include a degree of uncertainty. In an effort to be as accurate as possible, scientists are trained to avoid the language of absolutes, which by the general public can be perceived as ambiguous. As an example, consider an entomologist who studies the behavior of moths when exposed to artificial lighting at night. It may be that 100% of the moths tested move toward the light, but a trained scientist would hesitate to say, "all moths do this," because it is not possible to test every moth on Earth. There could be a subgroup out there somewhere that behaves differently. Graduate students in science are trained to use phrases like "the evidence suggests," or "the most likely explanation for ...," but to a general audience, these extra-cautious phrases sound as though the scientist is not thoroughly convinced of their conclusions. Worse, those who stand to gain by discrediting science could intentionally introduce such doubts. If One Health professionals wait until they have won over the skeptics and "proven" the risks and dangers of such things as habitat destruction, climate change, and pollinator decline before human behaviors change, we will have failed.

A second issue in communicating One Health information is in the area of understanding how people evaluate risk. The climate-denial research mentioned earlier categorized participants using two competing, cultural worldviews. The authors describe the first group as "persons who subscribe to a 'hierarchical, individualistic' worldview – one that ties authority to conspicuous social rankings and eschews collective interference with the decisions of individuals possessing such authority – tend to be skeptical of environmental risks." This group, they assert, would process information in the framework of other also valuable variables, such as potential restrictions on commerce and industry. The second group is more egalitarian and communal, described by the authors as "persons who favor less regimented forms of social organization and pay greater collective attention to individual needs – tend to be morally suspicious of commerce and industry, to which they attribute social inequity." These individuals evaluate scientific information from a broader and more collective perspective. The study found that not only does cultural perspective shape one's perception of risk, but also, the gap in acceptance of science increased as science literacy and numeracy increased. This tendency for science denial among hierarchical-individualist individuals was also seen if the risk presented to them was that associated with the use of nuclear power (although the authors note that this gap may have changed after the Fukushima Daiichi nuclear incident in Japan in 2011).

Moreover, the public is continually bombarded with information, and in some cases, there is intentional misinformation with which to contend. As discussed in Chapter 3, self-proclaimed "experts" can make arguments that seem reasonable, and information is presented to the public in a way that makes false evidence seem equal to, or as acceptable as, the fact-based evidence accepted by an overwhelming consensus of health experts and scientists. With climate change, the consensus among publishing scientists and relevant peer-reviewed articles is somewhere around 99%. However, the Yale Project on Climate Change Communication reports that the general public's *perception* of the scientific consensus on climate change is only around 60%. Misinformation is dangerous and difficult to displace. The cases made against HIV as the causative agent for AIDS led to a deadly delay in response to the epidemic in South Africa in the early 2000s, and the continuing anti-vaccination rhetoric in the USA has led to vaccine-preventable outbreaks and deaths.

## 9.3 Conclusions

There are many benefits to providing a strong One Health presence in elementary curricula when students are still developing their world views, and the skills of problem solving and critical thinking that accompany a science education are useful regardless of the future path a student might take. Moreover, children are naturally interested in animals and the environment, and One Health is a great way to engage young minds. In addition, there is a clear need to introduce One-Health to an interdisciplinary audience of undergraduate and graduate students who represent the professionals of the coming generation.

Concerning education of the general public, it is important to understand how adults consume and integrate information. Many see it in the context of what they already know or have heard, and the scientists who must educate and inform the public often fail to communicate engagingly. Overcoming these communication deficits is a focus in Chapter 10.

## End of Chapter Questions & Activities

A. Thought Questions:
   i) When was the first time you heard about One Health? Was it from a teacher?
   ii) Who was your favorite teacher? What did they do that impacted you?
B. In-Class/Guided Activities:
   i) Prepare a lesson about a One Health concern for various target audiences: children, non-science adults, and trained health professionals. What assumptions were made for each group?
C. At-home Activities:
   i) Volunteer to teach a lesson about One Health at a local school or scout club.
   ii) Consider the undergraduate, graduate, or online courses outside your field that would improve your skill set and sign up for one.
D. Long-term Action Steps:
   i) Commit to being a life-long learner.
   ii) Join a neighborhood book club and read environment-based books when it is your turn to choose.
E. Recommended Reading:
   Janovy, J. Jr. (2003). *Teaching in Eden: Lessons from Cedar Point*. RoutledgeFalmer.
   Kolbert, E. (2014). *The Sixth Extinction: An Unnatural History*. Henry Holt and Co.

# Interview

*An Interview with Louise Bradshaw, MSEd: the Fred Saigh Director of Education for the Saint Louis Zoo*

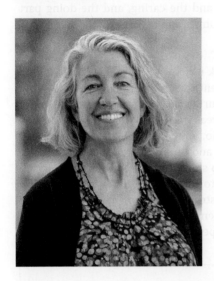

**Do you see yourself as a One Health practitioner?**

I think the word practitioner is very interesting to me. When I first read this question, I thought, well, of course not. I do not have a DVM, I do not have a PhD, I am not an MD, I have a master's degree in education, I have a biology degree, a bachelor's in biology, so I do not think of myself in that way. But on the other hand, the whole practice of One Health, the whole endeavor of One Health requires a lot of public support and understanding. So that's the sphere within which I am promoting the public support and understanding, being a champion for One Health both here internally at the Zoo and with external audiences. So, from that perspective, I would say, I am a practitioner in the support side of the One Health practice.

**How do your actions reflect One Health, personally or professionally?**

At home, certainly there are a lot of decisions that I am thinking of as I think about the footprint that I or my family leave on the planet. How are we operating in our lives to create the least harm for the environment, particularly in the animals and particularly as it has to do with health?

**What can an individual do to make a difference for planetary health?**

I think of the individual actions, what you can do … I think learning a lot, understanding and then figuring out what's important for me to know, what's important for me in my own life. Because conservation actions work best when they are operating at a community level, policy level; it's in that area where things really move forward.

**Where is One Health headed?**

I am very positive about where it's headed. I think on an intellectual level, where we all can frame things as interconnected and help people understand interconnectedness, is a really important underlying value to help people see their place and the importance of doing things at whatever level they can, whether that's knowing more or donating or whatever in this interconnected space. I feel really excited. It's exciting to work across disciplines. I think it's heading in an exciting direction, exactly where I do not know. But I think the future has lots of possibility and hope, which is really exciting.

**How can we encourage people to care about planetary health?**

Put more emphasis on it. Most of us, as human beings, have some level of care about our own health. To be able to then move out from self to family, to community of humans, then even up to the level of ecosystem services, I think most people can make some connection at one or more of those levels.

**As a zoo educator, how do you measure the impact that you have had?**

It's easy enough to say, people have learned things, that's very easy, content is very easy, but we know understanding something and knowing something is not directly correlated to doing something about it. It's not directly correlated to feeling strongly and passionately that something needs to be done. All these different pieces, the knowing, and the feeling and the doing, are interconnected but they also occur differently for different people, they occur differently at different times.

**Do you ever feel pressure between presenting science and the sensibilities of the general audience?**

I mentioned when we were talking about research in forming our practice; there's a lot of really interesting work being done in the area of empathy. How to create empathy and use empathy as a positive orienting device around establishing care for animals and wanting to make the knowledge, and the caring, and the doing part for animals and for the environment.

**Parting Thoughts?**

I think it helps to make sure there is that easy entry point for the average person. Box turtles are such an easy entry point, they really are. Everybody loves box turtles. So, you start with a real charismatic cutie, and oh my gosh, it's incredible. Try not to spend too much time stuck in the ivory tower part of it. But make sure there is a strong engagement on the public engagement side of things, and get help from people who do that for a living.

---

### Case Study: The Decline in Amphibians

Co-authored by Paige Stamps

In the early 1990s, scientists noticed a major decline in the number of amphibians with more than one-third of amphibian species now threatened with extinction, and about 7% of amphibian species are listed as critically endangered. There are many proposed reasons for these declines, but the major factors are thought to be habitat destruction, increase in disease rates, climate change, and the effects of introduced species. The simultaneous emergence of these four factors is having a large negative impact on amphibians all around the world.

Amphibians, mainly frogs, are very dependent on specific habitats, and since amphibians live part of their life in land and part in water, they feel the effects of alterations to both environments. Rain forests contain the greatest biodiversity of amphibians, but in the past 40 years, more than 20% of the Amazon rain forest has been cut down. The Amazon, as well as rainforests in Africa and Asia, are being cut down to make buildings, furniture, and paper, and therefore, efforts to reduce, reuse, and recycle could help amphibian survival.

Fungal attacks are another factor in amphibian declines. A fungal chytrid pathogen called *Batrachochytrium dendrobatidis* causes chytridiomycosis disease. This fungus infects amphibian skin, causing it to become very rough and thick. This is deadly to frogs because they absorb water through their thin, semipermeable skin. Some species of frogs, such as the bullfrog, are resistant to this pathogen, and scientists are hoping that learning the basis of resistance can lead to preventatives for all amphibians.

A 2009 study in salamander decline found that climate change was a bigger factor than habitat destruction or chytridiomycosis. The investigators compared surveys conducted between 1969 and 1978 in Central America, and during that time two out of three of the most common salamander species on the west coast of Guatemala have disappeared, and the third is difficult to locate. The authors speculate that increasing temperatures are driving salamanders to higher elevations on the flanks of the volcano Tajumulco, where they are experiencing low reproduction rates and high mortality.

Global warming and climate change are harming frog species, as well. Frogs come out of hibernation and breed when the environment factors, such as temperature, are right.

Since temperatures have been rising earlier in winter than usual, frogs are breeding earlier than usual, however, tadpoles cannot sustain life in these colder conditions.

Amphibian decline is a warning to us about our effects on the environment and the sixth mass extinction.

## Works Cited

Adhanom, T. (2016) Personal endorsement of One Health posted to http://www.onehealthinitiative.com/publications/One%20Health%20Endorsement%20Letter.pdf (accessed December 19, 2017).

Bonardi, A., Manenti, R., Corbetta, A. et al. (2011). Usefulness of volunteer data to measure the large-scale decline of "common" toad populations. *Biological Conservation* 144: 2328–2334.

Bosch, J., Martinez-Solano, I., and Garcia-Paris, M. (2000). Evidence of a chytrid fungus infection involved in the decline of the common midwife toad (Alytes obstetricans) in protected areas of Central Spain. *Biological Conservation* 97: 331–337.

Braman, D., Kahan, D.M., Peters, E. et al. (2012). The polarizing impact of science literacy and numeracy on perceived climate change risks. *Nature Climate Change* 2 (10): 732–735.

Cardiff, R.D., Ward, J.M., and Barthold, S.W. (2008). 'One medicine–one pathology': are veterinary and human pathology prepared? *Laboratory Investigation* 88: 18–26.

Fontbonne University Program in One Health http://onehealth.fontbonne.edu (accessed June 30, 2018).

Hayes, T.B., Falso, P., Gallipeau, S. et al. (2010). The cause of global amphibian declines: a developmental endocrinologist's perspective. *Journal of Experimental Biology* 213: 921–933.

IPSOS (2015) Global Warming Issue Unites World Opinion: 82% View Climate Change as Major Threat. URL: https://www.ipsos.com/en-us/ipsos-global-dvisor-global-warming-issue-unites-world-opinion-82-view-climate-change-major-threat (accessed December 29, 2017).

Kahn, L.H. (2011). The need for one health degree programs. *Infection, Ecology and Epidemiology* 1: 7919. doi: 10.3402/iee.v1i0.7919.

Kilgannon, C. Neighborhood Report: Bayside; At Fort Totten and Elsewhere, Crows Dying Mysteriously. *The New York Times* August 22, 1999.

Ludwig, G.V., Calle, P.P., Mangiafico, J.A. et al. (2002). An outbreak of West Nile virus in a New York city captive wildlife population. *American Journal of Tropical Medicine and Hygiene* 67 (1): 67–75.

Lueddeke, G.R., Kaufman, G.E., Lindenmayer, J. M., et al. (2016) Preparing Society to Create the World We Need Through One Health Education. Report of the Survey and Web Conference on One Health K-12 Education.

McConnell, I. (2014). One Health in the context of medical and veterinary education. *Scientific and Technical Review of the Office International des Epizooties* 33 (2): 651–657.

National Science Board (2016). *Science and Engineering Indicators 2016*. Arlington, VA: National Science Foundation (NSB-2016-1).

OECD (2016). *PISA 2015 Results (Volume I): Excellence and Equity in Education*. Paris: PISA, OECD Publishing. doi: 10.1787/9789264266490-en.

Pidgeon, N. and Fischhoff, B. (2011). The role of social and decision sciences in communicating uncertain climate risks.

*Nature Climate Change* 1: 35–41. doi: 10.1038/NCLIMATE1080.

Rabinowitz, P.M., Natterson-Horowitz, B.J., Kahn, L.H. et al. (2017). Incorporating one health into medical education. *BMC Medical Education* 17: 45. doi: 10.1186/s12909-017-0883-6.

Sodhi, N.S., Bickford, D., Diesmos, A.C. et al. (2008). Measuring the meltdown: drivers of global amphibian extinction and decline. *PLoS One* 3 (2): e1636. doi: 10.1371/journal.pone.0001636.

United Nations (2015) Transforming Our World: The 2030 Agenda for Sustainable Development. https://sustainabledevelopment.un.org/post2015/transformingourworld (accessed December 28, 2017).

United Nations Education, Science and Culture Organization (2015). *Education for all 2000–2015: Achievements and Challenges*. Paris: UNESCO publishing.

United States General Accounting Office (2000) West Nile Virus Outbreak Lessons for Public Health Preparedness. Report to U.S. Congressional Requesters. https://www.gao.gov/products/HEHS-00-180 (accessed December 21, 2017).

University of California – Berkeley. (2009) Salamander Decline Found in Central America. *ScienceDaily*. http://www.sciencedaily.com/releases/2009/02/090209205311.htm (accessed December 21, 2017).

Westminster College Program in One Health (2017) http://www.westminster-mo.edu/academics/degree-requirements/major-minor-summary-sheets/Documents/Majors/Majors_PDF/One%20Health%20Major.pdf (accessed June 30, 2018).

Zimmer, C. (2012) West Nile Virus: The Stranger that Came to Stay. *Discover*, August 17, 2012. http://blogs.discovermagazine.com/loom/2012/08/17/west-nile-virus-the-stranger-that-came-to-stay/#.WjprLzdG3IU (accessed December 18, 2017).

# 10

# Communication and Advocacy in One Health

*The single biggest problem in communication is the illusion that it has taken place.*

George Bernard Shaw

## 10.1 A Hole in the Ozone

In 1986, school children around the world, but especially in the USA, Europe, and Australia, lobbied their parents to stop supporting fast food chains until the companies ended their use of Styrofoam clamshells as packaging materials. Nightly, on local and national news broadcasts, children, their parents, and environmental activists called on these large fast-food chains, like McDonalds and Burger King, to reduce their **ecological footprint** and make their products more sustainable, moving away from long-term environmentally-stable polystyrene and toward environmentally-friendly recyclable and/or compostable packaging products. This was all in response to the discovery of a hole in the atmospheric layer of ozone approximately 10.5 million square miles in area above Antarctica (Figure 10.1). This hole, roughly two million square miles larger than the entire landmass of North America, threatened all life on the planet with exposure to rapidly increasing levels of cancer-causing ultraviolet radiation.

In 1985, researchers studying the atmosphere noticed a loss of atmospheric ozone above Antarctica. Publishing their findings in

the journal *Nature*, it was clear that the culprit was the rise of chlorofluorocarbons, or CFCs, in everyday, disposable products. These products included the polystyrene clamshell-shaped takeout containers that many fast food companies used as packaging for their foods. CFCs are extremely stable in the lower atmosphere, which makes them valuable for use as refrigerants, cleaning solvents, and to create the spaces in polystyrene which also makes it lightweight. However, as these chemicals make their way into the **stratosphere**, ultraviolet radiation breaks the bonds separating the molecules of chlorine from the remaining molecules of fluorine and carbon. These chlorine molecules then "bump" into free ozone molecules, binding with one of the three oxygen molecules. This binding of chlorine to oxygen results in the formation of an oxygen molecule ($O_2$) and a molecule of chlorine monoxide (ClO). However, ClO is not environmentally stable, and when exposed to a free oxygen atom, the oxygens bind together, freeing the chlorine atom to begin the process of cleaving ozone into oxygen again. A single chlorine atom can repeat this cycle many thousands of times. As CFCs amass in the stratosphere, the amount of chlorine atoms available to activate this ozone reducing cycle grew at an alarming rate, resulting in a massive hole in the ozone layer above Antarctica.

Once the hole and the cause were identified, a series of global actions unfolded, culminating in the signing of the Montreal Protocol in

*Introduction to One Health: An Interdisciplinary Approach to Planetary Health*, First Edition.
Sharon L. Deem, Kelly E. Lane-deGraaf and Elizabeth A. Rayhel.
© 2019 John Wiley & Sons, Inc. Published 2019 by John Wiley & Sons, Inc.
Companion website: www.wiley.com/go/deem/health

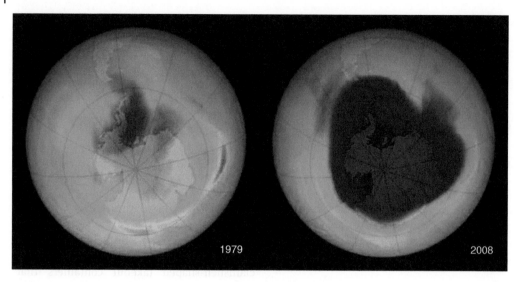

Figure 10.1 Evidence of the ozone hole above Antarctica in 1979 and 2008. The hole is evident in the deep blue and purples. *Source:* Courtesy of NASA.

1987. The Montreal Protocol phased out the production and use of the chlorofluorocarbons responsible for depleting ozone in the upper atmosphere. Even with this swift and global action, the atmospheric layer of ozone will not be fully recovered until 2070, assuming no future additional threats to the ozone layer. This slow recovery from a significant, but short-term, environmental threat suggests that damage to the environment can be overcome. However, the recovery occurs on the scale of environmental change, or in other words, at a glacial pace. As of 2017, the hole in the ozone has returned to pre-1985 sizes, suggesting that quick, global actions can have significant positive benefits for environmental health.

The global reaction to the development of a massive hole in the ozone layer in 1985, culminating in the signing of the Montreal Protocol in 1987, is hailed as one of the most important and successful responses to an environmental threat yet. Importantly, this success can also be hailed as a significant win for communication and advocacy of science to the general public and policy makers alike. In less than two years, a potentially catastrophic environmental threat was identified, actions were taken at local and international levels, including important actions taken by business and industry leaders, and governments across the planet mobilized and enacted legislation to resolve the problem. This was due, in large part, to effective messaging that disseminated specific action items for people to engage with and which they could easily share.

While the global response to the news of our damaged stratosphere is lauded as a communications and advocacy success – and importantly, a success for environmental health – it was, by no means, guaranteed at the outset. However, there are lessons to be learned from this environmental "close call" that can be applied to our current human, animal, and environmental health problems. For example, one reason for the ease and speed of the global move away from CFCs was already existing replacement chemicals: hydrochlorofluorocarbons (HCFCs) and hydrofluorocarbons (HFCs). These chemicals are structurally similar to CFCs and so can be used in many of the same ways but contain no ozone depleting elements. For many current environmental threats, no such easy fix exists or is waiting in the pipeline. As such, the strength of resolve of the global community is even more important in addressing these greatest threats to planetary health. Still, we know that our actions can rapidly change our planet, and the damage to planetary health as a result of our actions will likely be long-lasting, even if our path changes quickly. Clear accessible communication is the only way forward in solving global health crises; the significance cannot be understated.

## 10.2 Scientific Communication

Everything in your life has been communicated to you in some way. From your name to the details of the most cutting edge theoretical physics concepts, communication is a fundamental part of living today. Communication plays a critical role in education, dissemination of news and noteworthy items, from the finding out if your team has won the World Series to full and informed participation in a democracy. We have all experienced communication snafus. For example, most people have experienced a great joke ruined when the punchline is fumbled over or watched the main characters in a romantic comedy make horrible decisions based on one errant piece of information. While some unintentional slips of the tongue can capture the speaker's true thoughts, for example, any opinion voiced by a politician speaking while unaware that his or her microphone was live, most people strive to communicate clearly and honestly throughout their days. Clear communication is a hallmark of science. However, traditional scientific communication is not renowned for clarity but instead is considered dry, dense, and, for many non-scientists, an intentional obfuscation of potentially exciting scientific discoveries.

Scientific communication is traditionally done through the publication of peer-reviewed articles in scientific journals and conference presentations published in conference proceedings. The process of peer-review, however, can proceed excruciatingly slowly and is not without issue. For example, recent evidence has come to light demonstrating that the work of well-known scientists is frequently evaluated less critically, suggesting that the use of a double-blind system for author and reviewers could improve the process of peer-review. However, despite concerns of efficacy of the peer-review process, scientific publications must be held up for critical evaluation by at least three experts in the field, and despite the thousands of articles published daily, many more manuscripts fail to meet the threshold of scientific standards of the peer-review process. Rarely, a scientist with a penchant for and considerable ability to communicate complex ideas directly to the public rises to the forefront of our communal consciousness – Carl Sagan, Stephen Jay Gould, Neil deGrasse Tyson – and inspires a generation. However, for the vast majority of scientists, the media is something to be largely avoided, with many seeing their role as scientists as one of passive collector of objective data instead of as an active advocate for science or conceptual ideas based on evidence. Moreover, many scientists view journalists and the media with suspicion, with the expectation that interview language could be taken out of context or turned into a pithy soundbite, with the potential to misconstrue the details of their scientific findings. Complicating these interactions is the frequent, highly technical language of many scientists and scientific results, many of which do not translate easily into non-technical language accessible to the general public, especially when filtered through the lens of the media. As a result of this lack of communication with the public *writ large*, science and scientists face an increasing amount of skepticism outside scientific circles, with dire consequences resulting from diminished recognition of the value of science and expertise of scientists, especially to policy-makers. The evidence of this can be found among arguments for the denial of human-caused climate change, evolution, and even vaccine safety.

Writing in *The Demon-Haunted World: Science as a Candle in the Dark,* Carl Sagan said, "We've arranged a global civilization in which most crucial elements profoundly depend on science and technology. We have also arranged things so that almost no one understands science and technology. This is a prescription for disaster. We might get away with it for a while, but sooner or later this combustible mixture of ignorance and power is going to blow up in our faces." This statement is profoundly true and simultaneously identifies how the lack of accessible language and communication between scientists and the general public is the mechanism that underpins the growing global threat of **science denialism**.

## 10.3 Science Denial and the Cautionary Language of Scientists

Science denial is one of the greatest threats to planetary health today. Unfortunately, overcoming the inculcation that leads to the denial of science will not occur simply by providing more evidence or additional data. As we learned in Chapter 9, early exposure to critical thinking exercises, evidence-based science, and potentially taboo subject matters in educational programming can have lasting effects on student thinking. However, for most people over the age of seven, education does not result in a shifting conceptualization away from science denialism, which may have been nurtured previously by parents and other role models whose power to indoctrinate, intentionally or unintentionally, is substantial, into a reality of science acceptance. In fact, evidence has begun to show that contrary to what many assume to be the benefits of education, storytelling and the development of emotional connections are far more likely to change people's thinking when it comes to complex, emotionally charged, and/or controversial ideas. Environmental educators know this to be true. For example, Jeffrey Bonner, anthropologist and President

and CEO of the Saint Louis Zoo, has described one of the defining moments in his development as a conservationist, as occurring when, as a child, he visited the Belle Isle Aquarium and was given the opportunity to touch an electric eel, watching as it discharged enough electricity to power light bulbs. The emotional connection inherent in his "electric eel moment" inspired him to pursue a life dedicated to human, animal, and environmental health. The sharing of his story and the emotional connection of his "electric eel moment" has gone on to inspire and encourage other environmental educators in their use of **transformational learning** opportunities, which focus on building emotional connections and telling stories over regurgitating facts and data.

Transformational learning, driven by storytelling and emotional connections, is not traditionally the language of scientists. Scientists communicate directly with other scientists via peer-reviewed publications and conference presentations. However, storytelling is an important, if undervalued, tool of science and scientists. For example, Richard Primack, esteemed conservation biologist at Boston University and author of numerous peer-reviewed papers recommends that scientists write an op-ed or a brief review article for a local newspaper or topical magazine for every peer-reviewed manuscript they publish. Not only does this double a scientist's publication record, it allows individual scientists to tell the story of the science to the people, reaching a variety of interested audiences, including both funders and policy-makers. However, developing an emotional connection through storytelling is not the task of most scientific writing. In fact, the language of science is unique to science. It is a cautious approach to language. To the uninitiated, it may lack confidence and suggest there are questions or uncertainty where there is not. Scientists are trained to be judicious in their interpretations of data and to be open to alternative explanations while working to identify the most likely scenario. This approach, described eloquently by philosophers of science as **Occam's razor**, suggests that, given a number of possible explanations, the simplest is the most likely. In scientific terms, this is known as **parsimony**. Still, this linguistic caution frequently prevents scientists from communicating in absolute terms. For example, the use of "frequently" in the prior sentence is scientific training cautioning against absolutes.

Unfortunately, the cautious nature of science as a language can have potentially calamitous consequences. In 1997, Carl Sagan wrote in *The Demon-Haunted World: Science as a Candle in the Dark*, "Science is more than a body of knowledge; it is a way of thinking. I have a foreboding of an America in my children's or grandchildren's time – when the United States is a service and information economy; when nearly all the key manufacturing industries have slipped away to other countries; when awesome technological powers are in the hands of a very few, and no one representing the public interest can even grasp the issues; when the people have lost the ability to set their own agendas or knowledgeably question those in authority; when, clutching our crystals and nervously consulting our horoscopes, our critical faculties in decline, unable to distinguish between what feels good and what's true, we slide, almost without noticing, back into superstition and darkness." Dr. Sagan's concerns have begun to come to fruition. When communicating with non-scientists, the language of scientists is frequently misinterpreted. For example, in 2017, a panel of NASA scientists testifying about upcoming Mars Rover expeditions before the US House of Representatives' Committee on Science, Space, and Technology were asked about the possibility of now-extinct civilizations on Mars from thousands of years ago (Figure 10.2). The lead scientist on the project responded by explaining that "the evidence is that Mars was different billions of years ago, not thousands of years ago, but there is no evidence [of early Martian civilizations] that I'm aware

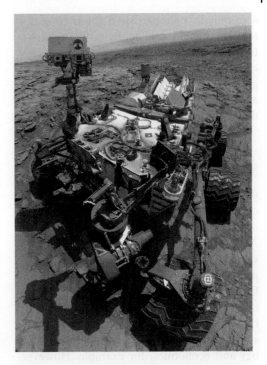

**Figure 10.2** Mars Rover Curiosity selfie from Mars. *Source:* Courtesy of NASA.

of." The dialogue between the NASA scientist and the congressman continued for a number of minutes, and yet, the strongest response offered by the scientist regarding the potential for early Martian civilizations was, "I would say that is extremely unlikely." For the record, there is no evidence of civilizations from any point in history on Mars. However, it is clear from this brief exchange that the cautious nature of scientific communication potentially leaves the discoveries and ideas of science open to interpretation by those without scientific training and/or by those who are interested in exploiting scientific ideas for their own financial benefit.

Ultimately, the denial of science and the loss of recognized expertise of scientists are bolstered by the language of science and scientists. As such, science denialism as a threat to global health will continue unimpeded until scientists and the public are better able to share a common language. This communication bridge will improve as training in scientific literacy improves, resulting in a society with a strengthened ability to evaluate claims, data, and sources, and as scientists engage in more and more increasingly creative programs to reach directly to the general public through outreach, advocacy, and **citizen science** programs, among other direct engagements.

## 10.4 Communication as the Bridge-Building Tool of One Health

As a truly interdisciplinary field, One Health synthesizes knowledge from across disciplines into one holistic, synergistic approach for solving the complex problems of planetary health. This situates One Health practitioners in the vital position of being able to speak across disciplines as disparate as virology and economics, for example. However, for far too long, relevant disciplines have not engaged in any meaningful discourse. Even in the significantly overlapping fields of human and animal medicine, academic training, disciplines, and institutional structures historically minimized and, at times, prevented engaging dialogue between health practitioners. However, human health (or animal or environmental health) does not exist in a vacuum, independent of planetary health. In order to effectively confront the perils facing global health today, it is imperative that health practitioners begin to reach beyond their respective silos and engage with the community and with experts from outside their own disciplines directly. In order to implement a One Health approach, it is necessary to engage with scientists from across multiple disciplines, economists, educators, activists, policy makers, and the local community. While field-specific jargon can present challenges, One Health practitioners understand that language must be able to transcend academic disciplines in order to implement solutions to complex problems that require input from multiple voices, each with a personal story, unique values, and

distinct motivations. Clear communication is also critical for building trust among scientists, policy makers, community members, and other relevant participants, which is essential for successful problem solving. Finally, clear communication is fundamental for advocating for the importance of addressing the greatest threats to planetary health and the value of utilizing the One Health approach. Truly, skilled communication that is clear and accessible is the bridge-building tool of the One Health practitioner.

## 10.5 Communication as Outreach

An increasing number of scientists are beginning to use non-traditional forms of communication to engage directly with the public in addition to publishing and presenting in traditional venues. Indeed, even scientists who are not interested in engaging with the public are, as a requirement of many funding opportunities, obliged to consider opportunities for outreach. For example, the National Science Foundation – one of the most significant sources of funding for US scientists, along with the National Institutes of Health – has, as part of all grant proposals, required scientists to develop an outreach program through which they will engage the public. This requirement has been in place for well over two decades and is evaluated along with the merits of the proposed science and plans for traditional scientific dissemination of knowledge. Still, the extent and enthusiasm with which scientists engage in outreach varies dramatically. Scientific outreach is as diverse as the scientists that engage in it, ranging from promoting their own work and the work of others on social media platforms; contributing to and promoting scientific advocacy groups, such as professional organizations, the Union of Concerned Scientists, and/or 500 Women Scientists; **blogging**; developing competitive online games for people across the country, such as March Mammal Madness; podcasting; writing pieces for newspapers, magazines, and online news sources targeting general audiences; "adopting" classrooms from across the country, wherein scientists guest lecture, share data, visit classrooms from remote field sites via Skype; and creating programming targeting traditionally underserved populations of school-aged children, among others.

The rise of social media platforms has had a profound effect on science communication. As more and more scientists and health practitioners have embraced social media as a tool for communicating science directly to the public, the use of these platforms as a means for quickly and clearly disseminating the importance and relevance of scientific findings has expanded dramatically. This encourages scientists to distill down the complexities of their work into digestible, accessible messages suitable for the general public and allows scientists to promote their own work and the work of others to audiences who might not otherwise learn of it.

As a social media platform, Twitter, in particular, allows scientists the ability to converse directly with the public in a way that, in the days before Twitter, was unthinkable. For example, scientists now routinely share the results of their peer-reviewed work on Twitter through the use of one or two short, accessible take-home messages, shared directly with the world. This allows other scientists to discover the work and cite their findings more quickly than ever before. And it encourages the general public to follow scientific trends and respond directly to and converse with scientists. For example, it is possible to follow #OneHealth on Twitter and routinely interact with scientists and other One Health practitioners (Figure 10.3). Twitter also provides a platform for scientists to advocate for science easily and directly with policymakers and other relevant, interested parties. For example, while activists and water protectors were fighting to protect the Standing Rock Water supply from an oil company's plan to construct the Dakota Access Pipeline, routing it across the Missouri River and the drinking water supply and other waters sacred to the Standing Rock Sioux, #NoDAPL was trending on Twitter. For the duration of the protests, #NoDAPL allowed supporters from across the planet to follow actions in North Dakota in real time and respond to both the needs of the protesters, by sending supplies and messages of

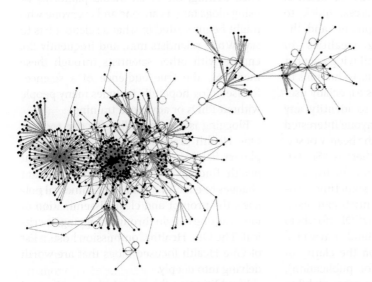

Figure 10.3 Connections between individuals tweeting #OneHealth on One Health Day 2017, created using the program NodeXL. Nodes represent individual twitter users. Network spans the entire globe.

support, and to government actions through calls to Congress. In another example, advocates of marine ecosystem health have begun to call for reducing the amount of disposable plastic bags used every day and replacing them with reusable bags, due to the perils they create for our oceans and ocean wildlife. These advocates have begun promoting their efforts by tweeting relevant science to followers, using the hashtag #ByeToBags. This has resulted in a growing, searchable database of support for this movement with which advocates can physically map to identify both hotspots for and gaps in support over time. Importantly, the growing use of Twitter by scientists can also highlight the day-to-day work of scientists and personalizes, like never before, highlighting not just science, but the funny, witty, challenging sides of science and scientists. For example, the hashtag #FieldWorkFail promotes the hard work and entertaining perils of scientists who do field work, documenting field cars getting stuck in the mud, important sample tubes stolen by study animals, accidentally gluing oneself to a crocodile, and many more of the amazing challenges of field work. Likewise, the use of #OverlyHonestMethods allows scientists levity in describing the very real challenges associated with the methods of science: working with limited resources, quick to expire reagents, fickle equipment, and the general, but entertaining, realities of experimental science. #ActualLivingScientist should be searched for brief introductions to actual living scientists; this is especially useful for anyone still unable to identify any actual living scientists. For anyone interested in the connections between the beauty of science and the beauty of art, there is #SciArt, #SpaceArt, and #BioArt. And finally, as a nod to the collaborative, yet sometimes isolating, nature of science, scientists can reach out for help using #ICanHazPDF (for help with access to papers behind paywalls), #FigureClub (for feedback on the clarity of figures before submission for publication), and #ShutUpAndWrite (for accountability and motivation to write).

In addition to the use of social media by scientists, academic blogging is now considered an essential tool for scientists and other academics. Blogging, while initially the domain of conspiracy theorists and soccer moms, has blossomed into a mechanism to reach the general public that affords scientists the ability to tell the stories of their science and their own experiences, while thoughtfully constructing a longer narrative than available through other social media platforms. Importantly, this also allows scientists the ability to provide evidentiary support in the form of citations. Blogging has become a vital part of science outreach and the dissemination of research findings. However, even in the linguistically casual world of blogging, clear communication is necessary in order to engage with people about the importance of science generally and One Health specifically. The most significant difference between these traditional forms of scientific writing and blogging is audience, even if there is overlap among readers. Academic writing, in the form of peer-reviewed, published manuscripts targets fellow scientists, including frequently people from the specific field who also have doctorates or are in graduate school. Alternatively, writing about science, or science writing, on social media platforms or using blogs targets anyone and everyone who might be interested in what a scientist has to say. While scientists may, and frequently do, engage with other scientists through these mediums, the true audience of a science-focused blog hopefully includes many people without PhDs or advanced training.

Blogging is an especially effective tool for One Health practitioners. As an interdisciplinary field where the impacts of important health findings could result in significant changes to economic and environmental policies, the prompt and clear dissemination of ideas, as one can do through blogging, is critical. The One Health Commission hosts a list of One Health focused blogs that are worth delving into deeply.

In addition to the use of blogs and social media, communication with the traditional news media – through interviews with media outlets, op-ed pieces written for local and national newspapers, and columns or articles written for appropriate science magazines – can all be used by scientists and other One Health practitioners to communicate directly with the public and advocate for science generally and the One Health approach specifically. These tools, while traditionally met with skepticism by scientists, should not be overlooked or discounted as a valuable tool. Clear communication, using accessible language that connects through an emotional story, is sometimes most effectively done through trusted journalists.

## 10.6 Citizen Science as One Health

Citizen Science projects are unique collaborations between scientists and members of the general public who have a passion for and a commitment to science that goes beyond simply reading about the efforts of scientists. As such, they are an incredibly valuable, albeit challenging to implement, form of outreach with the public. Not exclusive to One Health projects, citizen science programs engage community members like no other scientific outreach program, enlisting the public as participants in the collection of raw data. The interdisciplinary nature of One Health is ideally suited to the collaborative nature of Citizen Science programs. Community members with a variety of areas of expertise can contribute to projects in a significant, meaningful way, resulting in the potential for scientific advances and discoveries that might not otherwise be possible. Some of the best known Citizen Science programs include the Audubon Christmas Bird Count and FoldIt. In both of these projects, citizens from across nations work together to provide valuable on-the-ground data to scientists. Examples of One Health-specific Citizen Science programs include the Saint Louis Zoo's Box Turtle Project, Project Monarch Health, and GoViral. The Box

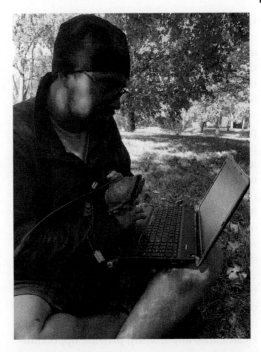

Figure 10.4 Esteban, a box turtle residing in Forest Park, and Will Condit, research assistant monitoring her health with the Saint Louis Zoo Institute for Conservation Medicine's Box Turtle Project. *Source:* Photo credit to Jamie L. Palmer, Saint Louis Zoo.

Turtle Project, developed and driven by the Saint Louis Zoo's Institute for Conservation Medicine (ICM), monitors the movement and health of box turtles in Forest Park, Saint Louis's largest urban park. Citizens contribute sightings of box turtles through the Project's social media websites, and volunteers can then work with ICM scientists to collect turtle health samples (Figure 10.4). These volunteers include, frequently, school children from throughout the St. Louis metropolitan area. Project Monarch Health tracks monarch migrations and the spread of the parasite *Ophryocystis elektroscirrha*, or OE. This protozoan parasite infects only monarch and queen butterflies and can devastate populations by causing irreparable damage to the pupal stage of the butterfly. Citizen scientists can assist the program by capturing and raising wild monarchs and sampling them for parasites by using a safe-for-monarch scotch tape technique. Finally,

GoViral is a Citizen Science project that engages citizens from mostly North America, although this is expanding globally, to sample the viral load of people and track the spread of viruses in the community. Engaged Citizen Scientists can request a sample kit from their website, perform a nasal swab according to provided instructions, and return their sample. Data provided can help scientists better understand how viruses spread in communities. And, importantly, because participants register for this program, individuals who have submitted samples can evaluate their own results against the larger population, which can help individuals better understand their own personal risk of exposure to viruses. Citizen Science programs may not be suitable for every One Health project, but they are valuable tools for inclusion of community members and outreach for One Health and, importantly, provide opportunities to increase community awareness and support for ongoing One Health projects.

## 10.7 Communication and Advocacy as a One Health Tool

One important role of communication and One Health is advocacy. As discussed previously in this chapter, scientists have traditionally positioned themselves as objective disseminators of knowledge, as individuals who observe trends, design experiments, collect and analyze data, and finally, distill the findings into clear, logical results, contextualizing them in light of the existing literature. However, this objective role of scientists has frequently left the interpretation of scientific findings to others, creating the potential opportunity for a misuse or exploitation of scientific results for personal gain. Science, in this context, is able to remain the pure pursuit of knowledge, unencumbered by the constraints of ethical or moral quandaries, political fall-out, or consequences to human, animal, or environmental health.

The desire of scientists to remain objective at all costs is due, in part, to concerns over losing scientific credibility professionally, over losing the perception of being objective publicly, and over fears of alienating funding agencies, among a myriad of other personal reasons. However, at increasing rates, scientists are choosing to advocate for science and scientific findings by participating in political discourse through engagement with policy makers. While this seems a relatively new trend, Albert Einstein spoke out fervently against the rise of Fascism in Germany in 1933 and was chastised later by the Prussian Academy of Science for doing so. He later said of the event, "I do not share your view that the scientist should observe silence in political matters, i.e. human affairs in the broadest sense. The situation in Germany shows whither this restraint will lead: to the surrender of leadership, without any resistance, to those who are blind or irresponsible." His warnings were not heeded, and World War II erupted soon after. Still, the role of scientist as advocate has not been formally embraced by many in academia, and for many scientists, graduate training actively discouraged activism, suggesting that advocate is a label that was to be shunned.

However, the global threats to planetary health that have resulted from human actions can no longer be ignored, swept under the rug as progress. And, accordingly, activism by scientists has had a resurgence. For example, a study published in 2017 by the Pew Research Institute found that "76% of the public and 97% of scientists said it was indeed appropriate for scientists to become actively involved in political debates." Despite this, many scientists still prefer **stealth issue advocacy**, or the discrete approach to advocacy wherein scientists profess their focus on objectivity while seeking to covertly advance a specific agenda, to more overt actions, such as protests, canvasing, or lobbying. For example, in 2017, Jane Lubchenko, Administrator of the National Oceanic and Atmospheric Administration (NOAA) stated that "I don't view our role as trying to convince people of something. Our role is to inform people." This same Pew report suggests that this tendency to discretely advocate for issues may actually damage more than help scientific reputations. Many scholars are beginning to realize that their responsibilities as citizens are not because they are scientists. Paul Ehrlich, renowned biologist and Bing Professor of Population Studies at Stanford University, supports this idea. He was quoted in 2011 as saying, "You often hear people say scientists should not be advocates. I think that is bull." He goes on to say, "With society moving toward a collapse, the idea that scientists, especially ecologists, should just do their work, present their data and not do any interpretation leads to the kind of imbecility we have in Washington today, where you have an entire Congress that is utterly clueless about how the natural world works." Those are strong words in support of the role of scientists as advocates.

On April 22, 2017, scientists *en masse* stepped into their roles as advocates for science in the March for Science, a global protest that drew over a million scientists into the political arena. And this embracing of advocacy among scientists is one important reason that advocacy is a critical tool for One Health. As an interdisciplinary field that aims to address complex threats to planetary health, One Health is an inherently applied field of study. Practitioners must advocate for inclusion of a variety of stakeholders in their own work – from educators and economists to anthropologists and theologians. Moving beyond the local level, One Health practitioners must advocate for their work by broadly disseminating their findings in both peer-reviewed literature and more directly to the general public. The immediacy of the need of many global health threats suggests that social media and the traditional news media can provide needed connections and support for One Health concerns as they unfold. In the USA, a growing cadre of One Health advocacy groups are beginning to utilize the tools of lobbying and social activism. The One Health Commission hosts a listserv and acts as a repository for all One Health programs, including opportunities for activism.

Advocacy and activism can work. In 1962, when Rachel Carson published *Silent Spring*, which detailed how dichlorodiphenyltrichloroethane (DDT) enters the environment, remaining long beyond the duration of the application, bioaccumulates, and ultimately, poisons birds, fish, and children, it called to action an entire generation of concerned American citizens, including scientists. This activism resulted in the eventual ban of DDT for use in the USA and the creation of environmentalism as a movement.

More recently, the global response to the 2014 Ebola outbreak in Guinea, Sierra Leone, Liberia, and Ivory Coast reflects the success that is possible from advocating for and implementing a One Health approach. While far from perfect for a number of reasons, the global response to the outbreak of Ebola, coordinated by the World Health Organization (WHO), employed teams of anthropologists, community engagement specialists, medical staff, sanitation workers, social organizers, and dignified, safe burial experts across the outbreak zone. While the initial response to the outbreak was sluggish by outbreak response standards, WHO experts realized that the most effective way to respond efficiently and with the greatest care for the greatest number of people, was to utilize a One Health approach. In time, these teams were able to communicate effectively with community members, including affected survivors and family members, and organize a response that limited the spread of the pathogen before a global pandemic occurred and was able to treat great numbers of infected individuals safely.

Importantly, scientists and One Health practitioners are well-positioned to use evidence-based advocacy, supporting their positions with policy makers and community members with data from across disciplines and thus making effective, arguments for their positions. Moving beyond local advocacy, more and more scientists have realized that one of the best strategies for engaging with policy makers is to become a policy maker, and as a result, in 2017, there has been a significant rise in the number of scientists running for elected office. From mayoral races to US Senate seats, scientists are joining the political discourse at local, state, and federal levels in the USA. The time when scientists can exist independent of the results they generate is ending. Using outreach and advocacy tools, scientists and other One Health practitioners are ideally suited to communicate to policy makers, community members, and the public *writ large* by interpreting evidence and developing emotional stories to build bridges for the benefit of planetary health.

## 10.8 Conclusion

There is no guide or "best practices" for One Health advocacy or science advocacy more generally. However, communicating One Health messages via social media platforms and traditional news outlets is important for the success of science and One Health, including the ability to advocate for One Health. The most effective approach to communicating with the public is to tell a fair and accurate story, based on scientific evidence, which has the ability to connect with the public on an emotional level. According to David Ropeik, a risk educator with Big Think who is based at Harvard University, scientists should embrace **responsible advocacy** and the following guidelines for advocacy, as reported in 2016:

- communicate one's values fairly and truthfully;
- make the connections between one's values and policy choices explicit;
- make sure to distinguish personal conclusions from the scientific consensus;
- acknowledge that people with different values would have different policy choices;
- be aware of how your values might impact objectivity, and be vigilant.

Clear, concise, and impassioned voices are what are needed for all people to see the connections between our human health and the health of animals and the environment.

## End of Chapter Questions & Activities

A. Thought Questions:
  i) Why do you think communication is challenging? Identify 3–4 constraints to clear communication and propose solutions to overcome them.
  ii) How can you advocate for your chosen One Health cause? What are the pros and cons of your methods?
  iii) How can scientists and One Health practitioners better communicate with the public. Identify three–four strategies for improved communication. What are some impediments specific to improved communication between scientists and the public.

B. In-Class/Guided Activities:
  i) Using Twitter, search for #FieldWorkFail, #ActualLivingScientist, and #OverlyHonestMethods. Describe how your view of scientists and the inner workings of actual science have changed with this peak behind the curtains. What other science-related hashtag would you like to see trend on social media?
  ii) Do not print your emails. Tag your signature with a concern for environmental health and actively organize your emails using electronic folders not binders.

C. At-home Activities:
  i) Be a Citizen Scientist. Find information online about existing citizen science programs and get involved. Or, reach out to a scientist who is engaged in research you find compelling and volunteer.
  ii) Write to your elected officials. Choose a topic that is important to you and express your concerns over their lack of support or thank them for their support. Be polite but passionate.
  iii) Embrace #ByeToBags and use reusable shopping bags.

D. Long-term Action Steps:
   i) Introduce environmental education to elementary, middle, and high school curriculum where it is lacking. Work with your scientists and your local school board to insure accuracy in the curriculum and adequate training for teachers.
   ii) Vote. Your voice matters.
E. Recommended Reading:
   Hayes, R. and Grossman, D. (2006). *A Scientist's Guide to Talking with the Media*. Rutgers University Press.
   Knief, A. (2013). *The Citizen Lobbyist: A How-to Manual for Making Your Voice Heard in Government*. Pitchstone Publishing.
   Olson, R. (2015). *Houston, We Have a Narrative*. University of Chicago Press.
   Rosenberg, M.L., Hayes, E.S., McIntyre, M.H., and Neill, N. (2010). *Real Collaboration: What it Takes for Global Health to Succeed*. University of California Press.
   Sagan, C. (1996). *The Demon-Haunted World: Science as a Candle in the Dark*. Ballantine Books.
   Wolfe, N. (2011). *The Viral Storm: The Dawn of a New Pandemic Age*. Times Books.

## Interview

*An Interview with Natalia Reagan: Biological Anthropologist and Comedienne*

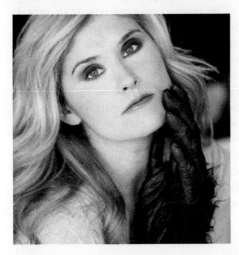

**When did you first hear about One Health?**

It's been fairly recent, like within the past year or two, which is unfortunate. I think it's one of those things that it seems so obvious, the idea that everything is connected.

**How is One Health important to your work?**

I just produced a lecture series at the American Anthropological Association (AAA), our big anthropology meeting, about the importance of biological anthropology in the public, and I just feel like my particular field has this really cool, unique opportunity to tackle social issues that affect health, like for instance, race, gender pluralities, sexuality. Social issues that you do not maybe think of as science issues, but if you look at understanding race and how there's very little genetic differences between individuals of the human species compared to, say, chimpanzees or other non-human primates, it helps promote tolerance. I think it promotes a better understanding that we are far more similar than different.

Diseases that are often times just sort of lumped into a box rather than looked at from a bigger picture. We have a propensity to want to compartmentalize. It's easy to put things in boxes, but unfortunately, that does not work, especially in terms of health, because the body is its own little ecosystem.

**Do you see yourself as a One Health Practitioner?**

Gosh. I mean ... A practitioner. I feel like that makes me sound like I am a doctor. I always joke that I do not have my PhD, so I introduce myself as "not Dr. Reagan."

I try to be as holistic as I can when I approach any sort of job in terms of science communication. Culture definitely plays a very important role in how humans behave, so, for me, I try to look at how I present a science story: is there anything I am missing, anything I am leaving out, anything that I think could better tell the story, whether it's including some backstory about context, about culture context? So I would like to think I am. We all lived in the same place, so to divide it up artificially is somewhat ridiculous.

### How do your actions reflect One Health, personally or professionally?

For me, activism is always going to be part of the job. One of the things I have to make decisions about when I am working with the public is how political will I be in the public. And for me, I have remained political because I find it vital just to remain active and resisting.

My decision-making is about how can I better inform the public but also make a difference. And again, everything is connected. And you could look at the Earth from miles away, and you can see how it's this peaceful-looking little blue, green, brown orb in the sky, and you do not see the divisions of countries, and races, and fighting, and warfare. We have this really cool, unique opportunity to tell the human story of who we are, and how we got here, our place in the universe. We are all very close, we are all very similar, and it does not have to be war, and pain, and suffering all the time.

### What can an individual do to make a difference for planetary health?

Well, I think having that difficult conversation: that conversation with people that might have different views. Listen, and then maybe respond. That's one of the things that I think is very important right now: to listen and hear what people need. And hopefully you can respond in kind.

I Am Big on Kindness

### How can we encourage people to care about planetary health?

Listening to folks is first and foremost, just to hear their perspective, because one of the biggest things, as somebody who's an entertainer and science communicator, knowing your audience is the first rule of thumb. In this particular case, knowing your audience will help you better inform them and give them information in a way that they will digest. If you are talking to a group of school students that might be from a more conservative religious town, obviously, they are not going to really respond to a little liberal rhetoric. You are going to want to say it in a way that speaks to them.

### Where is One Health headed?

It is imperative at this point. I think as climate is changing, as globalization is making us more connected now than ever, I think One Health is the only way to go in terms of just moving forward. We are connected so much these days. And with being able to jump on a plane and be clear across the globe in less than a day, staying connected is the only smart thing to do. Because we can jump on planes, we can also bring germs clear across the globe and spread those around, so, the more we know about just what's going on in other parts of the world, I think the better informed we can be about what's going on in our world.

### What is the best way to advocate for your cause?

Again, know your audience. And then that will give you the foundation on which to build your argument. And then from there, listen to what the audience is lacking and then respond in kind.

Take your work seriously, take what you research seriously, but do not take yourself so seriously. Have fun with it. People like that.

Scientists who want to become science communicators are often worried they are going to come off as silly, or if they are not having a stern face at all minutes of the day while talking about what they do, then they are all of a sudden losing some sort of street cred in the field, and that's just not the case. And if it is the case, then we need to rewrite the way we give street cred out to scientists.

**Humor is an important part of your communication style; can you speak more to the melding of comedy and scientific concepts? Is any topic off limits?**

I always read peer-reviewed articles and found myself giggling at something, even some of the most innocuous, silly things. I also have kind of an unfair advantage by studying monkeys.

I like to encourage people, if they are toying with the idea of adding humor to their science, to just read an article and try to find a funny spin on it. Try to write a little bit in their head, like a little comedy bit, and see how that plays out. As far as off-limit topics, I have done two talks on race, and there were elements of humor, but it's not funny, especially as a white cisgender female.

I am very self-aware of the fact that this is not a laughing matter. Generally, unless you are part of a culture, stay clear of the joke. The last thing you want to do is to alienate or turn off anybody you are trying to reach. I think it's very important when it comes to communicating science to just make sure you are using your best judgment.

**Parting thoughts for future One Health practitioners?**

Well, they matter.

One Health practitioners definitely matter and are important. In a time where we have got climate change, we have got a leader of the free world that basically has a war on science, is a xenophobe, and wants to build a wall. We know that building bridges works, and that's what One Health is doing, we are building bridges throughout the world, throughout different disciplines, which is exactly what we need. And I think that continuing to do that at all costs is important. And with globalization and just access to one another, it makes it a lot easier to share this information. And so I just would say keep going forward in doing what you are doing because the world is going to be a better place with it.

---

## Case Study: Endocrine Disruptors

Co-authored by Thomas Hood and Madeleine Smith

Plastics are ubiquitous in the global environment, used for packaging, flame retardants, insulation, plumbing equipment, and much, much more. Plastics now account for one-third or US$250 billion of the packaging industry, which is the largest single market for US plastics. Plastic has become the preferred choice for packaging materials due to its many advantages over other material choices – plastic products are lighter and use less energy to produce and transport. Unfortunately, plastics are frequently made with chemicals that can act as **endocrine disruptors**. An endocrine disruptor is a chemical that may interfere with, either by activating or repressing, the body's endocrine system, producing adverse developmental, reproductive, neurological, and immune effects in both humans and animals. One endocrine disruptor in particular, Bisphenol A (BPA), is under increasing scrutiny for its adverse effects on planetary health.

As early as the 1930s, BPA was recognized as an endocrine disruptor capable of estrogenic effects. However, as uses of plastics became more prevalent in time, the use of BPA in the manufacturing of plastics grew to an industrial scale, resulting in today's current market, in which millions of metric tons of BPA are created and used annually. BPA is used in the production of many water bottles, plastic food containers, and baby bottles, meaning that most people have had direct exposure to BPA via chemical leaching. In 2007, the US Centers for Disease Control found detectable levels of BPA in 93% of urine samples collected from more than 2500 patients aged six and older, with the highest levels in women and children.

BPA is harmful to humans, especially young children. It has been found to possess **reproductive toxicity**, having estrogenic and anti-androgenic effects and may be a contributing factor in the development of both breast and prostate cancers, early onset of female puberty, diabetes, obesity, and attention deficit disorders. BPA is a recognized **obesogen**, interfering with physiological weight control patterns. Childhood obesity, a contemporary endemic, is known to lead to cardiovascular disease in adulthood and is a major contributor to several non-communicable diseases such as metabolic syndrome, type 2 diabetes mellitus, coronary heart disease, stroke, some forms of cancer, and serious social and psychological consequences.

As an endocrine disruptor, BPA also has a profound effect on habitats and ecosystems. Exposure of male fish to BPA results in their feminization, resulting in production of a lower amount of sperm, the production of female hormones, and, in some cases, the production of eggs in male fish testes. Evidence has also demonstrated an increasing prevalence of induced feminization in frogs. In birds, BPA exposure can reduce comb and testes size, negatively affecting reproductive organ growth and spermatogenesis. And in mammals, exposure to endocrine disruptors, including BPA, has been shown to result in numerous health consequences, as described earlier. In addition to these, BPA exposure has been linked to a decrease in fertility in polar bears, cetaceans, such as porpoises, dolphins, and some species of whale, and pinnipeds, including seals and sea lions. Additionally, BPA has also shown evidence of passing through breastmilk to offspring, exposing young to a myriad of early-onset hormonal cascades.

In response to the now well-understood health effects of BPA on human, animal, and environmental health, a burgeoning advocacy movement has promoted the production of "eco-friendly" and environmentally-conscious plastics. Consumers can exert significant pressure on companies, heavily influencing the product market and what corporations decide to produce.

As a result of this grassroots activism and attention from major media outlets, including the *New York Times*, efforts are underway to reduce the impact of plastics on the environment, including through the use of bioplastics, which utilize biomaterials over petroleum products in the plastics manufacturing process. In response to activism and media attention, many corporations are conforming to societal demands by removing BPA from commonly used consumer products. For example, the Campbell Soup Co. announced that it would integrate a new, BPA-free can lining for all soups, resulting in BPA-free soup cans in 2017. Appleton, a specialty paper company, markets a BPA-free thermal paper that uses Bisphenol-S (BPS) instead. In a similar vein, one plastic resin distributor, Eastman Chemical, began marketing a new a product, Tritan, which they dubbed not only as BPA-free but free of any estrogen-like activity.

Unfortunately, new research is suggesting that BPA-free does not necessarily mean safe for consumption. BPS, considered the safe alternative to BPA, may be as harmful to brain development as BPA. In fact, recent research suggests that nearly all plastic products, including water bottles and food containers, have estrogenic activity.

The only true solution is an increase in awareness and consumer pressure and a reduction in our exposure to and reliance on plastics. Human action is capable of having profound effects and implications on the One Health Triad, and we must remain vigilant of the long-term, global effects of our actions.

# Works Cited

Bertoli, S., Alessandro, L., and Alberto, B. (2015). Human Bisphenol A exposure and the "diabesity phenotype". *Dose Response* 13 (3): 1–12.

Blakemore, E. (2016). The hole in the ozone was super scary, so what happened to it? *Smithsonian Magazine*. http://smithsonianmag.com/science-nature/ozone-hole-was-super-scary-what-happened-it-180957775 (accessed August 17, 2017).

Christmas Bird Count. http://audubon.org/conservation/science/christmas-bird-count (accessed September 14, 2017).

Flint, S., Markle, T., Thompson, S. et al. (2012). Bisphenol A exposure, effects, and policy: a wildlife perspective. *Journal of Environmental Management* 104: 19–34.

FoldIt. https://fold.it (accessed September 14, 2017)

GoViral. https://www.goviralstudy.com (accessed October 18, 2017)

Ike, M., Jin, C.S., and Fujita, M. (2000). Biodegration of Bisphenol A in the aquatic environment. 42 (7): 31–38.

Institute for Conservation Medicine, Box Turtle Project: http://stlzoo.org/conservation/institute-for-conservation-medicine/box-turtle-project (accessed June 12, 2017).

Jandegian, C.M., Deem, S.L., Bhandari, R.K. et al. (2015). Developmental exposure to bisphenol A (BPA) alters sexual differentiation in painted turtles (*Chrysemys picta*). *General and Comparative Endocrinology* 216: 77–85.

Levy, G. (2004). Bisphenol A induces feminization in Xenopus laevis tadpoles. *Environmental Research* 94 (1): 102–111.

Monarch Watch: http://www.monarchparasites.org (accessed September 16, 2017)

Moore, C. A. (1989). McTruth Fast Food for Thought. The Washington Post. http://washingtonpost.com/archive/opinions/1989/12/10/mctruth-fast-food-for-thought/88133f5b-ac81-4d4e-9505-e5d7c85dfbe3/?utm_term=.f615b7e7cb9d (accessed September 16, 2017).

Rochester, J.R. (2013). Bisphenol A and human health: a review of the literature. *Reproductive Toxicology* 42: 132–155.

WHO (2016). *Situation Report: Ebola Virus Disease 10 June 2016*. Geneva, Switzerland: World Health Organization.

Yong, E. (2017). Do scientists lose credibility when they become political? The Atlantic. http://theatlantic.com/science/archive/2017/02/when-scientists-become-advocates-do-they-lose-credibility/518157 (accessed June 13, 2017).

Part V

The Humanities of One Health

# 11

# Culture and Theology in One Health

A tale handed down through time by the Baila people of Zambia (retold):

*Elephant has always been a large animal, but long ago he had only small, curled tusks. Elephant often watched with envy as his nephew, Warthog, rolled in the dust with his beautiful, long tusks.*

*One day, Elephant said, "Nephew, I see that your long tusks keep you from getting up off the dirt. Let us trade tusks for the day, and you can see how it is to have small, easy tusks."*

*Warthog was suspicious and reluctant to swap, but Elephant insisted so Warthog gave in to his uncle, saying, "I will trade tusks with you, but only for the day. At dusk, we must trade back."*

*Elephant and Warthog swapped tusks, and Elephant spent the day happily pulling the bark off of trees with his new, wonderful tusks. Warthog, who knew he had been tricked, spent the day miserably waiting for dusk. But when dusk came, Elephant was nowhere to be found.*

*"I have been tricked," Warthog said to his friend Antbear. "I shall never forgive my Uncle Elephant."*

*"Come into my burrow and rest," said Antbear, "We shall dine on some roots."*

*Warthog's tusks had always been so big that he could not join Antbear in his lovely burrow, and once Warthog was inside, he was happy because he and Antbear could now pass the evening together.*

*Both Elephant and Warthog were happy with their trade, but Warthog would never trust his Uncle Elephant again* (Figure 11.1).

Elephants (*Loxodonta africana spp*) and warthogs (*Phacochoerus africanus*) have not lived happily ever after with their new tusks, nor have rhinos with their horns or big cats with their skins. Hunting and poaching, along with habitat loss have driven many of the world's majestic creatures to the brink of extinction. In 2014, Paul Allen, of Microsoft fame, began an effort to take an aerial count of the remaining elephants. He called it the Great Elephant Census. The Worldwide Fund for Nature (WWF) estimates that there were three to five million African Elephants at the beginning of the twentieth century. In 2016, the Great Census put that number at 352 000. Black rhinoceroses (*Diceros bicornis*) are in even worse shape, with a population estimate of around 5000 remaining in the wild.

Controlling wildlife crime in Africa is difficult for many reasons. Parts of Central and Northern Africa are encumbered by a history of war and upheaval and beset with marauding gangs like the Janjaweed of Sudan and the Lord's Resistance Army which patrols areas around the Central African Republic and the Democratic Republic of Congo. The illegal harvest and trade of ivory and rhino horn bankroll these brutal regimes, which have established sophisticated organizations to move their bloody haul to the coasts for transport to foreign markets. Leaders of

*Introduction to One Health: An Interdisciplinary Approach to Planetary Health*, First Edition.
Sharon L. Deem, Kelly E. Lane-deGraaf and Elizabeth A. Rayhel.
© 2019 John Wiley & Sons, Inc. Published 2019 by John Wiley & Sons, Inc.
Companion website: www.wiley.com/go/deem/health

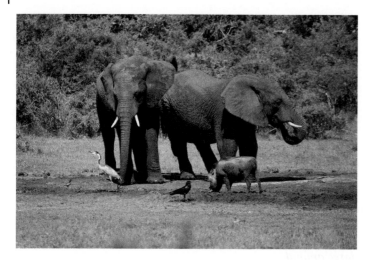

Figure 11.1 Two African Elephants with a Warthog. *Source:* Courtesy of Ron Porter.

poaching rings have been caught many times; however, the governments of the countries where this poaching occurs are often ill-equipped to deal with criminals that are so well financed. In a system where corruption extends to the highest levels of government, it is easy enough to purchase freedom, even for the worst of criminals.

The cargo is predominantly bound for Asia, where the rhino horn is ground into a powder used in traditional medicines, and the ivory is carved into religious figurines, art, chopsticks, and ornaments of cultural significance. In 2014 a survey was conducted by National Geographic and Globescan, assessing the attitudes of potential ivory consumers in five countries: China, Vietnam, the Philippines, Thailand, and the USA. Among confirmed and likely buyers of ivory products ("likely" being those who would buy ivory but do not feel that they could afford to do so at that time), the attributes given to ivory include respect, pride, confidence, and empowerment. Ivory is a status symbol in these cultures and is valued for the extreme respect shown when given as a gift. These attitudes do not bode well for elephants, given that China has a rapidly expanding middle class. Moreover, only half of the likely buyers believed that elephants are in immediate danger, and a third did not feel that

small purchases of ivory contributed significantly to the overall market demand.

St. Louis, Missouri, was founded on the trade of animal products: deer skins and beaver pelts. In many ways the ivory and fur trades are similar. In the early seventeenth century, the American wilderness was plundered for fur to meet the growing demand of an industrialized Europe. And while there is still a fur industry today, demand for fur has declined significantly after the animal-rights and anti-fur campaigns of the 1970s.

"I think the downslide is just going to continue and continue," said Christina Fox of the Canadian Anti-Fur Alliance, quoted in a New Your Times article in 1991. "It's not going to happen in a couple of years, but people are just becoming more and more aware that you don't have to wear a dead animal for decoration."

Today, many organizations are trying to effect similar change concerning the use of vulnerable-animal products like ivory, tiger bone, bear bile, and rhino horn. WildAid, a conservation group focused on ending illegal trade in animal products, has as its slogan, "when the buying stops, the killing can too." WildAid deploys celebrity ambassadors from within target cultures, like Jackie Chan, who fights to save endangered pangolins (*Manis pentadactyla* and *javanica*), and Yao Ming, and Lupita Nyong'o, who champion anti-poaching campaigns. These ambassadors are fully committed to the causes that they embrace. Several studies have shown that such social marketing can be a valuable approach to changing the preferences, and thus the culture, of consumers.

We consider culture and religion together in this chapter because they are both motivational forces, and in many cases, religion and culture are inextricably bound together. Culture, tradition, and religion underpin much of human behavior and can have both beneficial and detrimental effects on the health of people, animals, and ecosystems.

## 11.1 Culture

Culture is a complex concept, biased by historical and current understandings of knowledge, communication, and diversity. In this chapter, the term "culture" will refer to the learned behaviors and beliefs that are shared by all members of a society. These cultural characteristics might be shared values, traditions, and ideals that are taught to all incoming members of the group. Typically, this refers to ethnic groups whose culture is handed down from generation to generation, and examples of methods of teaching culture include storytelling, art, music, and observation. Of course, the term "culture" is often used differently in everyday speech, giving rise to such ideas as "counterculture," "culture of corruption," "corporate culture," or "social-media culture." In a One Health context, it is important to know that cultural behaviors can put the members of a given group at increased risk of violence and disease. Additionally, the discussion of the Ebola outbreak in Chapter 7 showed how cultural beliefs could lead an at-risk group to hamper healthcare interventions. Cultural insensitivity can also stymie the relationship of a well-meaning One Health practitioner with his or her colleagues.

## 11.2 Culture, Social Structure, and One Health

### 11.2.1 Poverty

Poverty and inequality put people at risk of disease and poor health. The constitution of the World Health Organization (WHO) states that "the highest attainable standard of health is a fundamental right of every human being." Yet, in many cultures and on all continents, exist subsets of the human population who are marginalized and do not enjoy the same right to health as their mainstream or wealthier neighbors. In December 2017, the UN's Commission on Human Rights concluded that the US state of Alabama had the worst poverty in the developed world, and a recent United Nations Children's Fund (UNICEF) study estimates that 33% of US children are living in poverty. Poverty deprives people of the ability to thrive, particularly children who are burdened with need during key developmental stages. However, methods of measuring poverty can vary from country to country and between reports of data. In the developed world, poverty is usually considered in relative terms, comparing the wealth of one individual to that of another. Because there is almost always someone wealthier, people who are fairly well off can feel relatively poor. In the USA, poverty is described as a family of four living on less than half the US median income of US $48 678 per year. While it is troubling that there is hunger in a wealthy country, the World Bank reports that worldwide, 767 million, or roughly 10.7% of the world's population lives on less than US $1.90 per day. For comparison, Alabama's poor could be living on up to US $65 per day. Just over half of the world's extreme poor live in sub-Saharan Africa, and another one-third are in Southeast Asia. To put this into perspective, this equates to an American citizen living on US $1.90 per day, or just under US $700 per year. Such poverty is evidence of social inequality, and these inequities are increasing. For the past several years the income disparity between the top 1% and the rest of society has grown in many countries, including Argentina, India, the Republic of Korea, South Africa, Taiwan, and the USA. Despite public health efforts, income inequality generates a healthcare gradient. Those at the lower end can find themselves in a self-perpetuating cycle of poverty and poor health. Poor health exacerbates poverty by usurping time and productivity from the sufferer, and poverty undermines health due to nutritional deficits, restricted access to clean water, poor indoor air quality in badly ventilated spaces, and increased exposure to infectious diseases due to overcrowded housing, including housing that is shared with animals.

### 11.2.2 Marginalization

Displaced populations represent another group that is at increased risk of disease. War, poverty, and increasingly ecological disaster are examples of circumstances that can create internally-displaced persons or groups, and refugees that flee from their homes seeking safety. Flight often means separation of people from their support systems of family and friends. The 2017 plight of the Rohingya refugees provides an example. The Rohingya have been occupants of the Rakhine State of Myanmar tracing back to the eighth century. However, they are seen as illegal immigrants by most of Myanmar, and persecution by the Myanmar army that began in 2012 has led to a mass migration of refugees into neighboring Bangladesh. Once across the border, they are cared for in camps set up by Médecins Sans Frontières and other aid groups. The survivors that arrive in these camps have endured unimaginable hardship. Most are severely malnourished, a situation that undermines the immune system and renders them even more susceptible to the infectious diseases of poverty, like tuberculosis, cholera, and malaria. To make it worse, the children arriving at the camps have not had medical care or the routine vaccinations that other children in Myanmar receive, making outbreaks of measles and polio more likely. A similar tale has recently played out for the people of northern Nigeria fleeing the Boko Haram and the Yazidi sect of Northwestern Iraq. The persecution of the Yazidi has resulted in an estimated 500 000 refugees now living in camps in neighboring Turkey. The predictions of continued climate change include loss of inhabitable land, which could result in geopolitical strife and the creation of more refugees. A One Health approach to this will include a strategy to accommodate homeless and marginalized people.

### 11.2.3 Women and Gender Equity

A report prepared by the Women and Gender Equity Knowledge Network in 2007 for the WHO Commission on Social Determinants of Health identified a gap in health care between men and women across many, if not most, cultures, stating,

> Only focusing on economic inequalities across households can seriously distort our understanding of how inequality works, and who actually bears much of its burdens. Health gradients can be significantly different for men and women; medical poverty may not trap women and men to the same extent or in the same way.

Women in many cultures are made more vulnerable to disease and ill-health by the roles that they are expected to fulfill. Pregnancy, labor, and parturition are risks that men, obviously, do not share; but the gap goes well beyond this biological role. According to the UN Statistics Division, there is no country in which women do not perform more hours of unpaid domestic work than men. Women are caregivers to children, the elderly, and the sick, duties which necessarily cut down on their ability to care for themselves or earn an income, perpetuating the health-poverty cycle for women. This standing as family caregiver also puts women at greater risk of exposure to disease. Moreover, women are more likely to marry young, adding to the work of caregiving, and women are more likely to be sexually and physically abused. All of these risks rise in low-income areas. Taken together, it is clear that if the poor have reduced access to health and healthcare, poor women bear the brunt of those burdens all the more.

Culture can affect the dynamics of disease emergence and transmission as well. For example, adolescent girls and young women account for one in four new HIV infections in sub-Saharan Africa. Several cultural traditions have been suggested to explain this discrepancy, including failure to educate girls, sexual promiscuity, rape, widow inheritance, female circumcision and infibulation, medicinal bloodletting, ritual scarring, genital tattooing, and rituals establishing a blood brotherhood.

Examples of other cultural drivers of disease include tradition-based interactions with animals, such as the live animal markets in Asia that provide areas where viruses mingle and mutate. These are known to give rise to new and potentially more virulent outbreaks. Further, animal-husbandry practices in developed countries include the use of antibiotics that encourage the growth of antibiotic-resistant strains of bacteria. Less global in effect, the dietary tradition of consuming raw pork in Southeast Asia is associated with cycles of parasitic and bacterial disease. In addition to animal interactions, healthcare traditions such as hygienic practices, nonuse of footwear, and reliance on traditional healers can be important drivers of disease, as well. All of these have been shown to exacerbate parasitic infection in rural Nicaragua. These are a few of the many examples of cultural practices that put people at risk, either directly or indirectly, and facilitate infectious disease emergence or re-emergence.

Interestingly, some conditions are specific to certain cultures. These include Anorexia Nervosa, an eating disorder that is limited to the Global North. Koro, a phobia common in Southeast Asia and Africa, is the intense fear that the genitals will recede into the body and cause death. Similarly, Dhat, or semen-loss anxiety, is thought to be limited to men from the Indian subcontinent. Finally, the Central-American disease Susto is the fear that the soul or spirit will leave the body after a sudden fright. Of course, with globalization and migration, these culture-bound syndromes will cease to be region-bound and should be recognized within the general medical lexicon, and human medical training should provide an understanding of the cultural links that can impact human health.

Despite the many examples of cultural practices and norms that are detrimental to health, culture can be beneficial to human health as well. Those cultures that promote a diet rich in fruits and vegetables are healthier than those that feature red meat. Some cultures discourage smoking, drinking, and other potentially unhealthy habits, while others promote a lifestyle that is relatively stress-free, which could reduce disease occurrence and severity. The WHO defines health broadly, stating that "health is not only the absence of infirmity or disease but also a state of physical, mental and social well-being." When both mental and social status are considered, a wider array of cultural characteristics emerge that may contribute to health.

## 11.3 Culture and Animal/Ecosystem One Health

Culturally linked human behavior has been a factor in animal and ecosystem health since human beginnings. Hunting, the domestication of animals, colonization of wilderness areas, urbanization, industrialization, and overpopulation have all left indelible marks on animal health and ecosystem ranges. How humans eat is particularly problematic. As was discussed in Chapter 5, a dependence on meat to provide protein was manageable when our population was small, but the UN's projected 10 billion people in 2100 cannot all be carnivores. In 2008, when the Earth's total population was ~6.7 billion, it took 1.5 years to restore the renewable resources consumed in that year. In that same year, 2008, we produced 1.5 years' worth of carbon dioxide.

This idea of Earth's Overshoot Day is mentioned in Chapter 2. Much like a food and water bank account, humans have been living on credit. Our dependence on cars, electricity-dependent gadgets, and non-renewable energy sources is key to climate change. Climate change, as covered in previous chapters is identified as one of the greatest threats to our continued, combined, planetary health. These are complicated problems that involve more than human culture, although the often-insatiable human desire to consume beyond their needs fuels much of it.

Poaching, overhunting, overfishing, and deforestation are human activities with clearly negative outcomes for animals and the environment. However, there are more nuanced ways in which humans control the well-being of the rest of Earth's life. Research published in 2010 shows one clear example of how human culture impacts animal health. The authors used datasets from previous studies to ask if the behavior of **pastoralists** concerning their domesticated dogs had had any implications for the health of African wild dogs (AWDs) (*Lycaon pictus*; Figure 11.2) in Botswana and Kenya. Responses to surveys suggested that cattle-ranging behavior varied distinctly between Kenyans and Botswanans. Kenyan herders (mostly of Maasai background) accompanied their cattle daily, and generally (88%) took their domestic dogs (DD) with them. In contrast, Botswanan herders (descended from various tribes) mostly (93%) allowed their cattle to graze free-range and left their domesticated dogs at home (Figure 11.3). The overall disease and mortality rates between DD in Kenya and Botswana were similar, but the same was not true for populations of AWD, an endangered canine species that roams in packs across ranges where these studies were completed. This seemingly inconsequential difference in human behavior which allowed the interaction of DD with AWD results in increased disease, mortality, and extirpation of AWD in the Kenyan region studied.

Just as there are positive cultural contributions to human health, there are abundant examples of cultures that include respect for- and benefit to the other components of the One Health Triad. Indeed, biologist Edward O. Wilson hypothesized an innate human **biophilia**, or "urge to connect with other forms of life," in his 1984 book of the same name. This connection to nature is evident in the ancient teachings in most

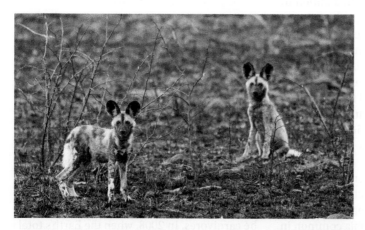

**Figure 11.2** African wild dog, *Lycaon pictus* (young) at uMkhuze Game Reserve, kwaZulu-Natal, South Africa. African wild dogs are red listed by the International Union for Conservation of Nature (IUCN), and considered one of Africa's most endangered carnivores. *Source:* Derek Keats, https://commons.wikimedia.org/wiki/File:African_wild_dog,_Lycaon_pictus_(young)_at_uMkhuze_Game_Reserve,_kwaZulu-Natal,_South_Africa_(15242425978).jpg. CC BY 2.0.

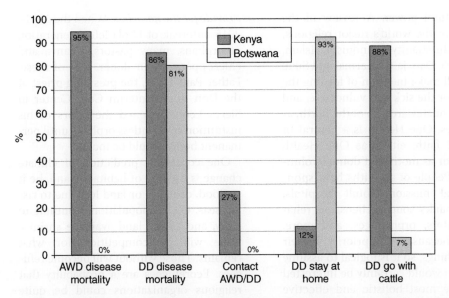

**Figure 11.3** The proportion of disease-specific mortality and contact between African wild dogs (AWD) and domestic dogs (DD) compared to domestic dog ranging behavior in the Kenya and Botswana study sites. *Source:* Figure courtesy of K. Alexander and J. McNutt.

cultures, having arisen during times when people were more aware of their dependence on nature for food and shelter and less aware of how nature worked. Texts going back as far as the Code of Hammurabi, of Babylon (1792–1750 BCE), include references to the connections between landscaping and floods and dog control and disease. The respect for nature evident among Native American cultures is well known as is the central place nature holds in many of the ancient Eastern beliefs. Indeed, our connection to nature is so deep and extends so far back in our diverse cultural pasts that it is present in most of the world's religions. According to the United Nations Educational, Scientific and Cultural Organization's (UNESCO) teaching and learning for a sustainable future,

It seems that people in all cultures have a set of beliefs that go beyond both the self and the natural world. We use these beliefs to help explain reasons for human existence and to guide personal relationships and behaviour. Part of the great diversity of humankind is the many different reli-

gions and belief systems we have developed – Animism, Buddhism, Christianity, Hinduism, Islam, Jainism, Taoism, and many more.

## 11.4 Religion and One Health

Many ancient societies, and a few that currently exist, believed or believe that illness was caused by evil spirits, was the result of spells of ill-will cast by others, or was the embodiment of the displeasure of the gods. However, improving health has been a component of most modern religions. Throughout history, advances of medicine and medical knowledge were associated with religious life. For example, Traditional Chinese Medicine (TCM) is rooted in the philosophy of the Tao; early Islamic medicine was built upon the principles of faith and trust found in the Quran; the Indian Ayurveda is said to have been delivered to sages by the gods; and in medieval Europe, medicine was largely the providence of monks and monasteries.

Religion, in this context, will mean any set of beliefs, practices, or attitudes pertaining to a supernatural power. A review of the sacred texts for the world's major religions, Buddhism, Christianity, Hinduism, Islam, Judaism, Baha'i, Dao, Jain Dharma, and Sikh, reveals that all make mention of feeding the poor, caring for the sick and vulnerable, and responsibility or stewardship of the Earth, as core principles. One Health is a natural fit for people of faith, either as One Health practitioners or as motivated donors/volunteers/voters. People of all faiths have sponsored medical missions, built hospitals, opened food banks, soup kitchens, and rehabilitation centers, orphanages, and more. They do this because it is a priority in their religious teachings, so it is logical to assume people of faith would certainly be interested in finding the most holistic and effective approach to world health. Four major areas of religious relevance to One Health goals are listed here:

1) *Feed the hungry and quench the thirsty.* How and what we eat, as well as access to water, is a major concern for the future. Food and water safety and security are human rights and areas where religious organizations have been active for some time. As an example, in Flint, MI in 2011 there was a crisis involving the leeching of lead into the city's water. The main points of the crisis are described in Chapter 3, but concerning the actions of the people of faith in this One Health crisis, the churches in and around Flint were providing bottled water to residents long before the State of Michigan acknowledged any problem.

2) *Care for the sick.* The convergence of factors that most encourage the outbreak of zoonoses including poverty, and increasingly the burden of climate change and infectious disease will fall on those least able to cope. Missionary aid groups have long been involved in mitigating this suffering. Indeed, many hospitals have religious affiliations, and the very concept of a hospital is credited to the Muslim physician Caliph Al-Walid I (705–715 CE).

3) *Provide for the homeless.* When the 2014–2015 outbreak of Ebola left a generation of orphans, many pastors, imams, and chiefs opened their doors. One of these, Father Paul Turay, the presiding priest at the Don Bosco Interim Care Center in Sierra Leone, opened the doors of his institution to countless orphans until permanent homes could be found.

One consistent prediction of climate change is the loss of habitable land, be it to flood, drought, or land loss due to rising seas. Global populations continue to grow, and as the land available shrinks, there will be competition for what remains. Those without will become refugees. Ecorefugees are a probability that religious organizations could be quite helpful in addressing.

4) *Stewardship of creation.* In all religions, there is a responsibility to live in harmony with nature and to care for the creation. During our time on Earth, we have exceeded the 350 ppm of carbon dioxide that the atmosphere can carry, we have acidified the oceans, and there is an island of plastic the size of Texas, or larger, in the North Pacific **Gyre**. Species loss is so rapid that we are in the midst of a sixth mass extinction, and the plummeting number of pollinators is concerning to all. As a species, we have not taken responsibility for our actions, and we have failed in recognizing our role in caring for the planet. **Ecotheology** is a growing field, and One Health theology could be as well.

The Alliance of Religion and Conservation (ARC) is a group that began as a subset of the WWF, with the goal of reaching out to religious organizations as collaborators in conservation efforts. Summarizing a statement made by Martin Palmer, the secretary general of ARC, religious organizations

own about 8% of the habitable surface of the planet, they contribute to or run about 50% of schools, worldwide, and they are the third largest investing group in the world. The question for conservationists isn't "why would you work with religious organizations; the question is why on Earth wouldn't you?"

There are some caveats concerning the role of the religion in One Health. It cannot be denied that religions have fueled war and human suffering and still today, intolerance can be a problem among the faithful. Also, some religions hold views that conflict with the need to counter overpopulation. In those cases, a religiously sponsored hospital or medical facility may not be the best place for patients in need of reproductive guidance. Thus, a One Health team should be wary of any religious organization that exhibits intolerance concerning national heritage, gender, minorities, sexual orientation, or any other personal characteristic. Health is a human right, with no contingencies attached.

## 11.5  Cultural and Religious Awareness and One Health

Working with collaborators of other faiths and cultures can be tricky, and unfortunately, most of us are blind to our cultural or social insensitivity. As an example, the authors of a 2017 paper suggest that One Health groups are displaying a Western bias by implying that there are strict boundaries between humans and animals. In many parts of the world, the relationship between humans and livestock form a porous and fluid border. Similarly, there are words, phrases, postures, and actions that are culturally-context dependent and have vastly different meanings depending on the audience. Such actions as making eye contact, using one's left hand, or displaying the "thumb's up," are offensive in some parts of the world, and failing to understand these norms can negatively affect collaborations. When working with international teams, it is important to be cognizant of the potential for cultural differences that come into play in One Health.

Awareness of cultural differences is important to effective communication of the One Health message and the formation of productive collaborations, but even more importantly, the benefit of including diverse points of view is one of the strengths of the One Health approach. We can build a One Health culture that takes root for the betterment of the planet that we all share.

## End of Chapter Questions & Activities

A.  Thought Questions:
   i)  How has your culture colored your view of health? Have you done anything unhealthy because it was culturally normalized?
   ii)  Can you think of something that you grew up believing, but you no longer believe? What made you change your mind?

B.  In-Class/Guided Activities:
   i)  Choose several cultures different from your own and study their values and beliefs concerning health.
   ii)  Study religious texts for mentions of the poor, the homeless, and stewardship of the planet.
   iii)  Visit the dollar-street website and explore how families in other places live. It is available at: http://www.gapminder.org/dollar-street/matrix?thing=Families&countries=World&regions=World&zoom=4&row=1&lowIncome=26&highIncome=15000&lang=en
   iv)  In class discussion-talk about your own culture and traditions.

C.  At-home Activities:
   i)  Educate yourself about other cultures by:
      1)  searching for websites that feature stories from other cultures. NPR's Goats & Soda is a place to start: https://www.npr.org/sections/goatsandsoda/

2) reading blog entries or posts by students from other cultures.
3) choosing movies produced outside your own country to watch, making note of the customs and culture.
ii) Look into the connections between health and culture in your own family. If there are any, are they beneficial or detrimental?

D. Long-tern-Action Steps:
    i) Examine your own belief system for motivation with respect to care for the Earth and for others.
    ii) Commit to learning a new language.

iii) Look for opportunities to travel outside your own country or community.

E. Recommended Reading:
Desmond, A. and Moore, J. (2011). *Darwin's Sacred Cause: Race, Slavery and the Quest for Human Origins.* University of Chicago Press.
Miller, K.R. (1999). *Finding Darwin's God: A Scientist's Search for Common Ground Between God and Evolution.* Cliff Street Books.
Wilson, E.O. (1984). *Biophilia: The Human Bond with Other Species.* Harvard University Press.

## Interview

*An Interview with Julienne Anoko, PhD: The Technical Officer of Risk Communication for Plague Outreach with the WHO*

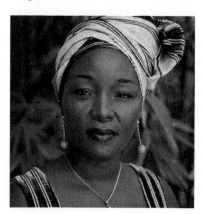

**When did you first hear about One Health?**

I first heard about One Health, I think it was in 2012. It was through my investigation looking at global health that I found One Health. And after that, in 2013, I was invited by Family Health International, the non-governmental organization (NGO), to participate as a speaker during the Prince Mahidol Award Conference in Bangkok. I was asked to speak on how integrating social sciences could greatly benefit One Health.

**How is One Health important to your work?**

I think that my work as an anthropologist and risk-communication expert during emergency outbreaks is important to One Health because it helps with understanding people in their multifaceted context. This is in order to influence outbreak response strategy to fit the community.

**Do you see yourself as a One Health practitioner?**

Yes and no. When I started intervening during outbreaks in 2005, I was not really conscious that I was a One Health practitioner because the concept was not existing at that moment. But after the One Health initiative arose, I consider myself a One Health practitioner because during each outbreak, I carry on research, provide the response team with first-hand knowledge on the context, and support both the strategy development and implementation in the field.

What I do is the human part of One Health. I see how people are living interconnected in their own environment and how they are managing their environment, how they are using the resources from their environment, and the sociocultural aspect of their life, their context.

## How can we encourage people to care about planetary health?

What I do in my own case, is try to change my children's minds and my relatives' minds. For example, I teach my children how to recycle garbage and batteries, not using plastic bags but to use the material bags that can be reused. I care about vaccinating all people who are around me and also advocating for vaccination; not using antibiotics, only when necessary and under a physician's advice; and following a healthy diet.

## How do you see people of faith fitting in to One Health?

Of course, people of faith are mobilizing a lot of millions of millions of people and this can be an audience where we can pass One Health messages. In the field we are already doing it. We are involving them. Here in Madagascar, we are involved with all the great faith organizations. We have something like 6979 young people who are mobilizing people to fight plague. So this has been mobilized in part by faith organizations and religious leaders. I think they are a very great audience and a friend that we can count on.

## Have you ever experienced any cultural or religious taboos?

We try every day to advocate, and sometimes some religious groups here believe that plague is because God is angry with people because people behave bad and they have to pray more than receiving the treatment. I have a big job in that case because we have to go again in the churches trying to convince people and to convince the religious leaders so that they can talk to their fellowship and so on. There are some new wave churches that believe that instead of having the medicine, what you can do is pray. And what I say to them is that perhaps God asks us to take care of our body and God will take care of our soul but it's not really easy to pass this message to them.

## Parting Thoughts?

Perhaps, I think from my point of view, always as a social anthropologist, I think that One Health professionals must be open-minded to understand the other people. If you are a One Health professional, you have to know that your culture is different from the culture of the other one, and to be a One Health practitioner or implementer you have to be open-minded. Be multicultural and be able to work in a multicultural environment. Be an empathic person, understand other people, and also not forgetting your own culture. One Health is the cross-sectoral meeting of three main disciplines, and I think people who are working for One Health must also have this capacity, the competencies of being multicultural and open-minded.

---

### Case Study: Bushmeat Hunting and Cheetahs

Coauthored by Christopher Graham

Bushmeat hunting, the hunting of non-domesticated animals, has serious implications for large predators in the African savannas. The most active hunting areas are located in central Africa, but the practice is spreading toward the borders of South Africa. With bushmeat hunting on the rise in these areas, large predators are running out of food and they are also becoming the unintended victims of different bushmeat hunting techniques. Cheetahs (*Acinonyx jubatus*), which are already at risk of extinction, are one group of predators impacted by this practice.

The surge in bushmeat hunting follows recent growth in African populations. As the number of people living near the African savannas increases, they begin to intrude into protected and wild areas. In the early stages of recent population expansion, bushmeat was used solely to feed the families and communities in the area, and in some remote locations bushmeat accounts for up to 98% of animal protein consumed. However, the popularity of bushmeat has led to what is known as the bushmeat boom in Africa. Today, bushmeat is also considered a luxury item, sold in nearby cities at premium prices. Hunting provides a living to the bushmeat hunters, but cheetahs, and numerous other species, are now suffering because of it.

One common method of bushmeat hunting that has proven particularly consequential is snaring. Snaring is detrimental to conservation efforts because it is highly effective, difficult to control, unselective, and extremely wasteful. Many animals, including cheetahs, get caught in these snares and are left to die. And while there is loss of life from the snares themselves, the larger factor for cheetah survival is the loss of natural prey. As natural prey populations decrease, the cheetahs are forced out of their protected areas to search for new food sources. This has led to a phenomenon known as Empty Savanna Syndrome, where the unregulated overhunting of large mammals causes them to leave their home areas in search of better environments. Although cheetahs can survive low prey densities better than other predators, they are still being forced to expand their ranges into human populated areas.

Farmers are a main group of people affected by the expanding range and increasing frequency of interactions with cheetahs. Because of the many cheetah sightings, farmers assume that their livestock are being hunted by cheetahs more frequently. However, cheetahs may be unfairly targeted, because they hunt in the day when they can be seen while many nocturnal predators also contribute to the problem.

Though absolute numbers are difficult to determine, current estimates of cheetah population are roughly 10 000 which, if accurate, indicate a 90% decrease over the past decade. Many of the issues stem from cheetahs being forced out of their protected areas. If something is not done to provide better control of how these areas and wildlife are managed, we could see the extinction of the cheetah along with many other large predators.

## Works Cited

Alexander, K.A. and McNutt, J.W. (2010). Human behavior influences infectious disease emergence at the human–animal interface. *Frontiers of Ecology and the Environment* 8 (10): 522–526. doi: 10.1890/090057.

Balosteros, C. Alabama Has the Worst Poverty in the Developed World, U.N. Official Says. *Newsweek*, 10 December 2017. http://www.newsweek.com/alabama-un-poverty-environmental-racism-743601 (accessed July 2, 2018).

Brown, K.S. (1997) Beavers and Boomtown: Remembering the St. Louis Fur Trade. *Missouri Conservationist Magazine*, February 1997. https://mdc.mo.gov/conmag/1997/02/beavers-and-boomtown-remembering-st-louis-fur-trade (accessed July 2, 2018).

Burniston, S., Okello, A.L., Khamlome, B., et al. (2015) Cultural drivers and health-seeking behaviours that impact on the transmission of pig-associated zoonoses in Lao People's Democratic Republic. *Infectious Diseases of Poverty* 4 (11). http://www.idpjournal.com/content/4/1/11

Burns, J.F. Fur Industry Shrinking With No End in Sight. *Special to The New York Times* February 26, 1991.

Cheetah Conservation Fund. *Race for survival*. https://cheetah.org/about-the-cheetah/race-for-survival (accessed July 2, 2018).

Christy, B. (2015) How Killing Elephants Finances Terror in Africa. *National Geographic*. https://www.nationalgeographic.com/tracking-ivory/article.html (accessed July 2, 2018).

Ember, C.R., Ember, M., and Peregrine, P.N. (2010). *Anthropology*. Upper Saddle River, NJ: Prentice Hall.

Ferrant, G., Pesando, L.M., and Nowacka, K. (2014). *Unpaid Care Work: The Missing Link in the Analysis of Gender Gaps in Labour Outcomes*. OECD Development Centre http://www.oecd.org/dev/development-gender/Unpaid:care_work.pdf (accessed July 2, 2018.

Gapminder. The Dollar-Street Project. http://www.gapminder.org/dollar-street/matrix?thing=Families&countries=World&regions=World&zoom=4&row=1&lowIncome=26&highIncome=15000&lang=en (accessed July 2, 2018).

Globescan and National Geographic (2015) *Reducing Demand for Ivory: An International Study*. http://press.nationalgeographic.com/files/2015/09/NGS2015_Final-August-11-RGB.pdf (accessed July 2, 2018).

Hance, J. (2012) Illegal Hunting Threatens Iconic Animals Across Africa's Great Savannas, Especially Predators. https://news.mongabay.com/2012/10/illegal-hunting-threatens-iconic-animals-across-africas-great-savannas-especially-predators (accessed July 2, 2018).

Hrdy, D. (1987). Cultural practices contributing to the transmission of human immunodeficiency virus in Africa. *Reviews of Infectious Diseases (Chicago)* 9 (6): 1109–1119.

Ingraham, C. Child Poverty in the U.S. is Among the Worst in the Developed World. *The Washington Post*, 29 October 2014. https://www.washingtonpost.com/news/wonk/wp/2014/10/29/child-poverty-in-the-u-s-is-among-the-worst-in-the-developed-world/?utm_term=.f73fbe199a12 (accessed July 2, 2018).

Karan, A., Chapman, G., and Galvani, A. (2012). The influence of poverty and culture on the transmission of parasitic infections in rural Nicaraguan villages. *Journal of Parasitology Research* doi: 10.1155/2012/478292.

Liu, Z., Jiang, Z., Fang, H. et al. (2015). "Consumer behavior" change we believe in: demanding reduction strategy for endangered wildlife. *Journal of Biodiversity and Endangered Species* 3: 1. doi: 10.4172/2332-2543.1000141.

MacGregor, H. and Waldman, L. (2017). Views from many worlds: unsettling categories in interdisciplinary research on endemic zoonotic diseases. *Philosophical Transactions of the Royal Society B* 372: 20160170. http://dx.doi.org/10.1098/rstb.2016.0170.

Medicins sans Frontieres (2017) *MSF Scales Up Aid to Rohingya Refugees in Bangladesh, Raises Concern About Conditions in Myanmar*. https://reliefweb.int/report/bangladesh/msf-scales-aid-rohingya-refugees-bangladesh-raises-concern-about-conditions (accessed July 2, 2018).

Mind Tools Content Team. Avoiding Cross-Cultural Faux Pas. https://www.mindtools.com/pages/article/cross-cultural-mistakes.htm (accessed July 2, 2018).

Mulaudzi, F.M. (2007). The cultural beliefs of the Vhavenda on the causes and transmission of sexually transmitted infections. *Health Sa Gesondheid* 12 (3): 46–54.

Poirson, J.M. (2015) Wild Meat/Bushmeat – Food Safety Implications. http://Fao.org. Animal Production and Health Division. http://www.fao.org/docs/eims/upload/298761/an321e00.pdf (accessed December 30, 2017).

Pyari, D. (2011). Environment stewardship and religion. *International Journal of Educational Research and Technology* 2 (1): 26–35.

Roberts, L. (2017). Nigeria's invisible crisis: hunger amplifies infectious diseases for millions fleeing the violence of Boko Haram. *Science* 356 (6333): 18–23.

Sen, G., Östlin, P., and George, A. (2007) Unequal, Unfair, Ineffective and Inefficient Gender Inequity in Health: Why it exists and how we can change it. *Final Report to the WHO Commission on Social Determinants of Health*.

Sims, L.D., Domenech, J., Benigno, C. et al. (2005). Origin and evolution of highly pathogenic H5N1 avian influenza in Asia. *The Veterinary Record* 157: 159–164.

Singh Balhara, Y.P. (2011). Culture-bound syndrome: has it found its right niche? *Indian Journal of Psychological Medicine* 33 (2): 210–215. doi: 10.4103/0253-7176.92055.

Star-Tribune. Quotes on feeding the hungry from world religions. *Minnesota Star Tribune*, 16 November 2007. http://www.startribune.com/quotes-on-feeding-the-hungry-from-world-religions/11402191

Stewart, D. (2004). *The Zebra's Stripes and Other African Animal Tales*. Cape Town: Struik Publishers.

The Great Elephant Census. http://www.greatelephantcensus.com/the-census (accessed July 2, 2018)

UNAIDS (2016) Prevention Gap Report. http://www.unaids.org/sites/default/files/media_asset/2016-prevention-gap-report_en.pdf (accessed July 2, 2018).

United States National Library of Medicine. Islamic Culture and the Medical Arts. https://www.nlm.nih.gov/exhibition/islamic_medical/islamic_12.html (accessed July 2, 2018).

Vaughn, L.M., Jacquez, F., and Baker, R.C. (2009). Cultural health attributions, beliefs, and practices: effects on healthcare and medical education. *The Open Medical Education Journal* 2: 64–74.

Verissimo, D. (2013). Influencing human behaviour: an underutilised tool for biodiversity management. *Conservation Evidence* 10: 29–31.

Weintraub, K. (2015) Finding Homes for Ebola's Orphans. *National Geographic*, 3 February 2015. https://news.nationalgeographic.com/2015/01/150203-ebola-virus-outbreak-epidemic-sierra-leone-orphans (accessed July 2, 2018).

Wide Range Conservation Program for Cheetah and African Wild Dogs. *Cheetah*. http://www.cheetahandwilddog.org/cheetah (accessed July 2, 2018).

Wilson, E.O. (1984). *Biophilia: The Human Bond with Other Species*. Cambridge, MA: Harvard University Press.

World Bank Group (2016) Taking on Inequality. http://www.worldbank.org/en/publication/poverty-and-shared-prosperity (accessed July 2, 2018).

Worldwide Fund for Nature. African Elephants http://wwf.panda.org/knowledge_hub/endangered_species/elephants/ (accessed July 2, 2018).

12

# Economics and One Health

*"There is no business on a dead planet."*
Yvon Chouinard, Founder of Patagonia

At approximately 10:00 p.m. on April 20, 2010, a combination of crude oil, gas, and concrete exploded up from the wellbore of an oil rig located 41 miles off the coast of Louisiana, killing 11, injuring 17, and destroying the rig (Figure 12.1). With this explosion, the Deepwater Horizon and its broken wellhead, 5000 ft. below the surface of the water, began spilling crude oil into the Gulf of Mexico at the rate of approximately 60 000 barrels per day, unabated for the next three months. The ensuing oil spill resulted in approximately 4.9 million barrels of crude oil spilled, which damaged 1300 miles of shoreline and more than 40 000 mile$^2$ of ocean, becoming one of the largest environmental disasters to date.

At the time of the explosion, the Deepwater Horizon and its crew were among the best in deep-water well-digging. It had been more than seven years since a major safety violation, and the Macondo Prospect, one of the deepest wells in the Gulf of Mexico, was nearing completion. In fact, the Deepwater Horizon and its crew had only months before completed the world's deepest well in the Gulf of Mexico. This combination of past successes resulted in a series of decisions made by executives at BP and Transocean – the rig's lessee and owner, respectively – to emphasize speed and efficiency over safety, ultimately costing lives and livelihoods of those on the rig and across the Gulf Shore states. The cost of the Deepwater Horizon explosion to BP was nearly US $62 billion; however, the story of the Deepwater Horizon actually began years before in a board room of one the largest oil companies in the world.

As early as 2009, BP's Environmental Impact Plan for the Murcado Projection well site, where the Deepwater Horizon was set to begin drilling, reflected the company's previous successes with deep water wells, stating that it was "unlikely that an accidental surface or subsurface oil spill would occur ...." The significant component of the plan, should a spill occur, was distance from the shore, which would, according to BP's plan, provide ample time for rescue and containment vehicles to be put in place and mitigate any potential harm to the shore. However, in that same year, a senior BP drilling engineer warned that a critical piece of the blowout preventer at the site could fail due to high pressure. Beginning in March and continuing through April 2010, as drilling neared completion, conditions around the well changed as evidence of shallow natural gas reserves were found. However, BP in an effort to save time and money – between US $7 and US $10 million dollars – reduced the number of redundant barriers and centralizers, minimized the amount of drilling mud circulation (done to remove air pockets), and canceled the final cement bond log test necessary before crude oil retrieval was set to begin. The canceled test was originally set for 7 a.m.

*Introduction to One Health: An Interdisciplinary Approach to Planetary Health*, First Edition.
Sharon L. Deem, Kelly E. Lane-deGraaf and Elizabeth A. Rayhel.
© 2019 John Wiley & Sons, Inc. Published 2019 by John Wiley & Sons, Inc.
Companion website: www.wiley.com/go/deem/health

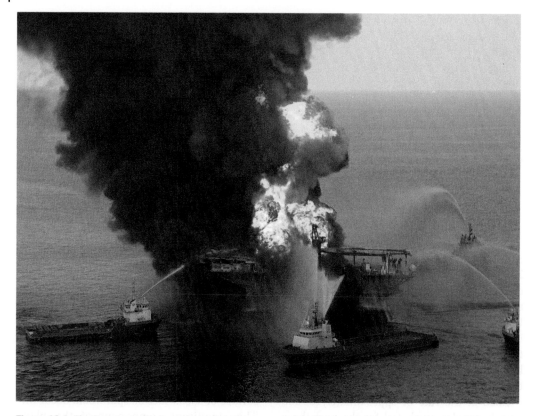

Figure 12.1 The Deepwater Horizon rig on fire. The uncapped wellbore spewed crude oil into the Gulf of Mexico for months.

on April 20; at 10 p.m. that night, the deck of the Deepwater Horizon was engulfed in flames.

Five years after the Deepwater Horizon explosion, the cost of the damage in settlements and penalties to BP reached US $61.6 billion dollars. In the aftermath of the explosion and subsequent clean up, BP has paid more than US $1 billion dollars to more than 400 local governments, US $4.9 billion dollars to the five Gulf Shore states – Louisiana, Mississippi, Alabama, Texas, and Florida – directly impacted for economic losses, more than US $8 billion dollars to the USA and five Gulf Shore states for loss of natural resources, and more than US $5 billion dollars to the US government for violations of the Clean Water Act.

While BP's economic cost included loss of revenue from lost oil and plummeting

market value, cost of clean-up, fines, and other legal penalties, the economic impact of the Deepwater Horizon reached far beyond BP. Gulf Coast fisheries were immediately and significantly damaged by not only crude oil contamination but by dispersant. The use of 4.9 billion gallons of a toxic oil dispersant, while critical to the cleanup efforts, resulted in the creation of additional concerns for fisheries and wildlife and ecosystem health. As a result, Gulf Coast fisheries operations lost an estimated US $95 million dollars in 2010 alone, more than US $168 million dollars between April 2010 and 2011, and more than US $247 million dollars by 2015. The long-term costs to Gulf Coast fisheries are harder to predict, but one study predicts economic loss to Gulf Coast fisheries could reach more than US $8.7 billion by 2020. Tourism in Louisiana, which normally accounts for approximately 400 000 jobs and more than US $34 billion dollars in revenue annually, was also significantly negatively affected, with three year losses reported at more than US $23 billion dollars. Across the Gulf Shore states however, the tourism reality was even more bleak, impacting more than 7.3 million businesses, more than 34 million employees, and resulting in a loss of more than US $5.2 trillion dollars in revenue, with small, local businesses the hardest hit. In addition to this, real estate values plummeted and remained at pre-2009 values for more than five years, and jobs across several industries were lost, including more than 300 000 oil industry jobs in Louisiana alone.

The direct economic fallout of the Deepwater Horizon disaster underscores the true cost of this environmental disaster. The economic valuation of more intricate systems, including wildlife populations and ecosystems, has long been challenged by how we interact with our environment. Throughout the Gulf Shores region, the cost to human, wildlife, and environmental health was high. For example, more than 5000 marine mammal deaths were reported after the Deepwater Horizon; a record number of dolphin illnesses were reported in 2010–2011; over 1000 sea turtles were found dead along Gulf Shore state beaches, approximately 2000 turtles were found stranded in the Gulf in the five years since the disaster, and evidence suggests that 10 000 or more turtles were exposed to oil in the year immediately following; as many as one million shorebirds were killed; fish populations declined by more than 50% and recovery is not predicted until well after 2020; lesions and heart defects were commonly found among large fish, including tuna and swordfish in the year following the disaster; deep sea coral communities were devastated as far as 60 miles from the spill site; and coastal seaweed communities, which provide home to shrimp, crab, lobsters, and many more unique wildlife species, were reduced by more than 85% in the year following the spill. In total, it is estimated that more than 22 000 tons of crude oil washed ashore in 2010. Even

five years later, tar balls continued to wash up on beaches across the Gulf Shore states. Research has shown that these tar balls are problematic for a number of reasons, including significantly, an increase in bacterial colonies found within – at the rates of 8–10 times normal bacterial incidence in seawater or sand. More troubling is these tar balls hint at the existence of larger, more environmentally significant tar mats found just offshore which suggest continued environmental damage well into the future. In addition to wildlife and human health impacts, entire ecosystems were devastated in the aftermath of the Deepwater Horizon disaster. Nearly 50% of Gulf beaches and 45% of coastal marshes were contaminated with oil; Gulf **benthic** communities have seen ecosystem die-outs in both abundance and diversity, with remaining species diversity reduced to approximately 10% of pre-spill levels; and small mangrove-dominated islands have begun to disappear entirely.

## 12.1 Economics: The Connection Between Values and Behaviors

Economics is, at its core, the study of decision making. In understanding how wealth and resources drive historic and current decision-making processes, economists can begin to understand future patterns of wealth, wealth distributions, resource allocation, and what these patterns can mean for people's decision making. The basis of economics, however, is the appreciation and examination of the true cost or the true value of a resource. And while it may seem straightforward to identify the true cost of a good or resource (e.g. a gallon of milk or a barrel of crude oil), the true value is often vastly different than its true cost. In order to understand or predict how people will make decisions or behave, it is critical to understand people's motivation.

**Behavioral economics** is the field of economics focused on examining the motivations of people behind their actions.

In behavioral economics, it is well documented that people consistently fail to act logically or rationally, and even more surprisingly, frequently fail to act in their own best interests. This is largely because of three reasons. First, people fail to properly take into account probabilities in their decision making. For example, in the classic example of failing to take statistics and probabilities into account: The Monte Hall problem. In this problem, an individual, let's name her Sue, must choose one of three doors – 1, 2, or 3 – and behind only one of the doors is an amazing prize (Figure 12.2). Sue, figuring that she has a one in three chance of winning, chooses door 1 as the door that is hiding the prize. As such, the host opens door 3, revealing nothing. The question is, then, if given a chance to change her choice of doors, should Sue stick with door 1 or change to door 2? At the time of the original problem, most people would say that it is better to stick with your original choice. However, Sue, being a probabilities expert, knows that she should change from door 1 to door 2. Door 1 – Sue's original choice – has a one in three chance of winning. However, because Sue has now obtained information about door 1, and by proxy door 2, she knows that door 2 has a two in three probability of being the winner. And so, Sue, of course, chooses door 2 and wins the prize. If your initial thought was that the new probability of winning was one in two for both door 1 and 2, you are not alone.

Second, people are typically risk-averse or risk-taking in surprising ways. This is, in part, because of our generally poor understanding of probabilities. For example,

many people fail to maximally invest (or invest at all) in their employer-matched retirement accounts. This risk-averse behavior is costing these individuals potentially thousands of dollars over their lives. However, the perceived risk of losing money through market fluctuations is, for some, greater than the potential of future economic gains. Finally, prices typically fail to include the true cost of an item, owing to the weight of negative externalities (explained later); however, people typically assume the price of the good accurately reflects the true cost. This creates a disparity between the intent and the reality of making spending decisions in accordance with one's values. In other words, while an individual may decide to invest their spending dollars with Company A because of the company's sustainability practices, religious ethic, or other value, due to the effects of externalities, Company A may not actually be the best company with which to invest in order to support those values. In reality, Company A may act to harm those values, be they environmental, religious, or other. Thus, many people intent on spending their money in accordance with their own values frequently fail to do so. This perceptional error between true cost and value lies at the core of behavioral economics and is fundamental to understanding the relationship between economics and questions of One Health.

## 12.2 Cost and Externalities

The true cost of a good, product, or resource is not the value or price of that item, although in common parlance, there is an equivalency between cost and price. For clarity, we will be using **price** as the price one pays for a good; the term most economists would describe as value. **Value**, we will be reserving mainly for the discussion of personally held beliefs and values related to an individual's personal ethic, and in this specific discussion, the ideas and motivations or belief that influence, positively or negatively, a person's spending.

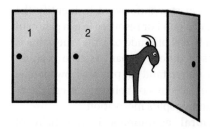

Figure 12.2 The basis of the Monte Hall problem. Should you choose Door 1 or 2?

And finally, the **true cost** of a good or resource is the price of an item if it fully included all of the hidden social costs and market failures, or what economists refer to as externalities.

**Externalities** can be thought of as hidden or external costs of a good or resource. In economic terms, externalities are a specific type of market failure that does not result in the complete collapse of a system of market or economy but instead results in costs borne by individuals not involved in the economic action. In this context, externalities fail to fully account for the true cost of the good or resource. As such, externalities can be positive or negative in their impact on the economic system. For example, individuals who commute by bicycle reduce congestion and pollution in their communities and improve their own personal health, contributing to lower healthcare costs. The cyclist may only be interested in saving on gas money, but the hidden costs of this decision are positive externalities. Alternatively, individuals who commute by personal car contribute to environmental pollution, including increases in smog-forming pollutants and greenhouse gas emissions. However, these individuals only pay for the price of the car, fuel, and maintenance. Society pays for the effects of automotive pollution, a negative externality.

As a result of the complexity of externalities, consumers looking to align their own personal values with the value of a good or resource will need to do a lot more work than simply comparison shopping by price. For example, if individuals are interested in identifying the best option for their commute – walking, bicycle, personal car, carpool, or public transportation – they could factor into the decision the value of their time, price of the bicycle or car, and perceived cost to the environment. However, the price of the bicycle, car, or train excludes the cost more broadly. Included in the true cost of these items are the cost of extraction of resources, infrastructure support and road building, engineering and development, loss of biodiversity and habitat to wildlife, and the clean-up and mitigation of pollutants resulting from all of these activities, including from the creation of fuel. However, because each of these is an example of an externality, and externalities are excluded from the price consumers pay, the disparity between price and true cost is exceedingly difficult to untangle. As such, an environmentally-conscientious consumer interested in minimizing the ecological footprint of his or her commute may find it challenging to truly know the impact of their decision. Pollution is one of the most commonly considered negative externalities. Unfortunately, in considering questions of One Health, the externalities of greatest concern are negative. Other examples of negative externalities that impact questions of One Health include, but are not limited to habitat and biodiversity loss, effects on economically disadvantaged communities, and social justice issues, including the effects of **environmental racism**.

## 12.3 The Cost and Value of Life

In economic terms, the value of a good is based on the price it would go for in an open auction. This concept of valuation works incredibly well for goods like a unit of coffee or a wooden chair and for services like an hour of childcare or a car wash. However, one consistent, long-term struggle for economics in consideration of the environment is how to value ecosystem diversity, non-human life, unutilized (by humans) land, and/or a forest? The oceans? A prairie?

The diversity of life in all its colors and variety has value. For example, a tree actively works to combat climate change and air pollution by absorbing carbon dioxide and other greenhouse gases, nitrogen oxides, ammonia, sulfur dioxide, and ozone. Trees also provide oxygen; cool cities by providing shade and breaking up urban "heat islands"; improve urban aesthetics by reducing road sounds, mask construction zones, or parking lots, and absorb dust; conserve water by slowing evaporation and contributing to atmospheric moisture through transpiration; slow runoff from rainstorms, reducing water pollution; slow soil erosion; and provide habitat for wildlife and food sources for many pollinators. Economically, a tree has value for the fruit it can provide (e.g. apples, oranges, mangoes), for the lumber it can become, and/or for the increase in property value it provides to homeowners through increase in "curb appeal" and for cooling. And, at least one tree owns its own land. Known as the Tree that Owns Itself, the Jackson Oak in Athens, GA, has legal ownership of itself and the ground surrounding its base for 8 ft in all directions. This list of potential values grows considerably when the effects of intact forest patches or networks of trees are considered. For example, an acre of mature trees can, in a single year, absorb the carbon dioxide equivalent of a single car driven for 26000 miles and provide enough oxygen for 18 people. Even in death, trees provide significant benefits. Dead and decaying trees provide homes for wildlife, return nutrients to the soil, and feed the **detritivore** community – including beetle larvae, wood lice, fungus, and snails and slugs. For every living thing on the planet, a similar assessment of the jobs, roles, and value could be calculated. What is the value of life? Answering this most fundamental question is at the heart of how we understand the economic motivations that directly impact environmental health, human health, animal health … One Health.

In a discussion of economics and conservation, and in consideration of how to value the diversity of life, one valuable, yet incomplete and much-debated tool, is the concept of ecosystem services. Ecosystem services are those benefits provided to people from ecosystems. These can include flood mitigation and control, clean water, pollution reduction, absorption of greenhouse gases and carbon sequestration, nutrient retention in soil, pollination, environmental health monitoring, and decomposition of dead organic matter. Ecosystem services typically fall into one of four categories: provisioning,

regulating, supporting, and culture. Provisioning services are those that provide resources directly; for example, food, fiber, or nutrients. Regulating services are global carbon sequestration and temperature control, flood control, and reduction of exposure to infectious diseases. Supporting services are those that support ecosystems more broadly, such as soil formation and decomposition of decaying material. Cultural services are spiritual, recreational, or educational benefits; for example, state and national parks used for backpacking or camping, the recreational use of lakes and rivers, or the creation of outdoor classrooms. However, all ecosystem services benefit human health directly or indirectly by providing security and stability in the face of natural disasters, providing reliable sources of food, and/or providing clean air, clean water, and medicines. Importantly, ecosystem services also are able to have a measureable price affixed to them. Current estimates place the value of ecosystem services at more than US $72 trillion annually, suggesting that ecosystem services provide a significant boon to the global economy. Notably, ecosystem services are also critical to the survival of human societies, which would cease to exist in a recognizable form if these services were to fail on a global scale. From a biodiversity conservation perspective, this is important because it works to value the ecosystem as a whole and provides some level of protection. From an economics perspective, the determination of the value of an individual ecosystem service is significant because it allows a price to be assigned to a specific component of nature, which can then be factored into calculations of true costs of goods and resources (Figure 12.3).

Ecosystem services, however, as a metric for the economic valuation of nature are not without concerns. For example, ecosystem services frequently fail to account for future value from services, or the **option value**. While this can be accounted for in models of existing known services, how science and technology will proceed or what needs

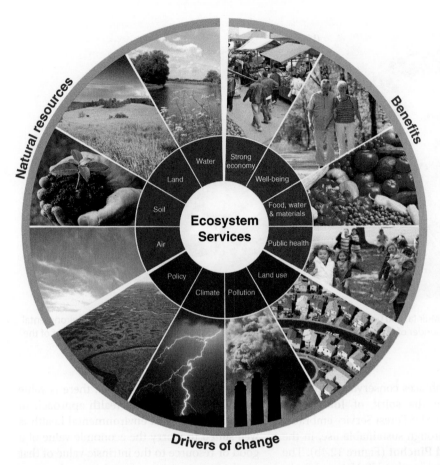

**Figure 12.3** Ecosystem services is a name for the variety of services provided for free by the planet.

humanity will require in 100 years or more, is unclear. As such, the assigning of accurate values to these services is unlikely to be accurate. Similarly, ecosystem services are also frequently incomplete. While large-scale forests may provide several tons of carbon sequestration annually for no charge, for example, these same forests also serve as habitats for a significant portion of the world's biodiversity. The focus on valuing these forests only as a source of carbon sequestration creates a significant gap in recognition of other, smaller-scale services with less direct economic benefit for people. Likewise, local or smaller-scale services are frequently undervalued as a contributing force in the calculation of ecosystem services relative to large-scale or globally-reaching services. Finally, one of the most important concerns regarding ecosystem services is the determination of value associated with ecosystem services, with many suggesting that assigning a price to ecosystem services undercuts efforts to work for planetary health entirely. The undervaluation or overvaluation of ecosystem services creates concerns not simply for the accuracy of specific occurrences but also for the value of the metric as a tool more generally.

How we value the environment is directly related to the values we hold sacred as individuals. For example, the US Forest Service and US National Park Service, whose missions are both conservation focused, act to support their individual missions through very different conservation ethics. The US National

(a)

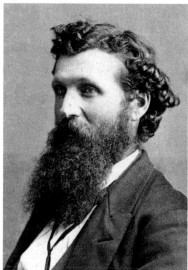

(b)

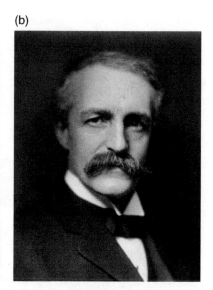

Figure 12.4 John Muir (a) and Gifford Pinchot (b) valued the environment but did not share an environmental ethic. Muir is the founder of the National Park Service, and Pinchot was the founder and first forest chief of the US Forest Service.

Park Service embraces conservation through preservation, in the spirit of **John Muir** (Figure 12.4a). The US Forest Service embraces conservation through sustainable use, in the spirit of **Gifford Pinchot** (Figure 12.4b). The resulting difference is that US National Parks are places untouched by industry while the US Forest Service promotes sustainable uses of resources such as logging, mining, and grazing. The difference in **environmental ethic** – use versus preservation – impacts all aspects of the global economy from personal habits to worldwide business decisions. Underlying this, however, is an important question about the **intrinsic value** of nature and its role in global health. Intrinsic values are the value of a species or biodiversity generally for their own sake, independent of the real or perceived value humans receive. The premise is simple: all life has value. From an economics perspective, however, this is a challenging concept to utilize. Because intrinsic values exist independent of an economic metric, economists frequently ignore these values in discussions of cost. The use of intrinsic valuation, additionally, is frequently considered to contribute only minimally to

conservation efforts. However, there is value in all life, and the One Health approach to human, animal, and environmental health is well suited to marry the economic value of a good or resource to the intrinsic value of that good or resource in profound ways.

## 12.4 The Conundrum of Economics and the Environment

Given what you have learned about economic externalities and the environmental health costs of negative externalities, in particular, for questions of One Health, it should come as no surprise that there is significant debate among scientists and economists on nearly all topics at this interface. Compounding these difficulties, valuation of specific components of the environment and/or human, animal, or environmental health is exceptionally difficult. Understandably, businesses do not typically choose to incur costs that others will bear, for example, clean up or mitigation of pollutants, in an effort to minimize price for consumers and maximize earnings. And, also understandably, consumers do not typically prefer to pay higher prices. However, the coalescence of significant costs hidden from consumer pricing, and ultimately paid by future generations, with the difficulty of truly capturing the economic and intrinsic value of nature, which includes human, animal, and environmental health, often results in business decisions to maximize short-term profits at the cost of human, animal, and environmental health. However, this is not always the case. It is possible, and frequently profitable, to create a successful business that values the health of human and animal life and minimizes impact to the environment.

## 12.5  Business and Sustainability: Patagonia

In the early 1950s, Yvon Chouinard spent his days climbing mountains in California. In 1957, he purchased the equipment needed to create reusable pitons, a small but critical piece of equipment which makes vertical ascents much safer, selling them for US $1.50 each. However, by 1970, it was apparent that reusable pitons, which needed to be hammered in and out of the rock face with each climb, were causing significant environmental damage in the very places that rock climbers cherished. This damage expanded small cracks, amplifying erosion potential, and left the rock face permanently marred. Thus, Chouinard made his first environmentally based business decision and introduced aluminum chocks to replace pitons. Soon after, through unintentional trend-setting, Chouinard found himself selling clothing to climbers as well.

Patagonia was born.

Patagonia has a long history of focusing on the values and traditions on which the company was founded. To this end, they have been at the forefront of employer-focused benefits, including opening an on-site child care center, promoting flexible hours and job-sharing, and promoting participation in the very activities – mountain climbing, surfing, fly fishing, camping – the company's gear was designed for. Aligning with this emphasis on cultural values, Patagonia has held an environmental ethic as one their core values since its inception. Annually, Patagonia donates 10% of their profits or 1% of total sales, whichever is greater, to small groups working to promote environmental health, advocacy, and conservation of habitats. The company has actively worked to minimize their ecological footprint, switching to organic cotton in 1996 and continually searching for even more environmentally friendly fabrics. Patagonia has reduced energy costs through switches to solar energy and radiant heat; eliminated colors that necessitated toxic metals for dyes and created fabric made from recycled plastic bottles; and promoted transparency throughout their supply chain.

> I know it sounds crazy, but every time I have made a *decision* that is best for the planet, I have made *money*.
> -Yvon Chouinard

Patagonia is a global company, bringing in US $750 million in sales in 2015. The environmental ethic of Patagonia, in synergy with its environmental activism and philanthropy, demonstrate that business considerations do not require policies for the destruction of environmental, human, and animal health. Business leaders, whose focus is sustainable practices and an environmental ethic, can make a profoundly positive impact on planetary health.

## 12.6  Business and Sustainability: New Belgium Brewing

In a Fort Collins, Colorado basement, in the early 1990s, New Belgium Brewing began. Inspired by a ride through Belgium on a "fat-tired" bicycle, with stops in small towns famous for beer, New Belgium brewing was willed into being by Jeff Lebesch and Kim Jordan. Lebesch – a home brewer at the time – handled the original brewing while Jordan – a social worker – managed advertising, distribution, bottling, and financial planning. From these auspicious beginnings in 1991, New Belgium Brewing has grown into the fourth largest craft brewery in the USA, with estimated sales of US $225 million and just under 700 employees in 2015. The company's core values and beliefs were penned by the co-founders before the first bottle of Fat Tire was ever sold, and these values have guided the company as it has grown ever since. Not surprisingly, New Belgium Brewing's first three values prioritize beer. However, the next two core values of New Belgium Brewing focus not on beer or profit but on environmental sustainability, responsibility, and stewardship. Learning and culture, employee quality of life, especially the maintenance of a work/family balance, trust, innovation, and fun round out the values established by the company's founders in 1991 and continue to drive the company's growth and development strategies. For New Belgium Brewing, profit is a goal, not a value.

At New Belgium Brewing, decisions about growth are anchored in the company's core values – emphasizing quality of life for all employees over profit. Strategic growth and transparency are important. This focus on transparency maintains not only the quality of the product, but means that employees, who are also owners, know exactly how much it costs to brew each bottle of beer, how much waste is generated, how much energy is consumed, and how much savings are generated (and morale boosted) by providing child care centers and free medical centers on-site. It also means that data on the carbon emissions, waste generated, water consumed, and energy utilized is publicly available, as is the company's plan for reducing greenhouse gas, waste, and water and energy consumption. For example, New Belgium Brewing, through a partnership with Waste Not Recycling, has reduced the amount of waste entering landfills by 99.9% and generates about 20% of its electricity on site. New Belgium Brewing is a **certified B Corporation**, or a corporation that has met rigorous standards of social and environmental performance, accountability, and transparency, and Platinum certified Zero Waste Business and actively looks for opportunities to continue to improve both product and environmental impact.

New Belgium Brewing continues to value waste management, including management of greenhouse gas emissions, and reducing water pollution. Partnerships with Waste Not Recycling, The Wetlands Initiative, Protect Our Winters, and other community groups focused on sustainability and advocacy support the philanthropic philosophy of the company while simultaneously protecting the resources that enable them to brew a quality beer. The profitability of New Belgium Brewing is as reliable as the quality of their beers (which are, for the uninitiated, delicious). It is clear that profit need not come at the cost of human, animal, and environmental health, and if considered from the beginning as a core value, planetary health and outstanding products can thrive together.

## 12.7 Global Economics and Planetary Health

The interconnectedness of the human health, animal health, and environmental health should be evident by now (Chapters 4–6). However, the interconnectedness of our One Health and the economy, while just as connected, intricate, and critical, is frequently overlooked or poorly understood in discussions of global health and conservation. Decisions about how we value the environment and the services the environment provides underpin major economic decisions, potentially without our being aware. Externalities abound, linking simple everyday purchases to some of the greatest threats to planetary health via a large, complex web of hidden costs, each with the potential to devastate the health of humans, animals, and the environment. However, global concerns require global solutions, and using a One Health approach to capture more accurately the true cost of our decisions and to develop a holistic strategy for minimizing the health costs for humans, animals, and the environment is critical. Externalities have a cost, and we, the people of the world, pay with our finances and with our health. Businesses can be profitable and value environmental sustainability and health. We must make individual economic decisions responsibly and support businesses that behave in a way that is responsible to the planet and planetary health.

## End of Chapter Questions & Activities

A. Thought Questions:
  i) What is the power of the dollar for One Health?
  ii) What would scaling costs to truly represent all costs for the One Health Triad do for the cost of health care, business, and so on?
  iii) Are there economic motivations that can incentivize behavioral changes for the betterment of planetary health that are as powerful or more than intrinsic factors? How can we better use economic motivators?

B. In-Class/Guided Activities:
  i) You live in a small community with only one road to its nearest neighbor. Your mayor has proposed building an additional road, which has the possibility to increase job growth locally. Explore the potential externalities of road construction. How many can you identify? How would the price of the proposed road construction change if these externalities were included?
  ii) Investigate greenwashing. Corporations, aware of public sentiment, can use marketing efforts to make their actions appear more environmentally palatable. What are some companies that have used greenwashing in the past? What are the strategies that were most successful? How can you be more aware of greenwashing practices?

C. At-home Activities:
  i) What is the true cost of a pencil?
    1) Identify all the parts of a pencil. Where does each part originate? Were they mined? Harvested? Other? What were the costs associated with producing the raw component of each part of the pencil?
    2) How was each raw part brought together into a pencil? Were there transportation costs? If so, what were the costs associated with truck or plane building, fuel production, and the nationwide infrastructure for transportation?
    3) Who built the pencil? Are there hidden costs associated with the design and construction of the pencil?
    4) How did the finished product reach the store? Identify the externalities associated with moving the pencil from factory to store, marketing and advertising, and selling the pencil.
    5) How does the true cost compare to the price?
  ii) Identify one product you currently use that has a significant hidden cost to planetary health and look for alternatives.

D. Long-term Action Steps:
  i) Resolve to be an environmentally conscientious consumer. Before you purchase anything, identify how it was made. What waste was created as a part of its construction? What are the long-term health impacts of the product and its waste? Is this necessary? You'll likely save money and the environment in doing so.
  ii) Identify B Corp certified companies and work to support them through investments and purchasing power.

iii) Urge your local municipalities to upgrade buildings in your community to LEED certified environmental standards.

iv) Make socially and environmentally responsible investments.

E. Recommended Reading:

Chouinard, Y. (2016). *Let My People Go Surfing: The Education of a Reluctant Businessman*. Penguin Books.

Honeyman, R. (2014). *B Corp Handbook: How to Use Business as a Force for Good*. Berrett-Koehler.

O'Brien, C.M. (2006). *Fermenting Revolution*. New Society Publishers.

Oreskes, N. and Conway, E.M. (2010). *Merchants of Doubt: How a Handful of Scientists Obscured the Truth on Issues from Tobacco Smoke to Global Warming*. Bloomsbury Press.

## Interview

*An Interview with Martin Meltzer, PhD: Senior Health Economist and Distinguished Consultant. He leads the Health Economics and Modeling Unit in the Division of Preparedness and Emerging Infections within the National Center for Emerging and Zoonotic Infectious Diseases at the Centers for Disease Control and Prevention.*

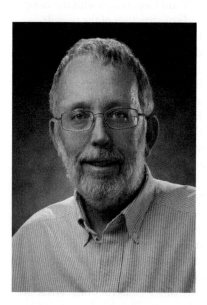

**When did you first hear about One Health?**

I heard about One Health about 10 years ago. I spent a large part of my career working on One Health, at the interaction, or the boundary, between human and animal health. I study what happens when diseases spill over from the animal world into humans, what you can do to either prevent or reduce that risk, and, how to best react to outbreaks when they occur.

**How is One Health important to your work?**

Our projects are in the emerging infectious disease domain, and one of the biggest threats to public health is dealing with infectious diseases. How do you deal with diseases that emerge from the animal kingdom? Or, what do you do when you have increasing human populations, particularly in developing countries, and there are not enough public health resources to ensure early detection of infectious disease outbreaks and rapid and effective responses?

When humans and animals interact, whether it's wildlife or domesticated, there is a risk of the transmission of infectious diseases that can have a dramatic and immediate impact on human communities. We do not always label it as One Health, but you cannot address just the human side of infectious diseases without thinking about the risk due to diseases in animals. For example, if you are going to worry about influenza pandemics in humans, you should be monitoring the changes, the variety, and the availability of influenza viruses circulating in chicken flocks, which is exactly what public health and animal health people do globally.

**How do you actions reflect One Health, personally or professionally?**

Many of the problems we work on, where diseases have spread into humans from animals or insects, we look at numbers to get a correct sense of the risk of further outbreaks before they happen. We constantly think beyond the human, about the risks that humans face because there are disease reservoirs in animals and vectors that can spill over into human communities. And, to me that is the One Health concept. I do not stop at only the humans.

**What can an individual do to make a difference for planetary health?**

That's a tricky question in many ways. One thing is to become educated to the degree to which we are globally connected. And, further, to understand that the conditions that increase the risks of outbreaks of infectious diseases in one country, however remote, is not somebody else's problem. I think it's reasonable to expect that, with the right amount of effort and conditions, we can reduce the risk of diseases moving from animals and insects into human communities by putting into place systems for earlier and more accurate detection, and earlier and more effective response.

**How can we encourage people to care about planetary health?**

As an economist, I always look for the motivation. For a person living in the USA, or Europe, or any developed country, the risk of an outbreak of infectious disease in their community becomes elevated when it goes from a small localized outbreak to a larger one that spreads across a country or region. And, even if the outbreak occurs overseas, there's the risk of that disease actually being imported into the country where you live.

An example of how disease outbreaks affect communities in other countries, the Ebola epidemic in West Africa in 2014–2016 reduced trade. The Ebola outbreak affected both the countries where this outbreak occurred and counties that export to those countries. In the USA, large outbreaks of infectious diseases in other countries could reduce our exports and impact our export economy without a single person in the USA becoming ill from that disease. And, with airplanes and expanding global travel, there's always the risk of a disease actually being introduced into an unexpected region or community. Responding to such outbreaks costs a lot of public and clinical health resources to be deployed to find and detect cases as they arrive.

**Where is One Health headed?**

I would like to see One Health come up with a clear, concise message that tells people who have not thought about this problem very much that there is a very good reason for people, communities, governments to consider the connection between animals, humans, and vectors. There are benefits to trying to get "ahead of the curve" and increase the resources given to early detection and rapid, effective responses. This is about markedly reducing the risk so that future outbreaks do not become national and international problems. I'd like One Health to really work towards producing a message that clearly transmits that to the rest of the public in simple terms.

**What is the power of the dollar for One Health?**

I think the One Health concept allows one, or encourages one, to look beyond the immediate cost of clinically treating somebody who becomes ill, and addressing the complete set of costs. For example, the Ebola epidemic in West Africa in 2014–2016, caused trade to be slowed down or even shut down for other parts of West Africa. In addition, we need to assess how much can we realistically reduce risk, and what are the economic benefits of risk reduction?

People respond to numbers, provided, of course, that the numbers are clearly explained. A lot of problems often occur when people throw around a dollar figure without explaining what it means, what was included and excluded. Expectations can become incorrectly set regarding what the burden or risk is, and what can and cannot be done, and what risk reduction would or would not cost. Dollars help convey the message, both regarding burden of disease, and the cost of an intervention to reduce that burden, and the benefits of actions to reduce the risk of that burden occurring. Dollar values are a tool.

**What would scaling costs to represent all costs for the One Health Triad do for people?**

If we get a more realistic and more complete picture of what these outbreaks of zoonotic diseases really cost, people in business, governments, and everywhere else will begin to realize the magnitude of the problem, and to really understand the benefits of investing in systems that allow for earlier detection and effective response. And, putting dollar values on the costs of scaling up the scope and size of interventions, and the potential benefits of that scaling up, allows people who do not normally think of these things to begin to appreciate what's at risk.

**What is something that most people fundamentally misunderstand about the connection between planetary health and economics?**

Literally, a disease overseas, an outbreak of an infectious disease, can rapidly spread and impact your community just by arriving at your doorstep. And, even if it does not spread, the disruption caused by that disease in the region that is experiencing the outbreak can have ripple effects that do affect you, such as potentially reducing trade and thus the economy in the community where you live.

**How can we use economic motivations to better incentivize behavior changes for planetary health?**

As an economist, I firmly believe that assuming people change behaviors, or agree to spend their tax dollars, because of "warm fuzzy feelings" is a poor way to plan policy and implement changes needed to globally reduce the risk of zoonotic diseases. I think people have to understand it's in their economic benefit, one way or another, to encourage leadership to actually invest in improved systems for disease detection and rapid response. The One Health concept connects people to the idea that they are not immune to these risks of disease just because the risks happen at the other end of the world.

**Parting Thoughts?**

Pay attention. For those considering, a career in public health, devote your career to collecting data that clearly and unambiguously demonstrates the risk of infectious diseases. Spend time sketching out what interventions could be applied, and then provide estimates of the benefits of such interventions, using either experimentation or actually deploying them on the ground as test cases. Explore and test methods and systems that will improve the ability and probability of early and successful detection, and will increase the probability of early and effective rapid response.

Bottom line: worry about the numbers.

---

**Case Study: The Economics of Lead-Contaminated Drinking Water in Flint, MI**

Co-authored by Pascaline Akitani and Mary McDermott

In April, 2014, residents of Flint, MI, began to complain about the appearance, taste, and smell of their drinking water. As discussed in Chapter 3, in the previous year, Michigan Governor Rick Snyder had declared the city of Flint to be in a state of financial emergency and implemented a money-saving strategy for Flint to stop receiving water pre-treated with corrosion inhibitors through the city of Detroit, MI. Once the cost-saving measure of taking drinking water directly from the Flint River, a river so polluted it once caught fire, was complete, the water actively corroded the community's water pipes, leaching lead directly into drinking water. The water crisis of Flint, MI, resulted in lead contamination to the entire community's drinking water. This resulted in significant health effects for the people of Flint, MI, including the exposure of every child under the age of six to dangerous levels of lead, a potent neurotoxin, rising infertility rates, a spike in spontaneous abortions immediately following the switch to using the Flint River for drinking water, and an outbreak of Legionnaire's disease, which resulted in the death of 12 people.

Lead poisoning is extremely harmful to the health of children and adults. In adults, lead can increase blood pressure, induce fertility problems, and cause nerve disorders and arthralgia. As children's brains and nervous systems are still developing, lead exposure in children is much more devastating, resulting in difficulties learning, seizures and other neurological symptoms, abdominal pain, developmental delays, attention deficit, hyperactivity, behavior disorders, hearing loss, anemia, coma, and, ultimately, death. Lead in the environment does not only affect the health of humans. When deposited in the soil, it can remain there for up to 2000 years. It interferes with the binding of other metals onto organic matter, hindering the chemical breakdown of inorganic soil components, which makes lead more soluble in the soil. Increased solubility allows plants to absorb heavy metals easier, reducing the rate of photosynthesis and hindering respiration.

Flint, MI, is a predominantly black community, with a mean household income of US $24 679 and more than 40% of its population living below the poverty line. General Motors (GM), the dominant employer in the region, complained to state officials that the water was too corrosive and was interfering with the production of engine parts. While GM switched almost immediately to a different water source, the residents of Flint, Michigan did not have that choice. As of 2017, only one-third of the lead pipes in the community of Flint have been replaced. At the current rate of replacement, complete replacement is not expected to be completed until 2021 and cost more than US $1.5 billion. The cost to human, animal, and environmental health is even higher.

## Works Cited

Avery, H. (2010) The ongoing administration-wide response to the Deepwater BP oil spill. The White House, President Barack Obama. http://obamawhitehouse.archives.gov/blog/2010/05/05/ongoing-administration-wide-response-deepwater-bp-oil-spill (accessed February 14, 2017).

Batavia, C. and Nelson, M.P. (2017). For goodness sake! What is intrinsic value and why should we care? *Biological Conservation* 209: 366–376.

Briault, A. (2014). Economics and One Health. *Veterinary Record* 174 (11): 85–91.

Colias, M. (2016) How GM Saved Itself from Flint Water Crisis. *Automotive News*. Crain Communications.

Deepwater Horizon Claims Center: Economic & Property Damage Claims. http://deepwaterhorizoneconomicsettlement.com (accessed February 14, 2017).

Edwards, M.A. (2015) Why Is It Possible That Flint River Water Cannot Be Treated to Meet Federal Standards? *Flint Water Study Updates.*

Elzinga, K.G., Tremblay, C.H., and Tremblay, V.J. (2018). Craft beer in the USA: strategic connections to macro- and European brewers. In: *Economic Perspectives on Craft Beer* (ed. C. Garavaglia and J. Swinnen), 55–88. Palgrave Macmillan.

Flesher, J. (2015). *Study: Spike in Flint Children's Blood-Lead Levels Corresponds with Highest Water-Lead Levels*. The Canadian Press.

Fuchs, V.R. (2000). The future of health economics. *Journal of Health Economics* 19 (2): 141–157.

Greene, D. (1993). *Effects of Lead on the Environment*. Royal Melbourne Institute of Technology.

Gros, J., Socolofsky, S.A., Dissanayake, A.L. et al. (2017). Petroleum dynamics in the sea and influence of the subsea dispersant injection during Deepwater Horizon. *Proceedings of the National Academy of Sciences* 114 (38): 10065–10070.

Hanna-Attisha, M., LaChance, J., Sadler, R.C. et al. (2016). Elevated blood lead levels in children associated with the Flint drinking water crisis: a spatial analysis of risk and public health response. *American Journal of Public Health* 106 (2): 283–290.

Hein, L., Bagstad, K., Edens, B. et al. (2016). Defining ecosystem assets for natural capital accounting. *PLoS One* doi: 10.1371/journal.pone.0164460.

Holzman, D.C. (2012). Accounting for nature's benefits: the dollar value of ecosystem services. *Environmental Health Perspectives* 120 (4): A153–A157.

Lynch, S.L. (2016). *Business Case Studies in Sustainability Practices*. Honors in the Major Thesis: University of Central Florida.

MacKinnon, J.B. (2015) Patagonia's Anti-growth Strategy. *The New Yorker*. https://www.newyorker.com/business/currency/patagonias-anti-growth-strategy (accessed July 4, 2018).

Nakamura, R., Suhrcke, M., and Zizzo, D.J. (2017). A triple test for behavioral economics models and public health policy. *Theory and Decision* 83 (4): 513–533.

Packham, J.R., Harding, D.J., and Hilton, G.M. (1992). *Functional Ecology of Woodlands and Forests*. Berlin: Springer.

Panko, B. (2017) Scientists now know exactly how lead got into Flint's water. Smithsonian Magazine. http://www.smithsonianmag.com/science-nature/chemical-study-ground-zero-house-flint-water-crisis-180962030 (accessed October 22, 2017).

Powers, S.P., Peterson, C.H., Cebrian, J. et al. (2017). Response of nearshore ecosystems to the Deepwater Horizon oil spill. *Marine Ecology Progress Series* 576: 107–110.

Primack, R.B. (2013). *Essentials of Conservation Biology*, 6e. Sinauer.

Roberto, C.A. and Kawachi, I. (eds.) (2016). *Behavioral Economics and Public Health*. New York, NY: Oxford University Press.

Scholte, S.S.K., van Teeffelen, A.J.A., and Verburg, P.H. (2015). Integrating socio-cultural perspectives into ecosystem service valuation: a review of concepts and methods. *Ecological Economics* 114: 67–78.

Stark, S. W., and Milstein, R.L. (2016) Lead Poisoning. *Magill'S Medical Guide: Research Starters*.

Urbina, I. (2010) Documents Show Early Worries About Safety of Rig. *The New York Times*. https://www.nytimes.com/2010/05/30/us/30rig.html (accessed July 4, 2018).

Weick, K.E. (2017). Earl Boebert and James M. Blossom: Deepwater Horizon: a systems analysis of the Macondo Disaster. *Administrative Science Quarterly* 62 (2): 23–26.

Welch, L. (2013) The way I work: Yvon Chouinard, Patagonia. Inc.

Yang, T., Nigro, L.M., Gutierrez, T. et al. (2016). Pulsed blooms and persistent oil-degrading bacterial populations in the water column during and after the Deepwater Horizon blowout. *Deep Sea Research Part II: Topical Studies in Oceanography* 129: 282–291.

# 13

# Politics and Policy of One Health

*"There comes a time when one must take a position that is neither safe, nor politic, nor popular, but he must take it because conscience tells him it is right."*
Martin Luther King Jr.

At first glance, one may question why a chapter on **politics** and **policy** is included in an introduction to One Health book. We often associate politics with **power** and money, and as history shows, political actions may be nefarious or they may be for the common good. However, on closer inspection, it becomes clear that health, and the lack thereof, are both closely linked to politics. This is true whether we are talking about human, animal, or environmental health. It is safe to say when thinking about any One Health approach, "it is all politics." In today's globally connected world, we need politics and the associated policies and laws to provide the political actions necessary to offer health care across the One Health Triad.

The war on poverty is one example of the many political sides to health. The causes of poverty and wealth inequalities across the globe are often the direct result of political actions, and thus politics result in health disparities. The humanitarian causes of poverty and injustice have inspired many political interest groups to work to alleviate poverty, which may also help to alleviate the diseases of poverty, for example diseases associated with poor nutrition and poor hygiene. Alternatively, and just as important when

viewed through a One Health lens, we must think about the politics of overconsumption and the associated planetary costs, with direct and indirect impacts on environmental, animal, and human health. As discussed in Chapter 2, Earth Overshoot Day reminds us that humans are using resources at an unsustainable rate. A large part of this resource overuse may be in the overconsumption of calories, which has led to the current obesity epidemic and the negative human health impacts associated with obesity. In fact, worldwide, there has been a shift in disease research and interests from infectious diseases to the non-infectious, and often chronic, human-induced diseases (e.g. obesity, diabetes, heart disease), as these non-infectious diseases increasingly threaten public health. This shift, termed the **epidemiologic transition**, describes the changes in patterns of population age distributions, mortality, fertility, life expectancy, and causes of death. It is also associated with overconsumption. In addition to the direct costs to human health from overconsumption are negative impacts on the environment and all living things within it. The politics of overconsumption, including our inabilities to enact policies or laws that would limit overconsumption, due to the shortsighted interests of **economic** gains, are all part of the political landscape of One Health.

If you still question whether politics plays a role in your own One Health work, we recommend you work on any health initiative,

*Introduction to One Health: An Interdisciplinary Approach to Planetary Health*, First Edition.
Sharon L. Deem, Kelly E. Lane-deGraaf and Elizabeth A. Rayhel.
© 2019 John Wiley & Sons, Inc. Published 2019 by John Wiley & Sons, Inc.
Companion website: www.wiley.com/go/deem/health

whether for environments, animals, or people, in any country that is currently under dysfunctional government rule. It is apparent that health and health care suffers when there is politic uncertainty and/or instability. For example, consider the change in life expectancy for people living in the African nation of Zimbabwe during the early years of rule under Robert Mugabe, with his politics, known as **Mugabeism**. Life expectancy, a public health indicator, shifted downward significantly in those early years. In 1988, when Zimbabwe was still a young nation, following a civil war that led to Mugabe coming to power, life expectancy in Zimbabwe was 59.6 years for males and 63.2 years for females. In 2001, 13 years later and after 21 years of Mugabe's rule, life expectancy had dropped to 41 years for both males and females. In this example, the political ruling party used health care, or the lack there of, as a political weapon. Compounding this politically driven health outcome, the HIV epidemic was sweeping across Africa at the same time. Bad politics, which resulted in hyperinflation, food shortages, and a defunct health-care system, coupled with an emerging infectious disease, proved a lethal combination.

Politics may also be beneficial to One Health. When One Health is viewed as a public good, as it should be, politics that advance One Health should follow. We have seen that when people become aware of challenges that have significance on a global scale, local efforts are scaled up to national and international levels to meet these challenges. For example, the current state of our "plastic world," with plastics disposed of across the Earth, causing health issues for environments, animals, and people, has motivated anti-plastic activists. Their efforts have led to policies, laws, and actions to help handle this One Health challenge.

Plastics are a significant planetary health issue. Plastics have impacts to seabird and marine mammal populations from ingestion or entanglement. Plastics also have potentially more troubling impacts, which until very recently were unknown. As covered in Chapter 4, we are now aware of the chemicals in plastics and the magnitude of impacts they may have on both human and non-human animal populations. With the discovery of endocrine disrupting chemicals, such as bisphenol-A (BPA), which have the ability to feminize animals across taxa, including in humans, the world is ready to revisit where we stand with plastics.

First synthesized in 1907, plastics were not in widespread use until the mid-1900s with use accelerated by World War II. Shortly after, in the 1960s, people observed plastic debris in the oceans. Then in the 1980s, the **Great Pacific Garbage Patch** was discovered and is now estimated to be up to 8% of the Pacific Ocean, with small plastic particles suspended at or just below the surface. In some areas of the Great Pacific Garbage Patch, plastic is so thick it is possible to "walk" across the ocean (Figure 13.1). People started to take note and not just of this one patch. Plastics, and/or their chemical byproducts which leach out into the environment, are now present in all terrestrial and aquatic regions across the planet. This awareness has moved people to political action.

Like so many political mobilizations, this started at the grass roots level. Two programs, #strawsSUCK and #ByeToBags, along with numerous other programs in local communities, are leading the way to get plastics out of the environment. These initiatives are not limited to a few environmental organizations, but rather the movement goes all the way up to governmental politics. It all starts with understanding the problem: in the USA alone, 500 million plastic straws are discarded every day, equivalent to 182.5 billion straws per year. This is over 1500 tons of plastic, just from straws, that goes into landfills, or worse, into the ocean. This realization motivated a group of individuals to do something about it. Based on this awareness and gaining an understanding of the extent of the problem, specific action was implemented. Many local and regional municipalities have enacted laws that ban the use of

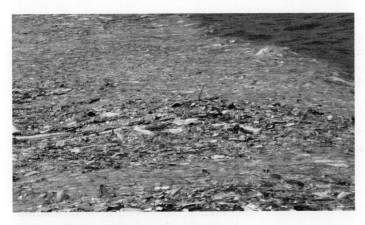

Figure 13.1 Pacific Garbage Patch.

plastic bags with Los Angeles, California being the largest city to have done so in 2012. In September 2017, Seattle, Washington was the first city to ban plastic straws. Grassroots moved governance for the good of One Health.

## 13.1  What Do We Mean by the Politics of One Health?

The modern globalized economy of the twenty-first century has resulted in an increased level of social, political, and economic interdependence due to the growing movement of people, produce, and other commodities across national borders. As we have entered the Anthropocene epoch with humans as the drivers of environmental changes today, planetary health is under the control of humans. Therefore, to advance the One Health view of a healthy planet, people must make decisions that support the health of *all* and then be able to turn these decisions into sustainable actions. We need politics to do this, even if the word politics conjures up different things for different people. How then do we define politics?

In its simplest form, politics is about making decisions that apply to a group. It is that easy. The group may be any human community, but we most often associate politics with the governance of a country or of countries.

Politics are hard to separate from power and allotment of resources. And, because humans often disagree about how to manage ourselves and our resources, politics often include debate, and increasingly, conflict, as individuals or parties strive for power. Politics, or perhaps more appropriately **political science**, the **social science** that deals with systems of governance, the analysis of political activities, political thoughts, and political behavior; is instrumental if we wish to turn human ideas and decisions into actions. Therefore, politics are key to the success, or failure, of the One Health initiative.

To make politics effective we must have the means to direct both the decision-making processes as well as the ability to turn decisions into actions. *Policies* are generally a course or principle of action adopted by a community, for example, a school district, city, state, or country. Policies may also be international agreements that help in decision-making and governance. Policies are a tool of politics. We may implement policies as procedures or protocols to ensure that the governance of the community is consistent with the intent of the community. *Laws* are the rules that regulate the actions of members within the community or governing body. To enforce laws, the imposition of penalties is often used. Determining the policies and laws in a community, at least in a democratic one, should reflect the people's beliefs. Therefore, one area of politics that One Health practitioners may pursue is **advocacy**. Advocacy is an activity by an individual or group aimed at influencing decisions. Covered in more detail in Chapter 10, advocacy may benefit the One Health approach within political, economic, and social systems and institutions.

## 13.2 How a Health Issue May Become a Political Issue

The management of disease threats to the One Health Triad has always been political. Humans make decisions and direct actions to prevent or handle these threats to health. To do this, we have policies and laws that help us decide how to handle diseases in any population. However, working on health challenges using a One Health approach makes the politics a little harder. For example, in a non-One Health scenario, managing environmental or animal health is often designed to provide human gain or profit, whereas managing human health is aimed at keeping people healthy and alive. Indeed, animal policies typically preempt concerns for the overall health of the animals, preferring instead to target animal cruelty issues and human food safety measures as top priorities. Therefore, in the global health crises of the twenty-first century that cross the human–animal divide, as so many EIDs do today, we see how politics may help or hinder how we handle these events.

One need only look at the politics that surrounded the 2014 Ebola epidemic, and especially after the arrival of the virus into the USA. By the time it arrived in the USA, Ebola had already killed over 4000 of the 8000 people infected in West Africa and had overburdened the health systems in the region, many to the brink of collapse. The initial slow response from the USA and other non-African countries may have been related to

the thinking that Ebola was a disease "over there" and therefore did not register as a "real" concern for the USA. In October 2014, things changed. By the time Ebola arrived in Texas, US soldiers, doctors, and nurses were rushing to help fight what the World Health Organization (WHO) was finally calling the largest and most complex Ebola outbreak in history.

Thomas Eric Duncan was the first Ebola patient in the USA. Duncan, infected with the virus while in Liberia, traveled to Dallas while his infection was still in the **incubation period**. Within days of arriving in Texas, following his international flights from Liberia to Brussels to Washington DC to Texas, he started to feel ill. On September 25, he first visited the emergency room (ER), but was sent home after being diagnosed with a low-grade viral disease. However, he returned on September 28 after clinical signs worsened. It was not until September 30 that the laboratory diagnostics confirmed that he was infected with Ebola. Mr. Duncan died in hospital on October 8.

In the days between the first clinical signs and death, Mr. Duncan interacted with numerous people both at the hospital and outside of the hospital between his initial ER visit and his return three days later. Everyone with whom he interacted was placed in quarantine until it could be confirmed that they had not been infected. In the end, two of the nurses that had cared for him did contract the disease but did not succumb to infection. Mr. Duncan was patient zero for Ebola in the USA, and had human-to-human transmission occurred at $R_0 > 1$, the Ebola epidemic would have quickly turned into a **pandemic**. EIDs should never be viewed as a disease only of importance "over there."

Once Ebola entered the USA, it became an even hotter political issue and added fuel to a divided political landscape that was already ablaze with blame and mistrust. The method by which the virus entered the USA added heat to conversations about immigration and border control as well as contributing to ongoing criticisms of the Obama administration and the government in general. While **politicians** were using this potential pandemic as a political weapon, there was a lack in comprehension of why and how the US health care system was so inexperienced to handle this zoonotic pathogen. There was an almost complete lack of understanding of how pathogens can be global and not just a "disease over there," or indeed how zoonotic diseases like Ebola have serious implications not just for human life, but also for biodiversity.

At the first visit to the hospital, the nurse that saw Mr. Duncan knew he had been in Liberia, the epicenter of the epidemic, but did not convey the information to others at the hospital. Further, during the debates that followed, in which this virus was used as a political weapon, almost everyone in the USA missed the significant fact of the virus's disastrous impact on endangered wildlife species, including mortality of up to 80% of gorillas in Ebola regions. In fact, Ebola, along with illegal hunting, is driving these animals, one of humans' closest relatives, towards extinction. Politics made this disease about border control and human movement, but it would have been much more effective to take a One Health approach and recognize that we can no longer afford to think of human health as separate from animal and environmental health: a disease in one nation poses risks to all nations.

The Ebola epidemic of 2014 would have been a perfect time to use politics to incorporate a One Health approach for more effective management of emerging wildlife and human health issues. The Ebola crisis offered an opportunity to raise awareness about the ways humans and wildlife share changing ecosystems. While we need to gain a better understanding of zoonotic diseases, we also must accept and address the role of humans in their development. EIDs, like Ebola, increasingly challenge wildlife conservation efforts and public health capabilities. This opportunity, lost to the politicians using it as a political pawn, could instead have led

to policies, actions, and laws based on the principles of One Health and not directed by politically fueled fear.

## 13.3 Political Differences, Realities, and Challenges

Politics are the mechanism that humans have devised for governance of a community, whether that community is a neighborhood district, a nation, or across nations. As mentioned earlier, the social side of One Health is key to political actions and the culture and **society** of the local community is key to political success. We dive deeper into cultural aspects of One Health in Chapter 11, but with the diversity of cultures and societies across the globe, the astute One Health practitioner is cognizant of a need for cultural and societal awareness. In recent years, One Health has gained some ground in guiding international research and policy that takes the One Health Triad into consideration, with many organizations working across platforms. However, there have been fewer gains in individual institutional traction. There remain a number of challenges impinging on our abilities to incorporate a One Health lens into policy and by extension politics. These include power-laden professional hierarchies, **institutional lock-in** around single-sector approaches, questions of personnel capacity, education and training levels, influence of funding flows, convenient articulations and securitizations agendas, global turbulence and connectivity, religious obstacles, and greed.

In addition to these challenges, it is apparent that not everyone is concerned about improving health for *all*, with recent political decisions in the USA trending away from ensuring that health care is available for all Americans and the removal of health safeguards for the most vulnerable. Adding to these are the science deniers that do not accept that climate change as human driven or deny facts if they hinder short-term economic gains. A possible limiting factor of our work to advance One Health is the politics that hinder scientific advancements and health care at the cost of short-term profits.

## 13.4 Key Local, National, and International One Health Organizations and Movements

Many local initiatives, policies, politics, and politicians – think of Barack Obama and his rise from grassroots community organizer to the most influential political position in the world – shape the world we live in and will continue to be the drivers of future decisions that affect One Health. In Chapter 14, we go further into the global environment, emphasizing that the local is global and the global is local in our interconnected world. The global reach and influence of the local empowers an individual to make real political change. There is a growing awareness that we need local municipalities, cities, and regions to take on the health challenges of today, as the larger national governments and international organizations struggle to affect positive change. The #ByeToBags and #strawsSUCK campaigns are just two examples of grassroots programs that grew from the local to help spark global change including political actions.

Beyond the grassroots efforts, we see that until recently the large and globally significant institutions such as the WHO, Food and Agricultural Organization (FAO), and the World Organization for Animal Health (OIE) have functioned isolated and independent. Each of these organizations represented a silo with efforts directed at their piece of the One Health pie. This is changing, albeit incrementally, with collaborative efforts across governing bodies as well as growth in private–public partnerships. Both of these may provide opportunities for the One Health initiative. Here we provide examples of a few of the more well-known agencies that work on international policies to help

govern health care within the three domains of the One Health Triad.

## 13.5 Environmental/Biodiversity

As discussed in Chapters 2 and 3, two of the biggest challenges with far reaching negative impacts on health across species today, are climate change and the loss of biodiversity. Therefore, it is hopeful that many organizations and nations are working on these critical issues. Policies and laws will be necessary if we are to both avert the most catastrophic outcomes of climate change and to slow the increasing rate of species' extinctions. Here we touch on some of the work in these areas.

### 13.5.1 International Climate Accord

The International Climate Accord, also known as the Paris Agreement, Paris Climate Accord, or Paris Climate Agreement, is an agreement within the United Nations Framework Convention on Climate Change (UNFCCC) that deals with greenhouse gas emissions mitigation, adaptation, and finance to start in 2020. The language of the agreement, negotiated by representatives of 196 parties at the Twenty-first Conference of the Parties of the UNFCCC in Paris, was adopted by consensus in December 2015. Although the Paris agreement is a major breakthrough in climate diplomacy and governance, there is nothing in the agreement that is truly enforceable. In other words, there are no real penalties if a country does not honor their commitments. Additionally, with the USA backing out of the Accord in 2017, we see how tentative international agreements are when political leadership changes.

### 13.5.2 International Union for the Conservation of Nature

The International Union for the Conservation of Nature (IUCN), created in 1948, is the largest and most diverse environmental network, with 160 countries, 1110 non-governmental organizations, and

213 governmental agencies as members. Operating through six commissions with volunteer efforts of more than 10 000 experts, the IUCN assesses the state of the world's natural resources. The six commissions are: (i) Commission on Education and Communication, (ii) Commission on Environmental, Economic, and Social Policy, (iii) World Commission on Environmental Law, (iv) Commission on Ecosystem Management, (v) Species Survival Commission, and (vi) World Commission on Protected Areas. The IUCN provides public, private, and non-governmental organizations with the knowledge and tools that enable human progress, economic development, and nature conservation to take place together.

### 13.5.3 The Convention on International Trade in Endangered Species of Wild Fauna and Flora

The Convention on International Trade in Endangered Species of Wild Fauna and Flora (CITES) was formed in the 1960s as an international agreement between governments with the aim to protect endangered animals and plants. It does this by ensuring that the international trade in wild animals and plants does not threaten their survival. First drafted by members of the IUCN in 1963, it went into effect in 1975. Today there are 183 parties (states and regional economic organizations) that agree to adhere to the convention, which works to protect some 35 000 species. Although CITES is legally binding, it does not have the place of national law, so individual parties must adopt their own legislation.

Within the USA, one means for enforcing CITES is through the Endangered Species Act (ESA) of 1973. This Act was designed to protect critically imperiled species from extinction in the face of unfettered economic growth and development. Currently, the Act is administered by the US Fish and Wildlife Service (USFWS) and the National Oceanic and Atmospheric Administration (NOAA).

### 13.5.4 United States Environmental Protection Agency

The United States Environmental Protection Agency (EPA) is a Federal agency created to protect human and environmental health by writing and enforcing regulations based on laws passed by the US Congress. The EPA, established in December 1970 under then President Richard Nixon, was a direct result of the seminal work of Rachel Carson in *Silent Spring* and her presentation of the worsening environment. Since it was founded the EPA has enacted numerous laws and regulations aimed at protecting water, air, and the land (Figure 13.2). For example, the Clean Water Act (CWA), which was first the Federal Water Pollution Control Act set forth in 1948, was reorganized and expanded in 1972 and under the EPA ensures pollution control programs. These include setting wastewater standards for industry and water quality standards for all contaminants in surface water. These are important standards across the One Health Triad.

The administrator and regional administrators of the EPA are appointed by political leadership, which can influence its focus. Administrators can determine when to be flexible to favor economic gains and when to be stricter with regulations to protect the environment as well as human and animal health. Unfortunately, in 2017, the USA witnessed a weakening of the EPA in its ability to protect environmental and human health based on evidence-based science. However, it is fortunate that we do not yet have to trade off pollution control for economic growth, as they may go hand in hand (Figure 13.2).

## 13.6 Animal and Human Health

### 13.6.1 World Health Organization

The WHO, established in 1948, is a specialized agency of the United Nations that is concerned with international public health. It is a member of the United Nations

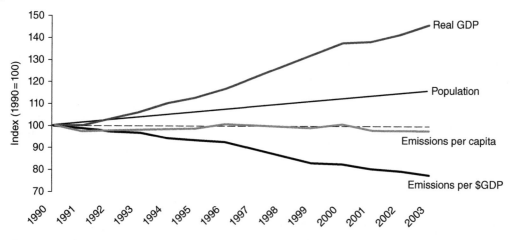

Figure 13.2 The EPA has enacted numerous laws and regulations aimed at protecting water, air and the land. US Greenhouse Gas (GG) Emissions per capita and per US dollar GDP.

Development Group and consists of 194 member states, with the current Director-General Dr. Tedros Adhanom, a One Health practitioner, in this position until July 2022. The primary role of WHO is to direct and coordinate international health within the United Nations' system. Main areas of their work include (i) health systems; (ii) promoting health throughout life (aging, reproductive health); (iii) non-communicable diseases (gun issues, addictions, obesity); (iv) communicable diseases (Ebola, HIV/AIDS, TB); (v) corporate services; and (vi) preparedness, surveillance, and response. The WHO was instrumental in 2000 in the eradication of smallpox- the first known disease ever intentionally eradicated.

### 13.6.2 Food and Agriculture Organization of the United Nations

The FAO is a specialized agency of the United Nations that leads international efforts to defeat hunger in both developed and developing countries. With 194 member states, the FAO acts as a neutral forum where all nations meet on equal footing to negotiate agreements and debate policy. The FAO acts as a source of knowledge and information on things such as agriculture, forestry, fisheries, and includes concerns related to nutrition and food safety.

### 13.6.3 The World Organization for Animal Health

The OIE is an intergovernmental organization coordinating, supporting, and promoting animal disease control. Currently, it comprises 181 member states and has relations with 45 other international and regional organizations, but maintains autonomy. The main objective of OIE is to control epidemic diseases. The OIE seeks to promote veterinary services and to ensure animal welfare and food safety. The OIE is extremely important in the context of One Health when we consider the health of food animals, the necessity to minimize zoonotic disease transmission, and the health of non-domestic animals to ensure the maintenance of ecological services.

### 13.6.4 Centers for Disease Control and Prevention

The Centers for Disease Control and Prevention (CDC) is the leading public health institution of the USA. It is a federal agency under the Department of Health and Human Services. The main goal of the CDC is to protect public health and safety through the control and prevention of disease, injury, and disability in the USA and internationally. Similar to the WHO it looks at communicable and non-communicable diseases. One department within the CDC is One Health, established based on the recognition that the health of people is connected to the health of animals and the environment.

## 13.7 Approaching Health Policies Through the One Health Lens

We need to align policy, programs, and political infrastructure to fight the health challenges of the twenty-first century, from zoonotic infectious diseases to climate change and pollution. We need to do this through unified political platforms and synergies between the three arms of the One Health Triad. Although many global health policies continue to lack a One Health foundation, there has been progress in recent years, as the need for a holistic approach has led to increased appreciation of shared risks. Slowly the walls of some silos are beginning to crumble. In fact, there are some health and conservation policies and laws currently in place to protect human health and the health of shared environments at both national and international levels. For example, we may view the Paris Climate Accord this way. Additionally, the three large international organizations – WHO, FAO, and OIE – although they have differing mission statements for human health, food production, and animal health, respectively, these organizations are often referred to as the One Health Tripartite with the realization of how completely connected each is to the other. This is all positive from a One Health perspective.

There are a number of examples embracing One Health global health policies. This includes the **Global Health Security Agenda** (GHSA) which was launched in 2014 to create a world safe and secure from infectious disease threats, to bring together nations from all over the world to make new, concrete commitments related to global health, and to elevate global health security as a national leaders-level priority. Another example is the **manifesto for planetary health**. This manifesto calls for a social movement to support collective public health action at all levels of society – personal, community, national, regional, global, and planetary. The aim of this manifesto is to respond to the threats we face: threats to human health and well-being, threats to the sustainability of our civilization, and threats to the natural and human-made systems that support us. The vision of this manifesto is for a planet that nourishes and sustains the diversity of life with which we coexist and on which we depend. Lastly, the **Stone Mountain Policy** of 2010 was an effort to operationalize One Health with a policy perspective that would allow a roadmap for implementation of One Health across all sectors of health. Although led by the CDC, whose mission has a clear human focus, this policy was written in close partnership with the OIE, FAO, and WHO. The Stone Mountain meeting – attended by the signatories of the policy – was part of a series of One Health meetings organized by diverse global institutions with the intent of providing a forum for national and international specialists to focus on policies and implementation of a One Health approach to improving human and animal health. The specific goal of the Stone Mountain meeting was to identify clear and concrete actions to move the concept of One Health from vision to implementation. All good for One Health.

## 13.8 Call to Action – Advocacy, Policy, and Politics

True of most everything today, a One Health approach will not succeed if there is no political will. We live in a complex world of bio-politics, special interest groups, funding flows, professional hierarchies, power relations, and the politics of governance. This combination of factors may all complicate efforts to protect and improve health across the One Health Triad. Therefore, it is fortunate that although politics are often the key to move large groups along, political movements often start small. It is a necessity for

One Health practitioners to be part of the political landscape if we wish to be successful. Each of us may be the key to moving policies and laws that support One Health. As the old Taoist saying goes, a journey of a 1000 miles begins with a single step – so too does political action start with a single idea.

The world of politics has changed immensely in recent decades due to the changing nature of communication, travel, and trade. Political decisions that were, until recently, only felt in one place on the planet may now have ramifications on the other side of the world and in a matter of seconds. This is both scary and empowering. In many ways, individuals today have more political power than ever before.

It should now be obvious that to be an effective One Health practitioner a person must be political. Political in the good sense and in the simplest meaning of the word, political in that decisions made apply to a group. As evident throughout the chapters of this book, One Health will be possible only if people work together for solutions to the current health challenges facing the planet. Now is not the time to be apolitical. To be apolitical – truly without politics – is to avoid interactions with people and the responsibility that you have as a global citizen. As we identify the technical skills that fit our niche within One Health, we must then turn to the political side of the job. We must position our ideas in a favorable light, know what to say, and how, when and to whom to say it. We must be political if we are to influence on the local or international stage.

We each have control, however small that may sometimes feel, to impact political decisions. Politicians have one overarching guide and that is to be re-elected. In democracies, to be re-elected politicians have to implement the will of the people. Individual One Health practitioners have the power to influence politicians and effect changes to policies. However, we must remember that to be effective in the political arena one must be able to communicate effectively and have that communication lead to actions. Politics is about influence and decision making for groups. Fortunately, there are a number of courses and books that can help advance a One Health practitioner in the political arena. Some key self-assessment questions may help one determine where their current political strengthens or weaknesses exist. Questions that each of us may ask ourselves include: (i) Can you effectively influence and manage people's perceptions of you and your ideas? (ii) Are you able to convert enemies to allies? (iii) Can you manage outcomes long before they are in sight? (iv) Do your ideas get a fair hearing? (v) Do you know when and how to present them? (vi) Are you in the loops that you wish to be included within?

Grassroots advocacy often leads to new policies and laws. The steps for making this happen may be looked at as a recipe – awareness, understanding, sharing, the "ask," and action. To care about anything, people must first be aware of it. We must present the issue in a way that people can both be aware and understand. Only after people are informed and understand the consequences of the issue will they feel inspired to share their new understanding. Such sharing spreads outward and leads to further awareness and growing concern for the issue. Any movement requires repetition, repetition, and repetition. After this awareness and understanding reaches a large number of people, we can make the call to action. One should always have ready the "ask" of your work. Have in mind, at all times, that elevator speech to give, should you have one minute to tell the world or that one person in the elevator with you, of what you are asking of them to do. Each of us, as individuals, can take our One Health concern and move it into group think (remember that influencing groups is politics) which is then turned into group action. Finally, this action, turned into a policy, may move us into the political position we wish to see; with laws enacted in response. As Dr. Keith Martin (see Chapter interview) states "We the people should be the puppet masters of politicians – not vice versa." Understandably, this is not easily accomplished and in many regions of the world, the ramifications for even discussions on this could be imprisonment. Still, again as our world becomes more connected, we may be able to effect change. One person at a time.

In any Democracy, the right to vote may be among the most powerful political tools we have for advancing One Health policies. As such, citizens of democracies must be informed and help to inform. They must know the politics in the local region, state, nation, and the world. They must remember that all good political moves start by making people aware and providing understanding of the issue. This starts by sharing an issue with one person at a time and then repeat ad infinitum. Following information sharing is the "ask" that ensures the persons' new-found knowledge is turned into policy, which can lead to laws centered on One Health principles. We can all advocate for those health and environmental concerns that fuel our passions. In today's connected world, most of us have in the palm of our hand a platform for change. Change comes from #BlackLivesMatter to #Metoo to #96elephants. We can reach out and share solutions to the global health inequalities and conservation challenges of the day. We must all be political.

## 13.9 Conclusions

The dichotomy of approaches for human versus non-human health care may lead to tensions and competition for political decisions on how best to provide health care to different populations. However, as we increasingly appreciate the link of shared disease issues threatening life across the One Health Triad, we may garner political will to move ahead with policies that help to ensure health for all. The greatest impacts happen at the policy and legislative levels, from internal policies and laws of each nation to international efforts and policies. These may include anything from laws that protect air and water, access to health care, animal welfare, and wildlife conservation. Individual One Health

practitioners must pay attention to policy; we must know who the actors are in the agencies making policies; we must get our voices into the political arena.

The good news is that individuals, especially in democracies, can and do impact policy. We have mechanisms that allow us to shape policies that will govern health across the One Health Triad. It is empowering to know that we each have a role in the politics of One Health today. Whether that role is to vote for health care, to advocate for health care, or to be one of the politicians that drive the changes. The "one" in "One Health" is each one of us as individuals. One person's actions add up and as Margaret Mead reminds us "Never believe that a few caring people can't change the world. For, indeed, that's all who ever have."

## End of Chapter Questions & Activities

A. Thought Questions:
   i) Do you know the positions of your elected officials on One Health issues? If not, find out.
   ii) Consider how a health topic for which you are passionate. Put together your "elevator" speech to defend a policy your local politician should support. Remember the steps of moving something into political action. Use them in your speech.
   iii) Can you name one health issue that is currently on the international, national, and state level? For each of these three issues, can you describe whether they are being approached through a One Health lens?

B. In-Class/Guided Activities:
   i) Have the class divided into four sides for a debate. Then discuss a One Health topic with the four groups with three groups representing a tunnel vision human health, animal health, environment health view, and the fourth group a holistic One Health

view. Capture what this discussion looks like and get an understanding for all the stakeholder views.

ii) Have each student give their one to two minute, elevator speech on the One Health topic of their choice.

C. At-home Activities:

i) Watch the YouTube recording by Matthew Stone, Deputy General Director of the OIE (the World Organization for Animal Health), talking about One Health in the OIE and working with FAO and WHO. https://www.youtube.com/watch?v=f2BYRNE4YPw

ii) Visit the CDC One Health page and learn about their initiative across the One Health Triad. https://www.cdc.gov/onehealth/index.html

D. Long-term Action Steps:

i) Get political. Go to meetings of the local parties or activist groups.

ii) Develop a #hashtag on a One Health issue for which you have passion. Using one of your social media platforms, tweet, Instagram, or facebook on the #hashtag daily over the coming year and see if you can start a conversation.

E. Recommended Reading:

Bardosh, K. (2016). *One Health: Science, Politics and Zoonotic Disease in Africa.* Routledge.

Bloomberg, M. and Pope, C. (2017). *Climate of Hope: How Cities, Businesses, and Citizens Can Save the Planet.* St. Martin's Press.

Clinton, C. and Sridhar, D. (2017). *Governing Global Health: Who Runs the World and Why?* Oxford University Press.

Grant, W., Medley, G., and McEldowney, J.F. (2013). *Regulation of Animal Health and Welfare.* Routledge.

Reardon, K.K. (2006). *It's All Politics: Winning in a World Where Hard Work and Talent Aren't Enough.* Doubleday.

## Interview

*An Interview with Keith Martin, MD, PC who is the founding executive director of the Consortium of Universities of Global Health (CUGH). He is a physician who served six terms as a Member of Parliament in Canada.*

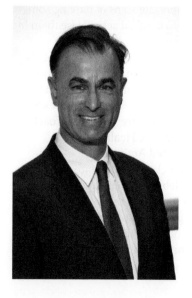

**How is One Health important to your work today?**

The health of people and the health of the planet are indivisible. One Health is a platform that enables us to aggregate the different disciplines needed to improve human and planetary health. Although it is not being fully utilized, One Health sits in a unique position within global health to address the existential challenge of our time: how we can live sustainably on Earth with a human population expected to top 9.2 billion by 2050. At CUGH, we work to find these opportunities to strengthen and mobilize the One Health community and apply what we know to address this challenge.

**What can an individual do to make a difference for planetary health?**

As individuals we need to reduce our environmental footprint. The summation of modest changes by the many equals a big impact. The other thing is to get politically active. We need to share evidence-based solutions with elected officials, communities, and individuals and collaborate to incentivize their implementation.

## Where is One Health headed?

One Health sits at a pivotal moment and will go in one of two ways. It can lose steam or it can drive forward and become much more mainstream and impactful. We need to do a better job of articulating what One Health is and how it can address development challenges. We need to aggregate good practices that improve human and environmental health, demonstrate their rate of return, and also the costs of inaction. The Global Health Security Agenda (GHSA) provides a platform that can be used to operationalize One Health practices. These practices can prevent the spillover of zoonoses through improving our management of ecosystems, protection of ecosystem services, and the care of livestock.

## Have you noticed change in receptivity to policies that fit within One Health and planetary health when US administrations turn over?

Very much so. In 2017, the current US administration is passing policies that will damage our environment and harm our people. In the area of environmental protection, we see the evisceration of the EPA and the removal of protections for large tracts of land and marine habitat including many monuments put in place by previous US administrations. We are also seeing the undermining of science and science capacity within the US Government. This is manifest by deep cuts to US agencies (CDC, EPA, USAID) and the removal of people with scientific backgrounds from those agencies replacing them with people without such backgrounds. Lastly, the ability of US government scientists to speak freely is being curtailed. This is an assault on science which deprives policymakers and the public of information they need to make informed, intelligent choices.

## Is there a coordinated Health Command Post in any of the global organizations or is their response to each emerging threat on its own, so to speak, for getting attention, and to garner support?

The WHO has the mandate to be the central agency in the area of pandemic preparedness and response. The OIE works globally to improve animal health. Each country is supposed to have a national focal point to prevent, detect, and respond to pandemic threats but many do not have the capacity to be able to have this system. The GHSA is a wonderful agreement to address this challenge but it will require us to do a better job of addressing the human resource deficits through training and of course identifying the resources to support the GHSA. There is not, unfortunately, any organization that I am aware of that can lead in terms of the sustainable environmental management that is necessary to manage ecosystems in a better way. Although, the United Nations Environment Programme (UNEP) has the mandate to work with nations to do this.

## Can you think of any policy-driven mechanisms that may help with Americans' approach to charity in terms of response to global crises?

The first thing is that people have a hard time wrapping their head around 250 000 people dying but they can relate to a child washed up face down on a sandy beach, dead. We have to communicate what we do through stories so a person may relate. We have to humanize the issues we are dealing with and make them relevant to the individual. Secondly, who pays? Official global development assistance is about US $148 billion a year. However, the amount that is lost to corruption according to the IMF is about US $1.5–$2 trillion a year. Low and middle-income countries are hemorrhaging resources via corruption and we turn a blind eye. But, by turning a blind eye we are allowing the massive loss of resources that could be used for public goods in the least advantaged countries in the world. We must sort this out.

### Parting Thoughts?

Get political, engage the public, translate One Health into stories. In the area of biodiversity loss, there is a real opportunity that is being missed and that is to mainstream conservation into development in a way that actually generates resources to both protect ecosystem services and improve the health of people. Lastly, since we are in the sixth extinction, there's a real opportunity to focus on the biodiversity hotspots. These are 25 identified biodiversity hotspots, about 1.4% of the earth's land surface. There is a massive urgency for us to focus on the protection of these biodiversity hotspots. We must also not forget the oceans, which are under severe threat from climate change, pollution, overfishing, and habitat destruction. As the oceans go so to do we.

---

### Case Study – $CO_2$ Emissions in Costa Rica

Co-authored by Zachary Carel and Justin Rujawitz

In recent years, the topic of climate change and global warming has become relatively controversial. Though there are skeptics who refuse to accept the current state of the environment, there is undeniable scientific evidence that supports the gradual elevation of $CO_2$ in the Earth's atmosphere. For instance, since 1998, the Earth has experienced seven of the ten hottest years in recorded history, and 2000–2009 yielded an unparalleled amount of record high and low temperatures when compared to previous decades. Along with the documented effects of climate change is the belief that human behavior is the leading cause for its existence due to their dependency on greenhouse gas emissions. Such emissions damage the environment, and the leading greenhouse gas emitted on Earth is $CO_2$. In fact, in 2013, 82% of all US greenhouse gas emissions involved $CO_2$. Unfortunately, we have no immediate action that is acceptable and that would eliminate $CO_2$ emissions. However, multiple countries have developed plans to become carbon neutral in the near future.

The first country to accept the challenge of becoming carbon neutral, and quite possible the most likely to succeed, is Costa Rica. Initially, the goal was to be neutral by 2030, but their government has stated they could potentially offset all $CO_2$ emissions by 2025. Historically speaking, Costa Rica has fallen victim to excess deforestation dating back to the 1950s; however, from 1979 to 2002 there were several incentivized reforestation plans that allowed 43% of their forests to recover. Furthermore, in recent efforts to control environmental waste, a tax is placed on tourists and businesses to offset their carbon emissions. For every ton of carbon-emitted, businesses are taxed 10 dollars and the money is used to fund further conservation and reforestation efforts. The emphasis on reforestation is key in the country's attempt to deal with excess $CO_2$ emissions due to the ability of trees to capture and store carbon emitted through human activity. According to a report in 2013, Costa Rica expects that of the 21 million tons of $CO_2$ emissions, 75% will be neutralized through carbon capture from reforestation.

Aside from reforestation, Costa Rica also has the added benefit of being in a geographically friendly location for alternative power sources. Not only is it a relatively tiny country (area = 19 730 square miles), but most of its area is bordered by water. Since Costa Rica's location provides it with a sufficient means to alternative power sources, it can combat the major cause for excess carbon emission. Where most countries rely on the use of greenhouse gases to power electricity, in 2013, 78% of Costa Rica's electricity came from hydropower and 18% came from wind and geothermal power; therefore, only 4% of their annual electricity is powered through greenhouse gas generating means. To put this in perspective, 39% of the US's electricity in 2015 was generated by burning coal.

It is undeniable that the world needs to take a more active approach to limiting greenhouse gases, even if a complete neutralization of $CO_2$ emissions is not likely to occur anytime in the near future. That said, Costa Rica has been successful in laying the groundwork that could ultimately lead to a united, globalized effort to diminish the world's reliance on carbon emissions.

## Works Cited

Allen, H.A. (2015). Governance and One Health: exploring the impact of federalism and bureaucracy on zoonotic disease detection and reporting. *Veterinary Sciences* 2: 69–83. doi: 10.3390/vetsci2020069.

Day, R.H., Shaw, D.G., and Ignell, S.E. (1988) Quantitative distribution and characteristics of neustonic plastic in the North Pacific Ocean. *Final Report to US Department of Commerce, National Marine Fisheries Service, Auke Bay Laboratory* Auke Bay, AK. pp. 247–266. http://swfsc.noaa.gov/publications/TM/SWFSC/NOAA-TM-NMFS-SWFSC-154_P247.PDF (accessed September 16, 2017).

Ebola highlights the link between human, wildlife health. http://www.stltoday.com/opinion/columnists/ebola-highlights-the-link-between-human-wildlife-health/article_aca7d3a8-7bcc-5614-aa89-5846daa5d33f.html (accessed September 16, 2017).

EPA. (2015a) Climate Change Indicators in the United States. In United States Environmental Protection Agency. http://www3.epa.gov/climatechange/science/indicators/weather-climate/index.html (accessed September 16, 2017)

EPA. (2015b) Sources of Greenhouse Gas Emissions. In *United States Environmental Protection Agency*. http://www3.epa.gov/climatechange/ghgemissions/sources/transportation.html (accessed September 16, 2017).

Ezenwa, V.O., Pieur-Richard, A.-H., Roche, B. et al. (2015). Interdisciplinarity and infectious diseases: an Ebola case study. *PLoS Pathogens* 11 (8): e1004992.

Herro, A. (2013) Costa Rica Aims to Become First "Carbon Neutral" Country. In *Worldwatch Institute Vision for a Sustainable World*. http://www.worldwatch.org/node/4958 (accessed September 16, 2017).

Horton, R., Beaglehole, R., Bonita, R. et al. (2014). From public to planetary health: a manifesto. *Lancet* 383 (9920): 847.

Index Mundi. https://www.indexmundi.com/facts/zimbabwe/life-expectancy-at-birth (accessed July 4, 2018).

Keenan, R. (2015). Costa Rica: lessons from 30 years of forest and environmental policy. *Revista Forestal Mesoamericana Kurú (Costa Rica)* 12 (28). ISSN): 2215–2504.

McKeown, R.E. (2009). The epidemiologic transition: changing patterns of mortality and population dynamics. *American Journal of Lifestyle Medicine* 19–26. doi: 10.1177/1559827609335350.

NPR In U.S., Ebola Turns From a Public Health Issue To A Political One. https://www.npr.org/2014/10/09/354890869/in-u-s-ebola-turns-from-a-public-health-issue-to-a-political-one (accessed October 15, 2017).

NPR Dallas Ebola Patient Thomas Eric Duncan Has Died. https://www.npr.org/sections/thetwo-way/2014/10/08/354577799/dallas-ebola-patient-thomas-eric-duncan-dies-hospital-says (accessed October 15, 2017).

Omran, A.R. (1971). The epidemiologic transition: a theory of the epidemiology of population change. *The Milbank Memorial Fund Quarterly* 49 (4): 509–538.

Samet, J.M. (2001). The science/policy Interface. In: *Ecosystem Change and Public Health: A Global Perspective* (ed. J.L. Aron and J.A. Patz), 100–115. Baltimore, MD: The Johns Hopkins University Press.

Sawin, J. (2013) Costa Rica and New Zealand on Path to Carbon Neutrality. In: Worldwatch Institute Vision for a Sustainable World. http://www.worldwatch.org/node/5439 (accessed October 15, 2017).

Stone Mountain Meeting. Operationalizing "One Health": A Policy Perspective – Taking Stock and Shaping an Implementation Roadmap. *Meeting Overview | May 4–6, 2010. Stone Mountain, Georgia.* https://www.cdc.gov/onehealth/pdf/atlanta/meeting-overview.pdf (accessed October 15, 2017).

Wikipedia: The Free Encyclopedia. Thomas Eric Duncan. https://en.wikipedia.org/wiki/Thomas_Eric_Duncan (accessed October 15, 2017).

World Health Organization. 2003. DAC Guidelines and Reference Series – Poverty and Health 90 pp. http://apps.who.int/iris/bitstream/10665/42690/1/9241562366.pdf (accessed October 15, 2017).

Part VI

Where Do We Go From Here?

14

# Working in a Global Environment

*"In today's world, bacteria and viruses travel as fast as money. A single microbial sea washes all of humankind. There are no health sanctuaries."*

Gro Harlem Brundtland (2001)
quoted in Brown et al. (2006)

Christmas Eve 1968 began the dawning of a new era in human history, and it began with what may be one of the most profound events in human history. It was on that day 50 years ago that an astronaut aboard the Apollo 8 flight took a picture of Earth from his spacecraft window while circling around the far side of the moon. People back on Earth first saw this picture, entitled "Earthrise" in January 1969: a photo that gave us a view of Earth through the lens of the Universe for the first time ever. This distant view, with the contrast of the stark moonscape and the blackness of space against the blue and green ball of life, showed us the Earth as both infinitely beautiful and infinitely fragile (Figure 14.1). The picture was instrumental in starting the environmental movement with the image cementing a sense of the Earth's vulnerability, which the publication of *Silent Spring* had awoken just six years earlier. This imagery helped us realize we all are living on one shared planet.

Following Earthrise, the 1970s marked a decade of greater understanding of threats to ecosystems across Earth, possibly triggered by this one photo and the holistic view from outer space. Earthrise may have been the spark that ignited many to view Earth as a living force for it was at this time that the Gaia Theory was proposed. The Gaia Theory, put forth by James Lovelock and Lynn Margulis, suggests that life on Earth was not only producing our atmosphere, unique in the Universe, to date, but also was regulating it. The theory also proposes that damage to the Earth, once done, is very difficult to undo. They described the Earth as a system of living organisms and inorganic material that are part of a dynamic system shaping the Earth's biosphere and maintaining the Earth as a fit environment for life. For many people, this theory came to mean that the Earth itself be regarded as an organism with self-regulatory functions. The theory of Earth as Gaia fits nicely with the knowledge that the maintenance of life of all organisms must have **homeostasis** for the continuation of life. We were now seeing the planet itself as self-regulating and "alive."

During this decade, great advances happened in the environmental movement with programs throughout the world directed at combating the growing environmental health concerns and the loss of biodiversity – issues that were becoming harder to ignore. In the intervening half-century, since astronaut Bill Anders took that history-changing photo, we have been witness to an ever-increasing list of global harms, many related to the mounting connections of people, animals, plants, and pathogens. At the time that Lovelock and Margulis were just starting to present their

*Introduction to One Health: An Interdisciplinary Approach to Planetary Health*, First Edition.
Sharon L. Deem, Kelly E. Lane-deGraaf and Elizabeth A. Rayhel.
© 2019 John Wiley & Sons, Inc. Published 2019 by John Wiley & Sons, Inc.
Companion website: www.wiley.com/go/deem/health

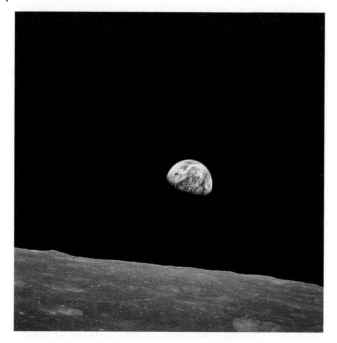

Figure 14.1 EarthRise. *Source:* Courtesy of NASA.

theory of Gaia and the fragile, living nature of the globe, we were becoming increasingly aware of the human-drivers changing the health of Earth and the animals and plants living in the global environment.

## 14.1 Think Globally, Act Locally, and the Butterfly Effect

You have probably heard the expression, *think globally, act locally*. This adage, first expressed in the early 1900s, urges people to consider the health of the entire planet while taking actions in their own communities and cities. Each of our local actions may have negative or positive impacts on planetary health. In the context of One Health, *think globally, act locally* reminds us that we should strive for local actions (and every action we make is ultimately local) that lead to positive results. At the very least, our actions should have minimal negative impacts. This statement should remind all of us to thinking about the whole planet – the globe – in all of our individual actions.

Today we might do better to think globally *and* act globally since everything we do can, and often does, have impacts on people, animals, and environments all over the world. Each of our actions are local and global in the connected world of today, and each of the One Health career paths we may choose have local and global implications. How then do our thinking and actions fit into the global environment? Do you remember the *butterfly effect?* This term, initially coined for theories of weather predictions, asserted that a butterfly flapping its wings in one part of the world might cause a hurricane in another part. Rather fitting today when we consider climate change and how actions on one side of the world, such as $CO_2$ release, has impacts on the other side. The premise is that small causes can have larger and remote effects. We may use the butterfly effect to explain events in systems other than the weather.

The ripples that flow out from local actions now have a global reach on a scale that makes the local quickly become global. The degree and variety of connections today ensure that each of us has a power extending from local to global. Examples may include how the social media revolution helped ignite the Arab Spring of 2010. Another example is the reach that the production of a new vaccine in one country, then shared across the planet, may have to stave off millions and millions of childhood deaths globally. Lastly, an all too common occurrence in the global environment is what may happen when an individual plant, animal, or person harboring a pathogen travels from one country to another. This is exactly what happened with the monkeypox virus when it arrived in Wisconsin, USA, in 2003 after having traveled inside an imported "pet" giant Gambian pouched rat (*Cricetomys gambianus*). A local action, such as placing a giant rat into a shipping container in West Africa, turned into a global health issue when the rat, along with the monkeypox virus it carried, arrived in the American Midwest.

Today we may more appropriately call the butterfly effect, the airplane effect. One airplane may carry a person harboring the Ebola virus out of an African nation and into other countries as happened in 2014 when it arrived in the USA and Spain. Alternatively, a plane with an illegal cargo of bushmeat that harbors a zoonotic pathogen may have its cargo offloaded in a country thousands of miles from its origin. It is estimated that at any one time there are one to two million people onboard an airplane and moving from point A to point B in this global environment. This does not include all the legal (and illegal) pets and agricultural products these millions of people may be carrying or the number of airplanes carrying only cargo. In this connected and global environment, we are moving people, animals, plants, and products by every mode of transportation that humans have devised whether in the air, land, or water. These travel connections have turned the local into the global. The true extent to which people and products crisscross the globe is hard to quantify, although the estimated global economy of US $74 trillion annually suggests it is enormous.

As covered in more detail in Chapter 2, we live in a connected world, and to be effective One Health practitioners, we must be prepared to work within the global environment. Just as the modern economy of the twenty-first century is now globalized from an increased level of social, political, and economic interdependence with growing movements of people, produce, and other commodities across national borders, health has also become globalized. In the post-Millennium Development Goals era, there is increasing recognition that health and sustainable development are inseparable in an increasingly globalized and interconnected world. The complex interplay between humans, animals, and environments; the dual burden of infectious and non-infectious diseases in all living things; emerging economies; and the expanded mobility of people are all having profound political, social, economic, and health consequences. These consequences demand of us to have a new concept of "global health." Global health must acknowledge that we are an interdependent global population, which requires that we determine which and whose health problems we tackle, and how we govern our collective efforts to protect and promote One Health – the health of humans, other animals, and environments. The One Health approach must be holistic, both across living species and across the planet, in today's global environment.

## 14.2 How a Global Environment Fits in One Health

We are each a global citizen, and we live in an increasingly global environment. People often refer to "global" as a concept of "over there," like when global health care professionals say they are off to country X to provide health care. However, as shown by the photo Earthrise, "global" is all of Earth, and it is just as global where these words are typed as where someone reads them. Our world is more connected than ever as humans, animals, plants, and products move from one country to the next, allowing disease causing agents – infectious and non-infectious – to have no borders. Whether it is a virus moving from one country to another, carried inside a Gambian rat traveling at 600 miles per hour in an airplane, or the BP Deepwater Horizon oil spill of 2010 leading to oil carried across the globe by ocean currents and within marine creatures, disease issues are global. Diseases are part of the global environment. Food-borne diseases may provide the best means to appreciate how a One Health approach fits into this global environment.

Many of the human emerging infectious diseases of the twenty-first century are associated with food supplies as we strive to feed a human population of 7.6 billion. We have moved from a time in which the majority of foods were produced locally and sold in local markets to a system in which foods are transported great distances and are often marketed through large chain supermarkets. This change in commerce also changes the pathogens to which humans are exposed through foods. For example, in a 24-hour period some estimates are that the food consumed by the average American originates in 20–30 different countries. This global food chain allows for animal and plant pathogens, and the chemicals and antibiotics used to produce them, to move rapidly around the world. For those zoonotic pathogens that humans acquire from food, but then have the ability to be transmitted from person to person (e.g. avian influenza [AI] virus), the entire globe has become a pathogen's potential playing field.

An example of this One Health connectivity at the dinner table is the Severe Acute Respiratory Syndrome (SARS) epidemic that occurred in the early 2000s. This public health crisis began in a city in southern China and quickly escalated from a local health issue to a health event with global economic, infrastructure, and health impacts. SARS was the first, of what has since been many, epidemic to occur so far in the twenty-first century.

SARS is caused by a coronavirus that, prior to the SARS epidemic, had never before been identified. This virus causes a severe respiratory disease with a **case fatality rate** of 9.6% in infected humans. The SARS global epidemic, which took place from November 2002 through July 2003, resulted in 8098 cases with 774 deaths in 37 countries ranging all the way to Canada, although the majority of cases were in China. As quickly as it started, it ended. No further human SARS case has been reported since 2003.

The contagious nature of this newly emerged coronavirus, which spread through respiratory droplets and fomites as well as through the fecal–oral route makes human-to-human transmission easy. However, the epidemic began with a zoonotic event from an animal reservoir in the **wet markets** of China. Wet markets are places of trade where all manner of wild and domestic animals are sold, living and dead, as food for humans (Figure 14.2). Although bats are the most likely natural reservoir for the SARS virus, the masked palm civet (*Paguma larvata*), which does not show clinical signs when infected, may have been the primary link of virus transmission to humans. These civets are sold commonly as a food source in the wet markets of Asia. Removed from the wild and held under unhygienic and stressful conditions, the civet was a perfect vehicle for the coronavirus to move out of the forest (e.g. bat reservoir) and into the global human population.

The economic cost to the global economy, associated with this one epidemic event, caused by one pathogen, that affected 37 countries but lasted for only nine months, was estimated at US $40–54 billion. In addition to the high economic costs and the loss of human lives associated with the epidemic, more than 10 000 masked palm civets were killed in Guangdong Province, China. Animal culling such as this is an all too common, but mostly ineffective, means for controlling a zoonotic pathogen. This one global human epidemic was a great reminder of how

(a)

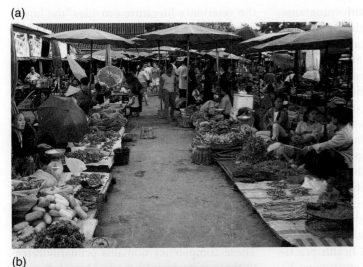

(b)

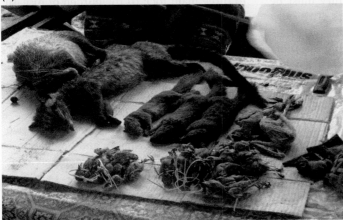

Figure 14.2 (a) A wet market in Laos showing all types of food being sold, including (b) wild animals such as the masked palm civet, bats, rodents and other species. *Source:* Photo credit Dr. Lucy Keatts/WCS.

interconnected we are and how all facets of life today – cultural, economic, societal, and physical – are functioning within a global environment.

## 14.3 Education and Skills Needed to Work and Thrive in a Global World

The One Health paradigm shift asks that we not focus our health care efforts on just humans, animals, or environments. Rather our efforts should be performed within the

framework of the One Health Triad, since we know that the health of each is related to the health of the others. Similarly, we must move away from global health being defined in the constraints of various professional groupings such as human or veterinary medicine, nursing, oral health, pharmacy, allied health, and other medical subspecialties, so that we may re-envision global health as simply One Health.

It is surprising of how often medical doctors that work in global health departments, after a lecture on One Health, say that they have not once thought of animal health in their global human health programs. Sometimes they often add they may have considered the environmental impacts on human health, both positive and negative, a little more often than animals, but even that link is often lacking in their day-to-day approaches to global health. It is hard to understand this lack of inclusion when we consider the connection that human patients have with animals. Many people eat animals (e.g. food animals), live with them (e.g. companion and working animals), or simply enjoy the ecosystem services that animals provide in their environments (e.g. free-living animals from bees to elephants). For true global health, the global health practitioners of the twenty-first century must be global One Health practitioners. To bridge health care across the One Health Triad, there are skills including communication, policy development, and technical abilities that are necessary to ensure a more holistic approach to global health.

As we covered in Chapters 8 and 9, there are core competencies and educational training that help advance all One Health practitioners. These One Health skillsets are necessary to obtain, whether you are a clinician in an inner city emergency room, a city planner working to develop a sustainable cityscape, a veterinarian responsible for animal welfare and food safety at a large commercial piggery, a social worker providing counseling for refugees, or the CEO of the Food and Agricultural Organization (FAO). However, some competencies may be more important for One Health practitioners to be successful in the global environment. Fortunately, in recent years, training in these core global health competencies is more accessible through a growing number of Global Health Departments in Medical and Veterinary Colleges and Schools of Public Health.

A number of global health professionals have provided competencies they consider most pertinent for the global health practitioner, with similarities presented across disciplines. For example, a 2006 publication in the veterinary literature provides "the how" of practicing veterinary medicine in a globalized world, and within it the authors provide 12 core domains that veterinarians should have proficiency in to succeed in global health (Table 14.1). Many of these competencies include the technical side of veterinary medicine, but they also include the social side of health care with the need for cultural and communication competencies high on the list. A second example from a 2017 publication directed at global human health workers lists 11 core competency domains that the authors gathered from 13 articles published on medical global health. These competency domains primarily refer to three main foci: (i) the burden of disease and the determinants of health; (ii) the core public health skills including policy development, analysis, and program management; and (iii) the "soft skills" that include collaboration, partnering, communication, professionalism, capacity building, and political awareness (Table 14.1).

The domains provided by these two examples – veterinary and medical – emphasize many of the same competencies that fit within the "soft skills" of global health care with a strong emphasis on communication and collaboration across transdisciplinary teams. However, there is a large difference in the recognition of human and animal involvement between the different groups of global health care providers. In the domains listed for global health veterinarians, the authors provide domains that include human dimensions such as the need to understand human cultural norms, the globalized food supply, world agricultural systems and trade, international organizations, and zoonotic pathogens. Whereas, of the 13 papers synthesized in the collated competencies for global human health care providers, there is no mention of the need to understand animal trade, agriculture, or health issues, even though the animals we eat may be one of the closest One Health links, binding humans and other animals.

**Table 14.1** Competencies for veterinary, public health, social/engineers and other discipline global One Health practitioners.

| Veterinary[a] | Public Health[b] | Social / Engineers (or other disciplines)[b] |
|---|---|---|
| Intercultural communication abilities | Communication skills (verbal and written) | Global burden of disease |
| Knowledge of disease surveillance technologies, including diagnostic tests | Strong Work Ethic | Globalization of health and health care |
| Familiarity with transboundary diseases | Teamwork skills | Social, economic and environmental determinants of health |
| Familiarity with infectious zoonotic diseases and bio-threat agents of concern | Initiative | Capacity strengthening |
| Knowledge of effective prevention and control strategies for animal and human health priority diseases | Interpersonal skills | Ethic and professionalism |
| Understanding of world agricultural systems | Problem solving skills | Communication, collaboration and partnering |
| Understanding world trade and international health regulations | Analytical skills | Health, equity and social justice |
| Educated perspectives on trade and policy | Flexibility / adaptability | Program management |
| Awareness of international organizations | Computer skills | Sociocultural and political awareness |
| Comprehension of globalization of the food supply | Technical skills | Strategic analysis |
| Working as part of multidisciplinary teams Interpersonal skills and flexibility | | Research competency |

[a] Data from Brown et al. (2006).
[b] Data from Sawleshwarkar and Negin (2017).

Of the 13 papers reviewed, a few mention the need for global health practitioners (i) to understand environmental factors and (ii) to appreciate natural diversity. Both issues speak to an understanding that human drivers on the environment, such as climate change and pollutants, play a role in human health. However, we must strive to better bridge all global health practitioners to be global One Health practitioners if we are to tackle the current health challenges.

One limitation that hinders a connection between the skills and competencies of the human, animal, and environmental health care providers is that many of these global health departments are themselves targeted to care for humans or animals. Just as schools of agricultural and environmental sciences may not consider health concerns beyond their fields either. As we move forward with planetary health, we may find it would be of great value to have schools of Global One Health that provide core competencies across the One Health Triad. Also with departments of One Health becoming more common at universities, this bridging may become easier to fulfill. Masters of Public Health programs may be one area where we see an increasing number of One Health courses that provide students a window into how global health care may happen across the One Health Triad.

## 14.4 How To Be a One Health Practitioner in a Global Environment

It is now clear that to be an effective global health practitioner, one must be a global One Health practitioner. Practitioners should still have an area of expertise, such as an economist, sociologist, forester, or dentist, but we must also have the mindset of One Health. Not only do we need to be inclusive of the health connections that link humans, non-human animals, and environments together, but we must also be cognizant of the connections that link all life on Earth and across the globe, for example travel and trade. It has been stated that global health overlaps with many other health disciplines, and there have been calls to explore similarities and differences between global health, international health, and public health. However, in discussions of the similarities among varied health fields, global almost exclusively implies worldwide or transcending national boundaries. To be most effective, it must also include all the categories of life and the need for a transdisciplinary perspective on health care that not only acknowledges our cohabitants on the planet that may make us sick, but also understands the importance of their health for ours.

There are, however, jobs within One Health that may provide a larger platform to ensure a more global outreach with direct influences working across national borders. These jobs might be in a clinical position with organizations such as Doctors Without Borders, Veterinarians Without Borders, or Dentists Without Borders. Many of the larger international aid groups, such as United States Agency for International Development (USAID) in the USA or the Department for International Development (DFID) in the UK, also provide opportunities in One Health with posts throughout the world. In the USA, the Peace Corps is a great chance for a One Health practitioner to, as

their motto says, "Make the most of your world," but also to provide health care in all its forms to people, animals, and environments across the globe. Additionally, many university professors lead One Health projects and programs. These professors may primarily focus on such areas as wildlife conservation, public health, or wildland restoration, but their work is often global or may provide templates on which local studies are then applicable to other regions. Now a growing number of these programs are presented as holistic One Health programs with positions in disciplines that span the One Health Triad (e.g. Health for Animals and Livelihood Improvement [HALI] and Animal & Health for the Environment and Development [AHEAD]). Additionally, a growing number of zoos (e.g. Wildlife Conservation Society, Saint Louis Zoo), aquariums, and conservation non-governmental organizations (e.g. EcoHealth, Conservation International, World Wide Fund for Nature (WWF)) have One Health practitioners working throughout the world.

As stated earlier, the interconnected, global environment today means that even the One Health practitioner working in a local capacity, such as a veterinarian at a small-town hospital, is part of the global One Health team. Every patient that enters a veterinary clinic may have a history that places the small-town practitioner on the frontline of global health. A dog rescued in Turkey, imported to the USA, and now sitting in an examination room in Alabama, could be infected with *Leishmania* spp. – the causative agent of Leismaniasis, a sometimes fatal zoonotic parasitic disease not present in the USA, or any other number of exotic pathogens. The veterinarian's diagnostic and therapeutic skills will quickly come into play not only for the immediate care of the patient but also to minimize impacts to human health. As introduced in Chapter 13, health care providers in 2014 at the Texas hospital were at the frontline of global health as their patient, recently returned from Liberia, was the first person in the USA with the Ebola virus.

The same may be true for professionals working for ecosystem conservation and/or agricultural production. Working for an agricultural organization or the National Park Service may place you on the frontline of global One Health, especially if one considers the costs of invasive insects and pathogens to the USA. The USA spends an estimated US $40 billion per year from the loss of crops and forest production associated with the introduction of invasive pathogens and parasites.

To ensure a global reach, regardless of where you work, it is important for One Health practitioners to identify a theme that ignites their passion and that is relevant throughout the world. There are many themes with global importance and that fit into a One Health approach. These themes may include poverty reduction and birth control, both significant health issues for humans everywhere. These themes are also important across the One Health Triad with the 7.6 billion humans, and the footprint we have across the planet, being the single largest driver of health impacts to environmental, animal, and ultimately human health. One may choose to work to conserve a highly endangered species, plant, or animal, so that the species may continue to provide its role in the ecosystem. Examples are the conservation of elephants, which are needed within ecosystems to provide their ecosystem engineer functions or the preservation of red mangroves to ensure coastal wetlands, and their roles as buffer zones from tropical storms and surges, are not destroyed for shrimp farming or other human enterprises. A One Health practitioner might work to better understand endocrine disruptor chemicals (EDCs), such as bisphenol-A (BPA) found in plastics, and their impacts on species. In fact, data collected by individual scientists on the negative impacts of BPA to non-human and human health were instrumental for the 2012 Food and Drug Administration ban of BPA use in baby bottles and sippy cups. By taking initiative and being an expert in a thematic health issue, a person becomes a One Health practitioner of value from Arkansas to Zambia.

## 14.5 International Programs, Policies, and Laws for One Health in the Global Environment

There are many international programs, policies, and laws in place to help lessen disease impacts on human and non-human animal populations and environments (Chapter 13). One example is the international whaling laws that have helped to minimize whale exploitation. These laws, when enforced, are good for whales but also for ocean environments since whales provide ecosystem services important to ocean health. Beyond whales, we now understand that there are limits to ocean resources, although enacting ways to protect this public good is hard, even as oceans make up about 70% of the Earth's surface. This too demands policies and laws to help with current One Health crisis, such as overfishing (See Chapter Case Study).

Many of the policies today focus on alleviating public health issues associated with the rise in EIDs, such as SARS, AI, or Ebola. For example, countries have put policies in place and/or made laws that limit the movement of animals and animal products during epidemics and in some, the use of temperature testing of people arriving at airports has been implemented. Although not always effectively enforced, these laws and policies provide international agreements to help avert public health pandemics. Unfortunately, as evident in 2017, international accords, such as the Paris Climate Accord, are at risk when governments, such as the USA, decide to pull out of global agreements.

An excellent example of a modern day health challenge necessitating international programs, policies, and laws are the AI pandemics of the late 1900s and early 2000s. These pandemics, starting with the first AI positive goose detected in 1996 in China to the swine flu scare that began in Mexico in

2009, are a reminder of global connections across the One Health Triad. Environmental changes coupled with the movement of animals and international travel and trade, led to a public health crisis on a global scale. Long before the current AI worries, influenzas have been on the health radar for over a century.

As early as 1918, J.S. Koen was able to determine that a flu virus in pigs was similar to the virus responsible for the Spanish flu pandemic in the global human population of that time. This discovery confirmed the zoonotic link of influenzas, although the high contagious nature and spread from human to human was of more concern. In fact, the Spanish flu pandemic of 1918–1919 lead to the death of an estimated 50–100 million people, or 3–6%, of the global population at the time and is one of the most important human epidemics of modern history. Influenza viruses have two core proteins: the hemagglutinin (H) and neuraminidase (N). In flu, the 9 H proteins and 16 N proteins can re-assort and recombine which leads to changes in the **pathogenicity** of the virus, one of the key concerns for AI. Some of these H and N combinations result in a virus of low pathogenicity while others are highly pathogenic and transmissible.

The epidemiology of AI includes low pathogenic avian influenza (LPAI) viruses that are commonly harbored in clinically healthy free-living and migratory species of water birds. This is where the global environment and the One Health of AI becomes evident and why there has been an increase in AI events in human populations in recent decades. Wetland destruction for poultry production plants has occurred across the globe and in many cases along **flyways** of water birds (Figure 14.3). With the replacement of these wetlands along these wild bird migratory routes with poultry plants, we have ensured the mixing of free-living and domestic birds, which allows the mixing of any pathogens they may carry. The natural LPAI viruses in the free-living birds may spill over into the domestic birds and with the ability of influenzas to re-assort and mutate, there is soon a highly pathogenic avian influenza

(HPAI) that is quickly carried across the globe in poultry products that may go from one country to the next within hours. With poultry as a top protein source for humans today, it is easy to see how widely distributed these potentially infected birds might travel and be traded in the global environment.

HPAI have largely not been able to transmit person to person at a high enough rate (i.e. $R_0 > 1$), and that to date has helped with the influenza epidemics of recent decades from becoming pandemic nightmares. Even so, the cost to wildlife, food security, and food production have been enormous. Some of the preventive and treatment methods utilized during the various AI events have included the culling of thousands of free-living birds and millions of poultry. AI may be a poster child of infectious diseases for One Health in a Global Environment. One Health practitioners have global impacts whether they are a chicken farmer in Thailand, the CEO of an international poultry production plant making decisions on where to place future operations, or a research scientist trying to keep up with vaccines through an understanding of the virus' ecology.

## 14.6 Conclusion

In the twenty-first century, it has become evident that the world is indeed connected, and that we live in a global environment with linkages making the health of one important for the health of all. Social media, and the internet in general, is one clear example of this connectivity. We reach far and fast through social media outlets when our words and actions spread across the globe. With the estimated 2.4 billion people using social media, we must take the power of the internet seriously in this global world and for us as global One Health practitioners. Social media has been responsible for relevant changes in both personal and community health, especially by making it easier for large numbers of people to rapidly share information, as discussed in Chapter 10. However, this rapid and far reach can be good or bad.

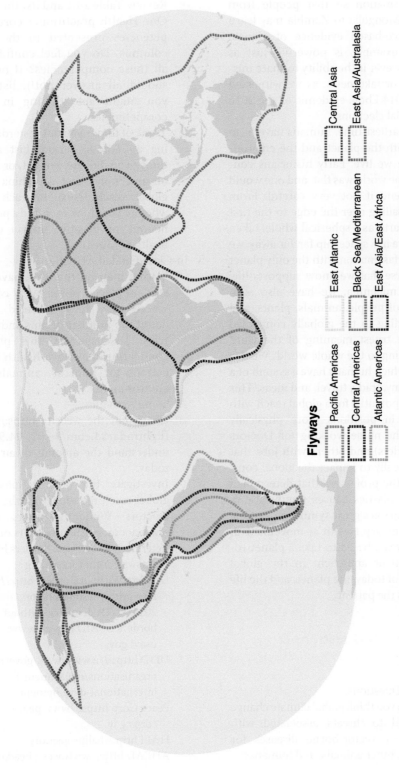

**Flyways**

Pacific Americas

Central Americas

Atlantic Americas

East Atlantic

Black Sea/Mediterranean

East Asia/East Africa

Central Asia

East Asia/Australasia

Figure 14.3   Avian influenza map of water bird flyways. *Source*: Map of major bird migratory flyways © BirdLife International.

Sharing information so that people from Australia to Mongolia to Zambia may learn of the science-based evidence of climate change, for example, is powerful. Just as powerful, however is the ability to share misinformation, or fake news, as we witnessed during the 2014 Ebola epidemic or the 2016 US presidential elections.

From the earliest time, humans have been fascinated with the planet and the environments where we live. Early historians contended that the world was flat, and one would sail off the end if not very careful. From thoughts of sailing over the edge to the first view of the Earth as a spherical whole, taken from a camera in a spaceship far, far away, we continue our fascination with the only planet in the Universe that we know supports life. Throughout millennia, we have also seen connections of people, animals, plants, and products leading to the globally connected world in the truest meaning of the word global – relating to the whole world. We live in a time in which humans have a system of a global economy, trade, travel, and ideas. This allows us the potential for a global reach with some of us in positions more physically global (e.g. the nurse working for Doctors Without Borders) and others with jobs that extend out locally to impact the global community (e.g. the professors that determined how BPA in plastics causes feminization). The Gaia theory is a great symbol of the One Health – Planetary Health – movement in that we are well advised to take a planet-to-individual-patient approach. In the global environment of today, the planet, and the life it supports, is the patient.

## End of Chapter Questions & Activities:

A. Thought Questions:
  i) How do you think global climate change will add to threats associated with water- or vector-borne diseases for wildlife, other animals, and humans?

  ii) Review Table 14.1 and list the global One Health practitioner core competencies presented in the three columns. Do you feel confident in all these competencies? If not (we should all answer not!), list ways you might get training in these competencies.

  iii) Think of things you did yesterday during a 24-hour period. List all the things you did, ate, bought, or shared on an iPhone, that you think had a global reach. Next to each mark whether you think each had a positive, neutral, or negative impact on the health of others.

B. In-Class/Guided Activities:
  i) With a map on the wall, have each student place a pin in every country where they have traveled. Then count the number of pins and countries. Discuss how this physical connection may have health implications for humans, animals, and environments.

C. At-home Activities:
  i) Check out the website https://www.flightradar24.com/34.92,-24.9/3 to understand the amount of air travel today.

  ii) Investigate the organizations with global reach mentioned in the text – Doctors Without Borders http://www.doctorswithoutborders.org Veterinarians Without Borders http://vetswithoutbordersus.org Dentists Without Borders http://forworldwidesmilesinc.org/2014/02/19/dentistry-without-borders USAID https://www.usaid.gov DFID https://www.gov.uk/government/organisations/department-for-international-development Peace Corp https://www.peacecorps.gov HALI http://haliproject.org AHEAD http://www.wcs-ahead.org

iii) Check out this website and note the change in food sources since 1961 and by country https://www.national geographic.com/what-the-world-eats

D. Long-term Action Steps

    i) During the coming semester consider all the ways that your words and actions have a reach at the local, national, and global levels. Then consider these through a One Health lens.

    ii) During your career, whatever that shall be, be a One Health practitioner and remember the local is global.

## Interview

*Interview with Gary Vroegindewey, DVM, MSS, Director of One Health at Lincoln Memorial University's College of Veterinary Medicine.*

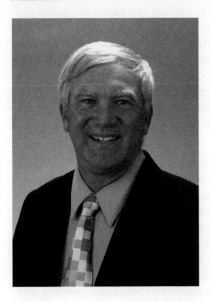

### Tell Us a Little About Yourself

I am a veterinarian who started in private practice. I was also in the United States Army Reserve during that time. I then went on to active duty with the Army Veterinary Corps. I became the Assistant Chief for the US Army Veterinary Corps

E. Recommended Reading:

Barry, J.M. (2004). *The Great Influenza: The Story of the Deadliest Pandemic in History*. Penguin Books.

Friedman, T.L. (2005). *The World is Flat: A Brief History of the Globalized World in the Twenty-first Century*. Farrar, Straus, and Giroux.

Lovelock, J. (2009). *The Vanishing Face of Gaia: A Final Warning*. Basic Books.

Sherman, D.M. (2002). *Tending Animals in the Global Village*. Wiley-Blackwell.

Wilson, E.O. (2016). *Half-Earth: Our Planet's Fight for Life*. Liveright.

and then the Director of the Department of Defense Veterinary Services. In that job, I had policy and oversight responsibility for everything that the Army did in the veterinary medical arena, including food safety, zoonotic disease control, care for government-owned animals, and army research and development.

### How is One Health important to your work?

I integrate One Health into the entire scope of my work at Lincoln Memorial University. I teach five courses in One Health, from the individual to population and global scales. This includes a course on the environment, which is unique in United States veterinary colleges. Prior to this position, my work with the military was based on One Health because as we sat on the Surgeon General staff, we came from all aspects of health; environmental health, public health, nursing, doctors, dentists, veterinarians and sat at the same table discussing issues. Before One Health had a name put on it, we were practicing it.

### How do your actions reflect One Health, personally or professionally?

The first time it came high on the radar screen was in the AI pandemic of the

1990s. It was very clear to all the people involved that we needed a One Health framework to understand this complex issue. Just by definition, it was AI, so birds were involved. We had wild bird populations, domestic bird populations, and the environment involved in terms of where the domestic birds and wildlife were, cultural aspects involved, and certainly human health. For me this was the first time we saw the convergence of multiple disciplines working together and solving a singular problem. The AI pandemic was also a watershed event in terms of One Health, as we got groups from academia, nonprofits, governments, and across governmental lines working together.

### Where is One Health headed?

We must remember that One Health all occurs within a sociosphere, beyond the ecosphere. It occurs within a cultural, political, economic, legal, religious context. We must understand these things if we are to be successful within the One Health arena. Moving forward One Health must include the sociosphere.

### What can an individual do to make a difference for planetary health?

Individuals must tell One Health stories to our audiences, however large or small. We must share stories on the interconnections of the health of environments, animals, and humans. By telling stories, individuals will spread the value of One Health. One individual can, and does, make an impact since One Health involves multiple individuals.

### How can we encourage people to care about planetary health?

We all have an aspect that we find important, whether it is infectious diseases, the environment, saving wildlife, biodiversity, antibiotic resistance, having food for the future. All of these elements effect all people, and if we find the touchpoint that is important to a person, that becomes the entry point for us to help deliver the One Health message.

### You touched on this cultural aspect previously, but how do you recommend that One Health practitioners advance this initiative across the globe?

I have been in situations on multidisciplinary teams that included doctors, dentists, veterinarians, and public health nurses going into areas in Africa where people would not have their children vaccinated unless we would vaccinate their animals first. Animals were critical in terms of sustaining that family and their community. There is an African proverb, "When the herds are gone, the end for human beings is not far." This is One Health. Not just the type of food they have, but their whole existence realized to be interdependent. This is a way we can approach global One Health through the combination of animal and human health.

### Parting Thoughts?

While we are looking at One Health, try to look at it outside the typical lens or box that you work with every day, and try to put yourself in the shoes of another One Health practitioner to see how they would approach the work. Then finally, One Health is not a fixed concept. One Health has been constantly evolving and as we evolve, we need to be adaptable to new challenges and opportunities in dealing with local, national, and global issues.

## Case Study: Overfishing

Coauthored by Pascaline Akitani

It has been stated "oceans are like a checking account where everybody withdraws, but nobody makes a deposit." This sums up well the state of the oceans and overharvesting of fish. Many people see fish as a limitless and renewable resource that, no matter how much we harvest, they will never be depleted. Sadly, many times over this has been proven untrue. The oceans, and animals of the oceans, have limits like all other resources. The overexploitation of fish throughout the world is real, and the severely depleted fish stocks with species extirpations, near extinctions, and extinctions, as its evidence.

About 80% of the world marine fish stocks, for which assessment information is available, are fully exploited to overexploited. Fish stocks assessed since 1977 have experienced an 11% decline in total biomass globally, with considerable regional variation. The average maximum size of fish caught declined by 22% since 1959 globally for all assessed communities. There is also an increasing trend of stock collapses over time, with 14% of assessed stocks collapsed in 2007. In 2006, more than 110 million tons (77%) of the world fish production was used directly for human consumption, which was approximately 4% of the protein source consumed by people. About 33 million tons (23%) was used for non-food products, in particular the manufacturing of fishmeal and nutritional supplements like omega3 and fish oil.

Oceans provide an enormous resource of protein for humans and are a major contributor to the world economy particularly, in developing countries. Although fishing began early in human history, it was not until the twentieth century that the impact we have on the oceans became dire, largely due to modern technologies. Marine resources are now under intense and non-sustainable pressure with negative impacts on the environment and biodiversity of the oceans. The use of advanced technologies in the fishing industry and the deployment of huge vessels and equipment is a major cause of overfishing. In addition, many fishing industries use unsustainable fishing techniques, such as long-line nets that catch excessive numbers of fish; but, more importantly they take **bycatch** that includes cetaceans, sea turtles, sharks, seabirds, and invertebrates. All are thrown back into the ocean either dead or soon to die due to the trauma of capture.

Scientists say the stocks of fish in the ocean will run out by the year 2048 if we continue with business as usual. This would be an economic, human health, and ecological crisis on many levels. In the short term, people reliant on fishing will lose their livelihoods. The loss of fish protein as a food source would create nutritional losses for populations throughout the world. Ecologically, pressure on terrestrial wildlife may escalate as shown previously in West Africa that when local fish stocks plummet, the terrestrial wildlife sustained increased harvesting pressures. As the great marine biologist Sylvia Earle tells us, "No water, no Life. No Blue, no Green."

## Works Cited

Bhandari, R.K., Deem, S.L., Holliday, D.K. et al. (2015). Effects of the environmental estrogenic contaminants Bisphenol A and 17 Ethinyl Estradiol on sexual development and adult behaviors in aquatic wildlife species. *General and Comparative Endocrinology* 214: 195–219.

Brashares, J.S., Arcese, P., Sam, M.K. et al. (2004). Bushmeat hunting, wildlife declines, and fish supply in West Africa. *Science* 306 (5699): 1180–1183.

Brown, C., Thompson, S., Vroegindewey, G. et al. (2006). The global veterinarian: the why? The what? The how? *Journal of*

*Veterinary Medical Education* 33 (3):
411–415.

Brundtland, G.H. (2001). Addressing the challenges of unequal distribution. *Plenary seminar, World Economic Forum* 29 January 2001.

Cook, D.C., Fraser, R.W., Paini, D.R. et al. (2011). Biosecurity and yield improvement technologies are strategic complements in the fight against food insecurity. *PLoS One* 6 (10): e26084.

Deem, S.L. (2015). Conservation medicine to One Health: the role of zoologic veterinarians. In: *Fowler's Zoo and Wild Animal Medicine: Volume 8* (ed. R.E. Miller and M.E. Fowler), 698–703. Saint Louis, MO: Saunders Elsevier.

D'Odorico, P., Carr, J.A., Laio, F. et al. (2014). Feeding humanity through global food trade. *Earth's Future* 2: 458–469. doi: 10.10022014EF000250.

Knobler, S., Mahmoud, A., Lemon, S., et al. (eds.) (2004). Forum on Microbial Threats. Learning from SARS: Preparing for the Next Disease Outbreak – Workshop Summary. ISBN 0–309–59433-2. 376 Pp. http://www.nap.edu/catalog/10915.html (accessed July 5, 2018).

Lovelock, J.E. and Margulis, L. (1974). Atmospheric homeostasis by and for the biosphere: the Gaia hypothesis. *Tellus. Series A: Dynamic Meteorology and Oceanography* 26 (1–2): 2–10.

Mbug, E.V., Kayunze, K.A., Katale, B.Z. et al. (2012). One Health' infectious diseases surveillance in Tanzania: are we all on board the same flight? *The Onderstepoort Journal of Veterinary Research* 79 (2): 500. doi: 10.4102/ojvr.v79i2.500.

Paini, D.R., Sheppard, A.W., De Barro, P.J. et al. (2016). Global threat to agriculture from invasive species. *Proceedings of the National Academy of Sciences of the United States of America* 113 (27): 7575–7579. doi: 10.1073/pnas.1602205113.

Pauly, D., Alder, J., Bennett, E. et al. (2003). The future for fisheries. *Science* 302: 1359–1361.

Pimentel, D., Zuniga, R., and Morrison, D. (2005). Update on the environmental and economic costs associated with alien-invasive species in the United States. *Ecological Economics* 52 (3): 273–288.

Porkka, M., Kummu, M., Siebert, S. et al. (2013). From food insufficiency towards trade dependency: a historical analysis of global food availability. *PLoS One* 8 (12): e82714. doi: 10.1371/journal.pone.0082714.

Rapport, D.J. (2004) Avian Influenza and the Environment: An Ecohealth Perspective. *A Report Submitted to UNEP.* https://www.k4health.org/sites/default/files/AvianFluEcoHealth.pdf (accessed July 5, 2018).

Sawleshwarkar, S. and Negin, J. (2017). A review of global health competencies for postgraduate public health education. *Frontiers in Public Health* 5: 46. doi: 10.3389/fpubh.2017.00046.

Vitousek, P.M., Mooney, H.A., Lubchenco, J. et al. (1997). Human domination of earth's ecosystems. *Science* 277: 494–499.

Worm, B., Barbier, E.B., Beaumont, N. et al. (2006). Impacts of biodiversity loss on ocean ecosystem services. *Science* 314 (5800): 787–790.

# 15

# The Past and Future of One Health

Imagine, if you will, the following scenario:

A small band of nomadic peoples roam a desert devoid of resources – previously verdant oases have dried completely, small patches of trees and other plants are dead and dying, and once abundant wildlife is scarce. Across the globe, formerly lush forests have been devastated – cut for timber, burned such that all that remains is charcoal, and left utterly devoid of life. Coral reefs have died and the oceans' waters are filled with massive, floating "islands" of waste, littered with degrading plastics that choke and kill ocean life from the tiniest krill to the massive blue whale. Animal life, bereft of habitats and food resources, is careening towards mass extinction, and those populations that remain are suffering the consequences of destroyed habitats, human overconsumption of resources, and decimation at the hands of pollution of the land, air, and water. Large-scale die-offs of amphibians, birds, fish, and aquatic mammals have occurred globally. Inland and coastal waters have been blackened with oil, spilled from enormous vessels or deep sea wells. Earthquakes have increased in both frequency and devastation, as a result of fracking, occurring in locations previously undisturbed by quakes. Droughts, floods, and hurricanes have become more frequent, more intense, and more devastating. The planet has become, in many respects, a wasteland.

While this might seem like an Orwellian future as described in a dystopian novel or film, the reality of the above scenario is playing out *today* all across our planet. We are potentially not long removed from a future that includes even more global environmental devastation, which includes the collapse of local and global economies and the rise of global violence and civil strife. In some nations, even these scenarios have become a reality with decades-long civil wars and rebellions and currency already so devalued that, much like in the dystopian film Mad Max, a barter system is used almost exclusively. Fresh water is rapidly becoming our most precious resource.

The collapse of civilization as we know it is hard to comprehend. Our technological advances have provided us the ability to feed billions of people with ease, explore the furthest reaches of our solar system, and communicate with individuals across the globe on devices we carry in our back pockets. Our civilization feels immutable. It is not. Consider ancient Rome, ancient Greece, or ancient Egypt. Recall early Mesopotamia, the early dynasties of China, and the Inca, Aztec, and Mayan civilizations. Going back even further into less well known early civilizations, remember Clovis people, the Mound Builders of the Mississippian cultures, the Silla, the Indus, the Nok, the Etruscans. The list of now-extinct cultures and civilizations is astounding. Certainly, during the time that Rome was falling as a globally dominant civilization, no Roman citizen predicted its fall.

*Introduction to One Health: An Interdisciplinary Approach to Planetary Health*, First Edition.
Sharon L. Deem, Kelly E. Lane-deGraaf and Elizabeth A. Rayhel.
© 2019 John Wiley & Sons, Inc. Published 2019 by John Wiley & Sons, Inc.
Companion website: www.wiley.com/go/deem/health

## 15.1  The Lesson of Easter Island

Easter Island is famous for being a very small, remote island in the Pacific where early Polynesians – the Rapa Nui – carved nearly 1000 massive stone *moai* before a drastic population crash all but eliminated the islanders (Figure 15.1). The story of the Rapa Nui is a complex one that is still unfolding as new evidence emerges. For a long time, the demise of the Easter Island Rapa Nui people and culture centered around evidence of a self-induced **ecocide**. Sometime around 800 CE, a small group of Polynesians arrived on the shore of the forest-covered island. In time, the islanders cut trees, implemented unsustainable farming practices, and expanded in population size. In subsequent years, the Rapa Nui population grew to its peak of 15 000 and resources from the forest began to fail. With no available trees for use as canoes, building materials, and fire, civil strife and starvation resulted in disaster for the Rapa Nui. In 1722, when Dutch explorers landed on Easter Island, the island was completely devoid of trees, and the population had dropped to between 2000 and 3000. *Moai*,

originally carved as a symbol of tribal strength, were frequently abandoned or toppled in the years just before the end – victims, too, of the warring tribes.

Recent evidence, however, has drastically changed how we understand the fate of the Rapa Nui. This evidence suggests that islanders arrived around 1200 CE, or 400 years later than originally proposed, and brought with them as stowaways the Polynesian rat (*Rattus exulans*). Rats reproduced quickly and spread rapidly, as they have on many other islands when introduced to a predator free environment. In addition to the ecological damage brought about by the islanders themselves, we now understand that rats contributed significantly to the decline of the trees of the island, expediting the process of island-wide deforestation. Once the environmental devastation was complete, the population of Rapa Nui declined to a small size of between 2000 and 3000, limited by the need to subsist in an environment with drastically depleted resources. This small population size, subsisting on extremely limited resources, ultimately made the Rapa Nui vulnerable to exploitation and infectious diseases brought

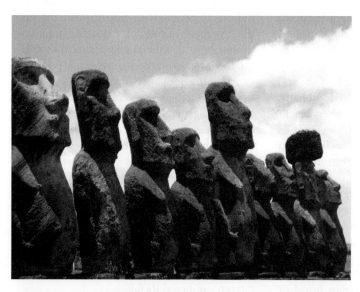

Figure 15.1  The moai of Rapa Nui (Easter Island). The Rapa Nui have long been considered to have suffered from ecocide. *Source:* Bradenfox, https://commons.wikimedia.org/wiki/File:Ahu_Tongariki_-_Rapa_Nui_(Easter_Island).JPG. CC BY 3.0.

by western explorers. By the time explorers began documenting their discoveries abroad, the Rapa Nui of Easter Island had been suffering from the effects of an ecological disaster, infectious diseases introduced by western explorers, and exploitation and capture for the slave trade for close to a century. These lines of evidence suggest that instead of an ecocide, or the intentional destruction of the environment resulting in the decline of a civilization, the Rapa Nui people likely suffered from a combination of factors, including environmental and ecological destruction. However, the fate of the Rapa Nui, who were meagerly surviving in a drastically underperforming ecosystem admittedly made depauperate through their own actions, ultimately collapsed at the hands of Western explorers.

This revised understanding of the fate of the Rapa Nui suggests that humans are easily able to survive in poor conditions for lengthy stretches of time. Unfortunately, this also suggests that humans, when faced with an environmental disaster of their own making, are not easily motivated to change their behaviors to their own benefit. We are now in a space and time to address a myriad of threats to planetary health. Using a One Health approach – collaborative, interdisciplinary, and holistic – is the best hope for the future of global health. Still, in order to understand how we should now proceed in the face of mounting threats to global health, we must first look to the past.

## 15.2 One Health in History

The concept of One Health is not a recent one. As early as the fourth century BCE, Hippocrates discussed the value of a clean environment for human health (Figure 15.2). Aristotle wrote prolifically on the intersection between human and animal health. Considered the father of medicine, Galen also experimented and wrote extensively on the human and animal health, noting the significant overlap in anatomy during the second century. Hippocrates, who is credited

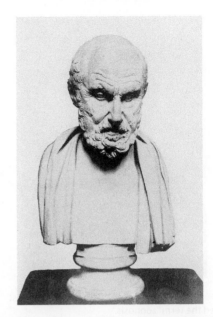

**Figure 15.2** Hippocrates. *Source:* Courtesy of Wellcome Images.

with issuing the edict adopted as the vow sworn by physicians and veterinarians today to "above all, do no harm," which when considered through the lens of One Health could be fully embraced by all One Health practitioners. By the mid-1700s, the One Health approach was being reinvigorated, with early epidemiologists and veterinarians emphasizing the role of the environment in spreading disease among humans and animals. Rudolf Virchow, a **pathologist** born in 1821, is credited both with coining the term "zoonosis" and with being the modern father of the One Health movement, arguing vociferously for the health of humans and animals being intimately connected and inextricably linked to the environment (Figure 15.3).

## 15.3 How One Health Became One Health

In 1964, the veterinary epidemiologist Calvin Schwabe coined the term "One Medicine" to demonstrate the shared knowledge and approaches of human and veterinary medicine and called for the continued

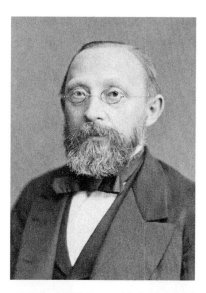

Figure 15.3 Rudolf Virchow, pathologist who first coined the term "zoonosis."

Health had emerged as an all-encompassing term for an approach to questions of planetary health that emphasizes not only the health of humans, animals, and the environment but the connections between them. One Health today is defined by the Center for Disease Control and Prevention (CDC) as "recognizing that the health of people is connected to the health of animals and the environment. The goal of One Health is to encourage the collaborative efforts of multiple disciplines – working locally, nationally, and globally – to achieve the best health for people, animals, and our environment." As we have covered throughout this book, physicians, veterinarians, conservation biologists, environmental scientists, politicians, economists, educators, science communicators, anthropologists, theologians, and other One Health practitioners are now coming together to advocate for collaboration.

integration of and focus on environmental health. By the mid-1990s, Conservation Medicine had also come to the forefront of awareness among the fields of conservation biology, ecology, and environmental science. Conservation Medicine focuses largely on the connections between animal and environmental health and on mitigating the damage to both from anthropogenic effects. Independently, both terms – One Medicine and Conservation Medicine – emphasize the holistic approach to solving complex health problems that should be embraced as a component of One Health. However, both terms are equally lacking in inclusivity in a critical way. One Medicine grew to be increasingly considered as a clinical specialty for veterinarians, unintentionally excluding physicians and environmental scientists in the process. Similarly, Conservation Medicine came to be considered largely in the context of health questions surrounding animals facing extinction. As such, human physicians were unintentionally excluded. In 2007, One Health appeared as an approach to examining questions at the interface of human and animal health. Soon after, One

## 15.4 Our Futures

We exist now at a critical juncture for planetary health. Decisions made today will have long-term consequences. As a result, we should consider a few potential futures and decide, by our actions, what future we would most like to inhabit. At the beginning of this chapter, we described what may seem like the consequences of continuing, unabated along the path we are currently on, but is actually the current state of some regions of the planet. Let us now explore a potential future that could come to fruition as a result of our current path, by exploring a future 100 years from now.

Climate change has continued unchecked, raising the global mean temperatures between 3°F and 8°F, with the number of days above 90°F increasing from 46 to 121 annually. This has shifted the agricultural growing season and range northward, reducing crop availability. Droughts have become more common, further compounding issues of food security. Rises in sea level, driven by the melting of polar ice caps, have resulted in large-scale flooding. Significant portions of the community as we know it today are underwater, unusable by humans or animals. As waters from the oceans intrude into river systems, salt water threatens the drinking water supply of communities across the planet. The combination of flooding, drought, and water contamination has resulted in a significant decline in biodiversity. **Extinctions** and extirpations will occur across biomes. Amphibian populations will be decimated, suffering both from loss of habitat and **desiccation**. Reptiles will struggle as both heat and increased exposure to estrogen-mimicking chemicals increases the rate of feminization, creating challenges to reproductive success. Bird populations will suffer as well, as both natives and migratory species struggle to find habitat and food resources. Invasive species will spread and limit economic growth and threaten food security across the planet.

The loss of usable land, both in urban and rural areas, threatens existing infrastructure and drives residents into increasingly exploited lands. Space and access to fresh water become the most important commodities. As resources dwindle and infrastructure crumbles, the health of humans, animals, and the environment is at constant risk. As water becomes increasingly scarce and ecorefugees flee the effects of climate change and civil wars, refugee camps become overfilled, densely populated wastelands, lacking enough food or medicinal resources for even a small portion of the residents within. Along the now-expanded banks of a river, a waterborne pathogen – a novel variant of cholera (*Vibrio cholera*) emerges in one ecorefugee camp. Completely resistant to antimicrobials, this novel pathogen spreads and kills rapidly. More than a million people in the region die as result of infection or collapsing infrastructure brought about by the stopping of critical services in the wake of a growing pandemic. Currently-marginalized human populations are devastated; individuals in the middle-class have become marginalized. Income inequality has further separated people, with the wealthy having consolidated even more of the wealth and resources available leaving virtually no resources available for the remaining population. The unchecked effects of environmental racism have left deep scars on the people and the land. The negative effects of science denial has left a population largely unable to do anything to resolve the problems. The problems experienced in the future, associated with our current behavior continuing unchanged, will result in a slow march towards global devastation.

It is hard to believe that it could get worse.

As covered in Chapter 3, there exist a number of significant threats to human, animal, and environmental health. As discussed above, the future as a result of our inaction is most likely a grim path. Our planet and health are threatened by unchecked climate change, the loss of biodiversity and habitat, increasing emerging and re-emerging infectious diseases in a world in which many people can travel to anywhere else on the planet in 36 hours, while others are marginalized due to income inequality, and the denial of science. However, in the USA in 2017, actions at the highest levels of government threaten even this grim future. Through limits on science funding, censorship at the highest levels – including of the US Environmental Protection Agency (EPA), the CDC, the US Fish and Wildlife Service (USFWS), and the National Institute of Health (NIH) – and the sweeping removals of environmental protections via executive orders demonstrate that the administration's values – unfettered, unregulated business practices over all other things. In addition, the funding of access to healthcare and to health research is under constant threat. If successful in these removals of protections for human, animal, and environmental health, the future of our planet and of all life will be in serious jeopardy.

## 15.5 Our Current Actions Establish the Path

More than any other time in history, the decisions we make today can take the planet in the direction of devastation or recovery. However, the future is both unknowable and as of yet, malleable. It is hard to comprehend the long-term consequences of our actions. de Soto, for example, while exploring the Mississippi River Basin intent on finding gold did not plan to devastate 95% of the native peoples whose path he crossed, via exposure to measles and smallpox; still, the damage was done. Similarly, the decisions we make and the actions we take will affect planetary health. For example, as nations around the world decide to implement the actions needed to uphold agreed upon reductions in greenhouse gases, as a part of the Paris Climate Accord, the planet's fate is in our own hands. If we decide to forego our responsibilities to planetary health, we will ultimately lose out. Decisions to rescind the environmental protections of unique and globally important landscapes cannot be undone. Once a landscape is damaged by our choices, it is damaged, and the recovery time needed for the planet will, in most cases, extend far beyond our lifetimes.

## 15.6 The Ethics of Our Decisions

The ethical considerations of any decision concerning human, animal, and/or environmental health are vast and complex. From how we obtain medicines for human and animal health to who has access to these life-saving products; from the locations of pollution-generating industries in poor, communities of color to the determination of responsibility for environmental clean-up associated with historic industrial operations, currently leaching toxic pollution into communities; from the use of confined animal feeding operations (CAFOs) for quick and easy access to meat for human food consumption to the consumption of animals as a food source at all. Ethical considerations underpin every decision we make. As mentioned throughout this book, One Health is an approach to solving complex problems of planetary health. The lens of One Health can truly be applied to any problem in order to consider a more holistic solution. This lens of One Health, however, is importantly also an ethical lens. Humans now number just over 7.6 billion people, and the human population is expected to continue growing for the foreseeable future. However, our unfettered population growth creates ethical dilemmas for all of human, animal, and environmental health. As a result, every decision, including to reproduce or not, should be considered through the lens of One Health. Ethical considerations are complicated, multifaceted issues of equity and inequality, and decisions made without regard to the ethical consequences are frequently also those made without regard for the consequences to planetary health, One Health.

## 15.7 Conclusions

Our decisions will come to affect the future in unknowable ways. Our past has shaped our today, and our current actions are setting the path forward for tomorrow. Some actions are permanent and irreversible. Irrespective of the path we, as a global community, choose, our actions will have lasting consequences for the health of our planet. Let us act for good. Let us act for One Health.

## End of Chapter Questions & Activities

A. Thought Questions:
  i) In this chapter, we painted a disturbingly grim future. However, the future is not yet written. What is the future that you would prefer? Consider the greatest threats to planetary health (see Chapter 3) and consider the implications of each. Describe how One

Health can create a more positive, vibrant, livable future.

ii) What do you think is the greatest threat to planetary health? What do you think is the greatest threat that you pose to planetary health? What actions could you take or could you influence others to take to remedy this specific threat?

iii) Describe in your own words how the history of One Health has or has not been human-focused. What evidence supports your claim? Has this hindered our ability to collaborate?

iv) What are the ethical considerations of both action and inaction for your greatest threat to planetary health?

B. At-home Activities:

i) Consider your home's landscaping now and in the future. Plant natives. Be OK without a well-manicured lawn. Consider converting your green space into a backyard wildlife area.

ii) Perform a home energy audit and address any concerns identified in the process. Make your home as energy efficient as possible.

C. Long-term Action Steps:

i) Downsize. Become a minimalist. For future purposes, really evaluate carefully whether or not you need whatever item you are considering purchasing. Is it really a need? Are there other ways to meet this need?

ii) Consider the ethical ramifications of your own health care choices.

D. Recommended Reading:

Alonso Aguirre, A., Ostfeld, R.S., Tabor, G.M. et al. (2002). *Conservation Medicine: Ecological Health in Practice.* Oxford University Press.

Alonso Aguirre, A., Ostfeld, R., and Daszak, P. (2012). *New Directions in Conservation Medicine: Applied Cases of Ecological Health.* Oxford University Press.

Atlas, R.M. and Maloy, S. (2014). *One Health: People, Animals, and the Environment.* American Society for Microbiology Press.

Cork, S., Hall, D., and Liljebjelke, K. (2016). *One Health Case Studies: Addressing Complex Problems in a Changing World.* 5M Publishing, Ltd.

Hunt, T. and Lupo, C. (2011). *The Statues that Walked: Unraveling the Mystery of Easter Island.* Free Press.

Zinsstag, J., Schellling, E., Waltner-Toews, D. et al. (2015). *One Health: The Theory and Practice of Integrated Health Approaches.* CAB International.

## Interview

*An Interview with Martyn Jeggo: PhD, DVM, Deakin University*

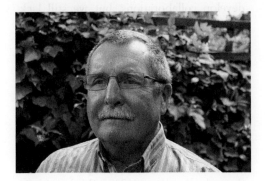

**When did you first hear about One Health?**

*EcoHealth Alliance* has pushed the process of One Health forward substantially in the last 10 years. Once I became an editor on that journal, or executive editor on that journal, I got interested in the One Health arena. I also was involved in a couple of major conditions here in Australia involving bat diseases that move from bats and affect livestock and then humans, including Hendra virus, which killed four veterinarians in Australia. A bat-borne virus that affects horses and subsequently, when it comes into contact with humans, causes a fatal human disease. This got me interested in host switching and the whole arena of One Health, which expanded as I started thinking about the environmental factors and increasingly, the social science which underpins One Health and is crucial for us making a serious impact in this One Health arena.

## How is One Health important to your work?

It's increasingly obvious that if we are going to tackle some of the bigger problems we have got in the world, we really need to take a much more multidisciplinary, multi-sectoral approach. In the health arena, it's clear that the environment, human health, and animal health are intrinsically linked. Until we start looking at it more holistically, we are not going to solve the problems, so it's crucial we take this broader approach. There are crucial problems facing the world that will not be solved unless we take a One Health approach.

## How do your actions reflect One Health, personally or professionally?

There's a fundamental science issue here that this interaction, unless we understand it properly, we are not going to solve these problems. When I am faced with a problem, I ask what's causing it? Is it multifactorial? Is it going to require a broad section approach that involves not just my discipline but a broader approach that understands the human context, the environmental context, and the social science context? Very often, the less we understand the societal context of a disease, we are probably not going to solve it. Many of the solutions to the problems we have got are not going to be reached by a narrow approach but a much broader approach. And again here, social science becomes a crucial dimension in trying to unravel these problems.

## What can an individual do to make a difference for planetary health?

An individual needs to appreciate the concept of One Health and how it can help, and decide if the problems that he or she is tackling as a scientist can best be dealt with by a One Health approach, by looking at it from a more multidisciplinary, multi-sectorial way.

Reaching out, particularly to the medical profession and to the social sciences to try and work out how we do this together in a way that's shared, cooperative, and collaborative, and not competitive, is what an individual has to do.

## How can we encourage people to care about planetary Health?

On the one extreme, we have got people who care passionately about the planet and environmental health. On the other hand, in the area of infectious disease research, there are those concerned more with human health than environmental health, and you are getting a feeling of panic focused on human health. People that work within government research tend to create change within. That change often is slow and beset by a huge amount of bureaucracy. Getting people to work as a team is the biggest challenge we have got. It's really important to appreciate the other point of view and what's driving an individual. All this is intrinsically linked, and unless we work as a team towards this, we are going to struggle. I think we have to have an approach that recognizes the different drivers and the different emotions that people have in occupying this One Health space.

## Where is One Health headed?

I break One Health activities into three areas. First, in research we have started to develop collaborations, but we still lack funding in the One Health arena. Not many organizations specifically fund One Health but fund parts of it, which makes it challenging when trying to work in a team. The second area is policy development, and here, we are beginning to see One Health groups, departments, divisions within government that are starting to devise policy based on One Health and then work out ways to implement that through regulation. The third area is operational activities, and there we still have a long way to go. Ministries of agriculture and health do not work well together. In fact, they work almost competitively. Working out how we can get a much more operational partnership is a bit of a challenge and that usually boils down to just simply resources. From research through to policy, to operation, the future of One Health is slightly different, and the challenges are certainly different.

### Parting Thoughts?

Currently, the veterinarian profession has got One Health and is doing well. Social scientists, environmentalists, ecologists have always got it and they are there. But we have a vast number in the medical profession who just simply do not understand where we are at with this, and that is doing us a disservice, particularly when large amounts of funding are available in this area that could be more effectively used if we could get the medical profession to adopt a broader One Health approach. It's getting there but it's very slow. I heard recently that if you ask 95% of medical practitioners what One Health is, they will not have a clue. We have a gap there.

## Works Cited

Blake, D.P. and Betson, M. (2017). One Health: parasites and beyond. *Parasitology* 144 (1): 1–6.

Cowen, P., Currier, R.W., and Steele, J.H. (2016). A short history of One Health in the United States. *Veterinary Heritage: Bulletin of the American Veterinary History Society* 39 (1): 1–15.

Deem, S.L., Kilbourn, A.M., Wolfe, N.D. et al. (2000). Conservation medicine. *Annals of the New York Academy of Science* 916: 370–377.

Gyles, C. (2016). One Medicine, One Health, One World. *Canadian Veterinary Journal* 57 (4): 345–346.

Hunt, T. and Lipo, C. (2011). *The Statues that Walked: Unraveling the Mysteries of Easter Island*. Free Press.

One Health Initiative Task Force (2008). *One Health: A New Professional Imperative*. American Veterinary Medical Association.

Rapport, D. (1998). Defining ecosystem health. In: *Ecosystem Health* (ed. D.J. Rapport), 18–33. Blackwell Scientific.

Roman, S., Bullock, S., and Brede, M. (2016). Coupled societies are more robust against collapse: a hypothetical look at Easter Island. *Ecological Economics* 132: 264–278.

Schwabe, C. (1984). *Veterinary Medicine and Human Health*, 3e. Baltimore, MD: Williams and Wilkins.

West, K., Collins, C., Kardailsky, O. et al. (2017). The Pacific rat race to Easter Island: tracking the prehistoric dispersal of *Rattus exulans* using ancient mitochondrial genomes. *Frontiers in Ecology and Evolution* 31: doi: 10.3389/fevo.2017.00052.

Whitmee, S., Haines, A., Beyrer, C. et al. (2015). Safeguarding human health in the Anthropocene epoch: report of The Rockefeller Foundation – Lancet Commission on planetary health. *The Lancet* 386: 1973–2028. doi: 10.1016/S0140-6736(15)60901-1.

## Glossary

**abiotic** physical rather than biological; not derived from living organisms

**advocacy** an activity by an individual or group aimed at influencing decisions

**allele** a variant form of a gene; in diploid organisms, two alleles are present at each gene

**animal** a living organism that feeds on organic matter, typically having specialized sense organs and nervous system and able to respond rapidly to stimuli

**Anthropocene** a proposed epoch dating from the commencement of significant human impact on the Earth's geology and ecosystems, including, but not limited to, anthropogenic climate change. As of August 2016, neither the International Commission on Stratigraphy nor the International Union of Geological Sciences have decided on the official starting dates or events for the Anthropocene

**anthropogenic** of, relating to, or resulting from the influence of human beings on nature

**anthropogenization** a state of becoming more human-altered or human-affected

**anthropozoonotic** an infection that is transmitted from human to non-human animals

**antigen** in immunology, an antigen is any molecule capable of inducing an immune response on the part of the host organism. Antigens are often associated with infectious-disease-causing agents, such as bacteria, viruses or fungi, but they may sometimes be part of the host itself as in an autoimmune disease (e.g. Lupus). In other words, an antigen is any substance that causes an immune system to produce antibodies against it.

**anti-helminthics** medicines that rid the body of parasitic worms

**antimicrobial resistance** the ability of an organism to evolve resistance to antimicrobial treatments, resulting in ineffective treatments and persistent infections

**bacillus (Pl. bacilli)** rod-shaped bacterium

**background extinction rate** the rate of extinction experienced by all of life that occurs through normative, natural processes

**behavioral economics** the field of economics that focuses on understanding how human actions impact economic outcomes

**benthic** the ecological zone at the deepest levels of a body of water, including an ocean, that includes the sediment surface and subsurface

**bi-directional pathogen transmission** the spread of an etiological agent of disease between two (or more) species, in which the agent may go in either direction

**biodiversity** the variety and variability of life on Earth

**biomagnification** the concentration of toxins in an organism as one progresses up through a foodweb

**biomass** the mass of living biological organisms in a given area or ecosystem at a given time

**biophilia** the term coined by Edward O. Wilson to describe what he believes is humanity's innate affinity for the natural world

**bioremediation** process of treating or handling environmental pollutants by naturally occurring or introduced microbes in order to degrade or reduce environmental wastes

**biotic** relating to or resulting from living things, especially in their ecological relations

**blogging** an internet based form of communication that allows for long-form narratives on any topic the author chooses; not peer-reviewed or subject to editorial review

**bushmeat** meat from non-domesticated mammals, reptiles, amphibians, and birds hunted for food in tropical forests. In parts of Africa and other developing regions also called wild meat or game meat. Commercial harvesting and the trade of bushmeat is considered a threat to biodiversity.

**bycatch** the unwanted fish and other marine creatures caught during commercial fishing for a different species

**carbon sequestration** long-term storage of carbon dioxide that acts to mitigate or slow climate change

**carcinogen** cancer-causing agent

**case fatality rate** the proportion of deaths within a designated population of "cases" (people or animal with a medical condition), over the course of the disease. A CFR is conventionally expressed as a percentage and represents a measure of risk.

**certified B corporation** a for-profit company that meets rigorous standards of social and environmental performance, accountability, and transparency

**citizen science** collaboration between scientists and interested members of the general public in which the general public participates in data collection and sometimes data curation of scientific experiments

**clear cutting** logging practice in which an entire plot of forest is cleared, leaving no plants standing

**Colony Collapse Disorder** a multifactorial disease syndrome of bees – a pathological condition affecting a large number of honeybee colonies, in which various stresses (e.g. mites, viruses, nicotinamide pesticides) may lead to the abrupt disappearance of worker bees from the hive, leaving only the queen and newly hatched bees behind and thus causing the colony to stop functioning

**concentrated or confined-animal feeding operation (CAFO)** an animal feeding operation (AFO) that (i) confines animals for more than 45 days during a growing season, (ii) in an area that does not produce vegetation, and (iii) meets certain size thresholds

**congenital** present at birth

**Conservation Medicine** an emerging, interdisciplinary field that studies the relationship between human and animal health and environmental conditions. Also known as ecological medicine, environmental medicine, medical geology, or One Health

**coprolite** fossilized feces

**coral bleaching** a process whereby the coral colonies lose their color, either due to the loss of pigments produced by microscopic algae (zooxanthellae) living in symbiosis with their host organisms (polyps) or because these zooxanthellae have been expelled.

**culture** the arts and other manifestations of human intellectual achievement regarded collectively; the customary beliefs, social forms, and material traits of a racial, religious, or social group

**definitive host** an organism that supports the adult or sexually reproductive form of a parasite

**deforestation** permanent clearing of forests on a large scale in order to make the land usable for other purposes

**desertification** persistent degradation of dryland ecosystems by human activities such that the land loses its ability to hold water or sustain life

**desiccation** the state of extreme dryness or the process of extreme drying

**detritivore** an animal that feeds on dead or dying organic material

**dilution effect** an ecological hypothesis stating that increased biodiversity decreases disease risk; often applied to zoonotic pathogens

**disease risk analysis** a multidisciplinary process used to evaluate existing knowledge in order to prioritize risks associated with the spread or occurrence of diseases

**Earth Overshoot Day** previously known as Ecological Debt Day (EDD); the calculated illustrative calendar date on which humanity's resource consumption for the year exceeds Earth's capacity to regenerate those resources that year. Earth Overshoot Day is calculated by dividing the world biocapacity (the amount of natural resources generated by Earth that year), by the world ecological footprint (humanity's consumption of Earth's natural resources for that year), and multiplying by 365, the number of days in one Gregorian common calendar year

**ecocide** willful destruction of the natural environment to the point that that environment can no longer sustain human life

**EcoHealth** an emerging, interdisciplinary field that takes an ecosystem approach to human health, incorporating wildlife health, and social and economic environments

**ecological footprint** measure of the ecological assets a given population requires to continue to live as they are; calculations of ecological footprints suggest that certain populations use far more than their share of the Earth's resources annually

**economics** the branch of knowledge concerned with the production, consumption, and transfer of wealth

**ecorefugee** a person displaced following environmental change, notably land loss and degradation and natural disaster

**ecosystem engineers** any organism that creates, significantly modifies, maintains, or destroys a habitat. These organisms can have a large impact on the species richness and landscape-level heterogeneity of an area

**ecosystem health** is a metaphor used to describe the condition of an ecosystem. Ecosystem condition can vary as a result of fire, flooding, drought, extinctions, invasive species, climate change, mining, fishing, farming, logging, chemical spills, and a host of other reasons

**ecosystem services** the variety of benefits that are provided to people, animals, and the planet by the world's ecosystems. These include carbon sequestration, flood and erosion control, climate control, and much more

**Ecotheology** a discipline within the study of theology that focuses on the connections between religion and nature, particularly regarding environmental stewardship

**edge effects** changes in community structure at the boundary of a habitat; plays an important role in fragmented habitats

**emerging infectious disease (EID)** diseases that have increased in number, have spread to new regions, and/ or have occurred in new species

**endocrine-disrupting agent** a substance that mimics naturally occurring hormones and interferes with their actions

**environmental ethic** environmental philosophy that extends ethical concern beyond humans and into the remaining natural world; an environmental ethic informs how one interacts with the natural world

**environmental racism** socially marginalized racial minority populations are disproportionately exposed to and affected by pollutants and lack of access to ecological resources

**epidemiologic transition** describes the changes in patterns of population age distributions, mortality, fertility, life expectancy, and causes of death

**epidemiologist** an investigator who studies the occurrence of disease or other health-related conditions or events in defined populations

**epigenetic** an agent or event that modifies the expression of a particular gene or genes; heritable

**evolve** heritable change over time; the process by which all forms of life have diversified, in response to environmental change, from a single universal common ancestor

**exposome** the cumulative catalog of environmental substances that an individual has encountered

**externalities** the cost or benefit that affects a party who did not choose to incur that cost or benefit

**extinction** the process by which an entire species is lost

**extirpations** local extinction of a species (or other taxon) that ceases to exist in the chosen geographic area of study, though it still exists elsewhere. Local extinctions (extirpations) are contrasted with global extinctions

**flagship species** a species selected to act as an ambassador, icon, or symbol for a defined habitat, issue, campaign, or environmental cause. Think Panda and the World Wide Fund for Nature (WWF)!

**flyway** a route regularly used by large numbers of migrating birds

**fomites** objects or materials that may carry infection, such as clothes, utensils, and furniture

**food desert** communities or regions where access to fresh fruits, vegetables, or other healthy food is limited; typically impoverished or otherwise marginalized communities

**fracking** a natural gas extraction process in which a deep well is dug and then filled in with a high pressure mixture of water and oil in order to displace gas deep in the Earth

**Gaia** the ancestral mother of all life in Greek mythology

**Gaia Theory** proposes that organisms interact with their inorganic surroundings on Earth to form a self-regulating, complex system that contributes to maintaining the conditions for life on the planet

**Gifford Pinchot** 1865–1946; American forester and politician; founder of the US Forest Service

**Global Health Security Agenda (GHSA)** launched in 2014 to advance a world safe and secure from infectious disease threats, to bring together nations from all over the world to make new, concrete commitments, and to elevate global health security as a national leaders-level priority

**Global North** North–South divide broadly considered as a socioeconomic and political divide; generally, definitions of the Global North include the USA, Canada, Western Europe, and developed parts of East Asia

**glyphosate** a commonly used herbicide, usually marketed by the name Roundup®

**granuloma** a localized area of inflammation that is often contained within a nodule

**Great Pacific Garbage Patch** also described as the Pacific trash vortex; is a gyre of marine debris particles in the central North Pacific Ocean discovered between 1985 and 1988. It is located roughly between 135°W to 155°W and 35°N to 42°N

**greenhouse effect** process of warming by which radiation is trapped by the atmosphere and reflected back to Earth; the resulting lack of heat escape warms the climate

**gyre**  a large system of circulating currents

**H5N1 flu**  highly infectious, severe respiratory influenza that originated in birds and is commonly referred to as avian influenza

**health**  as defined by the World Health Organization, health is as a state of complete physical, mental, and social well-being

**hemochromatosis**  recessively inherited disease associated with excess storage of iron

**herd immunity**  a form of indirect protection from infectious disease that occurs when a large percentage of a population has become immune to an infection, thereby providing a measure of protection for individuals who are not immune

**heterozygote advantage**  the adaptive advantage given to individuals who are heterozygous for a particular trait, giving them better fitness then either of the homozygous forms

**homeostasis**  the tendency toward a relatively stable equilibrium between interdependent elements, especially as maintained by physiological processes

**hygiene hypothesis**  a theory that states that a lack of early childhood exposure to infectious agents, symbiotic microorganisms (such as the gut flora or probiotics), and parasites increases susceptibility to allergic diseases by suppressing the natural development of the immune system

**immunological memory**  the ability of the immune system to rapidly respond to an antigen that has been previously encountered. Memory involves the retention of an antigen-relevant population of lymphocytes

*in utero*  meaning "in the uterus," *in utero* generally refers to embryonic or fetal developmental conditions or events

**incidence**  the number of new cases that occur in a known population over a specified period of time

**income inequality**  the manner in which income is distributed unevenly, resulting in the creation of a significant gap between the wealthy and the remaining population

**incubation period**  the time interval between invasion by an infectious agent and appearance of the first sign or symptom of the disease in question

**index case**  the first documented patient with clinical signs (primary case) at the onset of an epidemiological investigation

**institutional lock-in**  the limitations of academic institutions for collaboration due to constraints on scholars' time, resources, and institutional flexibility

**intrinsic value**  actual value of a good or service based on underlying assumptions of tangible and intangible factors; in environmental economics, intrinsic value refers to the value of nature unrelated to economic valuation

**introduced species**  a species living outside its native range

**invasive species**  an introduced species that outcompetes native wildlife and/or spreads in a way that causes harm to the environment, human, and/or animal health

**invertebrate**  an animal lacking a backbone, such as an arthropod, mollusk, annelid, coelenterate, etc. The invertebrates constitute an artificial division of the animal kingdom, comprising 95% of animal species and about 30 different phyla

**island biogeography**  the study of the species composition and species richness on islands in order to explain the uneven distributions between, as originally posited, continental and insular communities of flora and fauna

**John Muir**  1838–1914; Scottish-American naturalist, author, philosopher, and conservationist; founder of the US National Park Service

**keystone species**  a species on which other species in an ecosystem largely depend, such that if it were removed the ecosystem would change drastically

**kwashiorkor** a form of malnutrition caused by lack of sufficient protein

**latent** dormant

**laws** a rule of conduct or procedure recognized by a community as binding or enforceable by authority

**life expectancy** statistical measure of the average length of life of a given organism

**macrophage** a type of phagocyte, which is a cell responsible for detecting, engulfing, and destroying pathogens and dead cells

**manifesto for planetary health** a call for a social movement to support collective public health action at all levels of society – personal, community, national, regional, global, and planetary.

**Mason-Dixon line** line resolving a border dispute between Maryland, Pennsylvania, and Delaware, surveyed between 1763 and 1767; in pre-Civil War USA, it also served as a border between slave states and free states

**methylate** the addition of a methyl group into a molecule

**microbiome** the microbial life that lives in or on an individual

**millennium development goals** eight goals with measurable targets and clear deadlines for improving the lives of the world's poorest people. To meet these goals and eradicate poverty, leaders of 189 countries signed the historic millennium declaration at the United Nations Millennium Summit in 2000

**morbidity** statistical measure of the rate of disease in a population

**mortality** statistical measure of death in a population

**Mugabeism** a form of populist reason, named for Robert Mugabe and his authoritarian leadership in Zimbabwe from 1987-2017. It can represent pan-African memory and patriotism as well as a form of radical left-nationalism dedicated to resolving intractable national and agrarian questions; it is most commonly associated with crisis, chaos, and tyranny in the name of nationalism

**multidisciplinary** combining or involving several academic disciplines or professional specializations in an approach to a topic or problem

**multifactorial** involving or dependent on a number of factors or causes

**necropsy** a dissection of a dead animal to determine the cause of death

**neonate** newborn

**non-point source** pollutant or infectious agent that is encountered from dispersed locations across a landscape, as opposed to a single point source of pollution.

**obesogen** chemical substance that interferes with fat production, synthesis, and/or metabolism and leads to obesity

**Occam's razor** problem-solving principle of parsimony, attributed to William of Ockham, that suggests that given two possible explanations for an event, the simplest explanation is the most likely to have occurred

**One Health** the collaborative effort of multiple disciplines – working locally, nationally, and globally – to attain optimal health for people, animals, and the environment

**One Health Triad** the three overlapping and interconnected groups of One Health, which includes humans, non-human animals, and the environment

**One Medicine** early variant of One Health that focused on the shared knowledge between human and veterinary medicine and emphasized the continued integration of and focus on environmental health

**option value** the value placed on an individual's willingness to pay to maintain a public asset

**organophosphate pesticides** chemical substances that are variations of phosphoric acid. Organophophates can be used as herbicides, pesticides, plasticizers, and solvents; some are known to be neurotoxins

**pandemic** an epidemic of infectious disease that has spread through a human or non-human animal population (or populations) across a large region; for instance multiple continents, or even worldwide

**parasite escape** the release of a host from its parasites upon its introduction or invasion into a new range

**parsimony** the simplest scientific explanation that fits the evidence; commonly used approach to understanding evolutionary relationships

**pastoralist** someone who tends to livestock that travel from pasture to pasture, such as sheep, camels, goats, and cattle

**pathogen introduction** the introduction of novel pathogen into a community through the introduction or invasion of a host; considered a competitive advantage for the introduced species

**pathogenicity** the ability of an organism to cause disease (i.e. harm the host). This ability represents a genetic component of the pathogen and the overt damage done to the host is a property of the host–pathogen interactions

**pathology** branch of medicine (human or veterinary) that is focused on understanding the cause, mechanisms, and course of disease typically through examination of body tissue and fluids

**patient zero** in medical science, the primary case or initial patient in the population of an epidemiological investigation

**personal protective equipment (PPE)** protective clothing (clothes, helmets, goggles), or other equipment designed to protect the wearer from infection or injury

**phyla** level of classification or taxonomy immediately beneath kingdom

**planetary health** refers to "the health of human civilization and the state of the natural systems on which it depends." In 2015, the Rockefeller Foundation and *The Lancet* launched the concept as the Rockefeller Foundation–Lancet Commission on Planetary Health

**PM$_{2.5}$** atmospheric particulate matter (PM) that have a diameter of less than 2.5 micrometers, which is about 3% the diameter of a human hair

**point source** pollutant or infectious agent is encountered at a single point in time and space

**policy** generally a course or principle of action adopted by a community (e.g. school district, city, state, country, international agreement) to help in decision-making and governance

**political science** a social science discipline that deals with systems of government and the analysis of political activity and political behavior. It deals extensively with the theory and practice of politics which is commonly thought of as the determining of the distribution of power and resources

**politician** a person who is professionally involved in politics, especially as a holder of or a candidate for an elected office

**politics** the activities associated with the governance of a country or other area

**popular sovereignty** the principle that the authority of a state and its government is created and sustained by the consent of its people, through their elected representatives (Rule by the People), who are the source of all political power

**population genetics** a subfield of genetics that examines the differences among and between populations in order to understand the effects of evolutionary pressures as a result of population dynamics

**power** the capacity or ability to direct or influence the behavior of others or the course of events

**prevalence** the number of instances of a given disease or other condition in a given population at a designated time

**price** the amount an individual is willing to pay for a good or service

**R₀** in epidemiology, the basic reproduction number is the number of secondary cases (affected individuals) expected to result from a single case of an infectious disease in a population that is fully susceptible to infection

**raptors** birds of prey; from the Latin word *rapere* – to grip or grasp

**redlining** racist housing policies at federal, state, and local levels

**re-emerging infectious disease** an infectious disease that had been previously eradicated or declined significantly within a region but is now resurging

**reproductive toxicity** a hazard associated with a chemical in which exposure interferes with normal reproductive function

**resilience** in ecology, resilience is the capacity of an ecosystem to respond to a perturbation or disturbance by resisting damage and recovering quickly

**responsible advocacy** advocacy that reflects a social conscience

**Rinderpest** a highly contagious viral disease of both domestic and non-domestic hoof-stock species

**science denialism** essentially an irrational action in which an individual denies the evidence and expertise of, in this case, science and scientists and acts in a way that conforms to the bias of their own existing beliefs

**selective logging** a form of partial forest removal in which individual trees are harvested while the larger forest is left intact

**selective pressure** a force that alters the reproductive success of a population, driving evolutionary selection of a phenotype

**senescence** aging, or the elderly period of life

**sentinel species** animals, plants, and/or microbes used to detect and provide early warning of dangers, typically environmental hazards or infectious diseases, to humans and/or the environment

**six degrees of One Health** the health of all life is connected such that there are six or fewer steps separating the health of all living things

**sixth mass extinction** the ongoing extinction event of species across plant and animal taxa that is mainly as a result of human activity. The current rate of extinction of species is estimated at 100–1000 times higher than natural background rates, with the vast majority of the extinctions most likely undocumented.

**skepticism** a questioning attitude or doubt over a claim

**slash and burn agriculture** a farming method, commonly used as a tool of deforestation, that involves cutting down all plants in a large-scale plot of land and then setting fire to the plot to destroy any remaining vegetation

**social media** networking platforms that facilitate the sharing of information, ideas, personal actions, and so on with a global community

**social sciences** a major category of academic disciplines concerned with society and the relationships among individuals within a society

**society** the aggregate of people living together in a more or less ordered community

**spillover** the transmission of a pathogen from a reservoir population with a high pathogen prevalence to a novel host population

**stealth issue advocacy** advocacy by scientists in which the claim is to be focused on issues but personal agenda items are also advanced

**stochastic event** an unpredictable event due to the influence of a random variable

**Stone Mountain Policy** part of a series of One Health meetings organized by diverse global institutions with the intent of providing a forum for national and international specialists to focus on policies and implementation of a One Health approach to improving human and animal health. The specific goal of the Stone Mountain meeting was to identify clear and concrete actions to move the concept of One Health from vision to implementation.

**stratosphere** the layer of the Earth's atmosphere that extends from above the troposphere (the atmosphere that connects to Earth) to approximately 32 miles above the Earth's surface

**Superfund site** any US land contaminated by pollutants and/or hazardous waste that requires government oversight for clean-up, as identified by the US Environmental Protection Agency

**sympatric** occurring within the same geographical area; overlapping in distribution

**tailings dam** earthenware dam to store mine waste

**taxa** (singular taxon) groups of one or more populations of an organism or organisms seen by taxonomists to form a unit, such as species, family, or class

**teratogen** a substance that can disrupt embryonic developmental processes

**theriogenology** the branch of veterinary medicine concerned with reproduction, including the physiology and pathology of male and female reproductive systems of animals and the clinical practice of veterinary obstetrics, gynecology, and andrology

**transdisciplinary** efforts by individuals from different disciplines working jointly to create new conceptual, theoretical, methodological, and translational innovations that integrate and move beyond discipline-specific approaches to address a common problem

**transformational learning** an approach to learning that advocates for experiences that engage an individual's psychology, convictions, and behavior

**translational medicine** a rapidly growing discipline in biomedical research and aims to expedite the discovery of new diagnostic tools and treatments by using a multi-disciplinary, highly collaborative, "bench-to-bedside" approach. In a medical research context, it aims to "translate" findings in fundamental research into medical practice and meaningful health outcomes.

**true cost** the cost of a good or service if the price reflected economic externalities commonly born by the people of the planet

**umbrella species** species selected as focal points for conservation efforts, typically because protecting these species indirectly protects the many other species that make up the ecological community of its habitat

**urban sprawl** the uncontrolled expansion of urban areas

**vaccine** a substance that can initiate artificially acquired immunity

**value** a person's principles or standards that inform behavior

**vertebrate biomass** mass of all vertebrates in a given area or ecosystem at a given time

**veterinary medicine** the branch of medicine that deals with the prevention, diagnosis, and treatment of disease, disorder, and injury in non-human animals. It also helps to maintain food supply through livestock health monitoring and treatment, and mental health by keeping pets healthy and long living

**viroimmunotherapy** (also called immunovirotherapy) is a strategic approach to cancer treatment in which the patient's immune system is modulated by viral and/or antigenic stimulation; this includes the use of antigen-bearing viral vectors as well as the use of oncolytic viruses that target the specific tumors involved.

**visceral gout** a disease of birds in which kidney failure causes a build-up of urates in the internal organs, leaving a chalky white coating on them. Symptoms include anorexia and emaciation

**wealth inequality** the disparity between the wealthiest and the poorest of the planet; in this context, wealth includes assets and other heritable goods, making it a far more accurate representation of the gap between rich and poor than income inequality

**wet market** a market selling fresh meat and produce, distinguished from dry markets which sell durable goods such as cloth and electronics; wet markets were traditionally places that sold live animals out in the open, including poultry, fish, reptiles, and pigs

**zoonosis/zoonotic** a disease that is transmitted between animals and people; often used to specify a disease that exists in animals but that can infect humans

# Index

*Introduction to One Health: An Interdisciplinary Approach to Planetary Health*, First Edition.
Sharon L. Deem, Kelly E. Lane-deGraaf and Elizabeth A. Rayhel.
© 2019 John Wiley & Sons, Inc. Published 2019 by John Wiley & Sons, Inc.
Companion website: www.wiley.com/go/deem/health

Printed and bound by CPI Group (UK) Ltd, Croydon, CR0 4YY

16/04/2025

14658464-0003